MW00611275

U18402 8090689

LIVER PATHOLOGY
An Atlas and Concise Guide

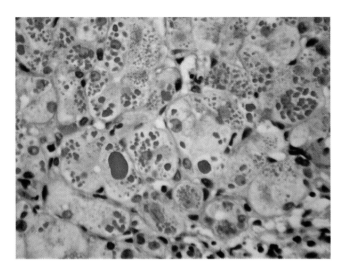
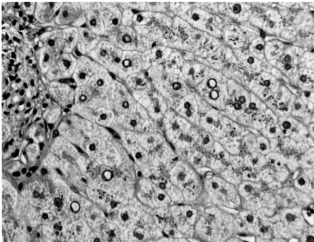

LIVER PATHOLOGY
An Atlas and Concise Guide

Arief A. Suriawinata, MD
Associate Professor of Pathology, Dartmouth Medical School
Hanover, New Hampshire
Department of Pathology, Dartmouth-Hitchcock Medical Center
Lebanon, New Hampshire

Swan N. Thung, MD
Professor of Pathology, and Gene & Cell Medicine
The Lillian and Henry M. Stratton–Hans Popper Department of Pathology
The Mount Sinai School of Medicine
New York, New York

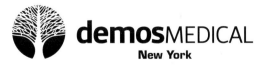
demosMEDICAL
New York

Acquisitions Editor: Richard Winters
Cover Design: Joe Tenerelli
Compositor: Manila Typesetting Company
Printer: SCI

ISBN: 978-1-933864-94-5
eISBN: 978-1-935281-48-1

Visit our website at www.demosmedpub.com

Medicine is an ever-changing science. Research and clinical experience are continually expanding our knowledge, in particular our understanding of proper treatment and drug therapy. The authors, editors, and publisher have made every effort to ensure that all information in this book is in accordance with the state of knowledge at the time of production of the book. Nevertheless, the authors, editors, and publisher are not responsible for errors or omissions or for any consequences from application of the information in this book and make no warranty, express or implied, with respect to the contents of the publication. Every reader should examine carefully the package inserts accompanying each drug and should carefully check whether the dosage schedules mentioned therein or the contraindications stated by the manufacturer differ from the statements made in this book. Such examination is particularly important with drugs that are either rarely used or have been newly released on the market.

Library of Congress Cataloging-in-Publication Data

Suriawinata, Arief A.
 Liver pathology: an atlas and concise guide / Arief A. Suriawinata, Swan N. Thung.
   p. ; cm.
 Includes bibliographical references and index.
 ISBN 978-1-933864-94-5
 1. Liver–Diseases–Atlases. I. Thung, Swan N. II. Title.
 [DNLM: 1. Liver Diseases–pathology–Atlases. 2. Liver–pathology–Atlases. WI 17]
 RC846.9.S87 2011
 616.3'6–dc22

                                                                        2011004289

CIP data is available from the Library of Congress.

Special discounts on bulk quantities of Demos Medical Publishing books are available to corporations, professional associations, pharmaceutical companies, health care organizations, and other qualifying groups. For details, please contact:

Special Sales Department
Demos Medical Publishing
11 W. 42nd Street, 15th Floor
New York, NY 10036
Phone: 800–532–8663 or 212–683–0072
Fax: 212–941–7842
E-mail: rsantana@demosmedpub.com

Made in the United States of America
11 12 13 14 15   5 4 3 2 1

*To my parents, Bing and Gien, my wife, Jenny,
and our sons, Michael and Matthew,
for their enduring support and encouragement.*
ARIEF A. SURIAWINATA, MD

*To Roy, Stephen, Arlyne, Rohan, Anduin, Andrew, Lisa and Maile Thung;
and my sisters Regina, Indah, Peni and Dewi
for their continuous and loving support.*
SWAN N. THUNG, MD

Contents

Foreword

Liver biopsy in the 21st century, for various reasons, is as much a challenge for the pathologists as for their clinical colleagues. The indications for liver biopsy continue to evolve. After the introduction of the 1-second technique by Menghini, liver biopsy had become popular as a very safe procedure with a considerable diagnostic yield. This was at a time when cross-sectional imaging was not available; until then, dangerous needles had made liver biopsy a risky procedure. The advent of cross-sectional imaging redefined the need for liver biopsy in a considerable number of patients and, particularly, obviated the need in many patients with cholestatic problems (1). Serologic testing for viral hepatitis A, B, and, later, Delta (D) and C, and other diseases further reduced the indications in a number of patients.

New opportunities brought new tasks for the pathologists. Liver transplantation became a viable option, with added inquiries on rejection pathology versus recurrence of chronic liver disease for which transplantation was performed versus opportunistic infections; while bone-marrow transplantation brought graft-versus-host disease as a challenge. However, improved immunosuppression subsequently reduced the indications for biopsies in transplant patients. With the introduction of many antiviral treatment agents, liver biopsies are now most frequently done for staging of fibrosis and assessment of disease activity in patients with chronic viral hepatitis B and C to assist management decisions. Metabolic syndrome is associated with fatty liver disease in epidemic proportions, and selection of these patients that may benefit from a liver biopsy continues to be a topic of debate.

Time has put a new pressure on clinicians to rethink liver biopsy because there are less invasive alternatives, including surrogate serum markers and advanced imaging technology. Devices and techniques that a few decades ago were considered a breakthrough in safety and acceptability are currently less so. Fibroscan, a device that translates a physical tissue property (elasticity) into a number as a reflection of more or less advanced liver disease, has emerged as an alternative to liver biopsy and may serve as a noninvasive device that helps in identifying disease severity and therapy indications in larger populations. We had discussed the benefits and limitations of this technology (2). Not performing a liver biopsy puts the burden on the clinician to be sufficiently sure about a diagnosis that

is clinically suspected. If a liver biopsy is done, the role of the pathologist becomes important. Key questions in respect to the findings on liver biopsy include:

- Is the specimen adequate to answer questions, including the stage of the disease and the grade of the inflammatory activity?
- Are the histopathologic findings consistent with the presumed clinical diagnosis?
- Has the histology improved because of or despite a therapy?
- Is it likely a single diagnosis or should multiple etiologies be suspected, for example, hepatitis C virus + iron overload + NASH or HIV + drug-induced injury in the context of coexisting HIV infection?

The diagnostic challenges include the recognition of the predominant pathology and then critically tailor the options to a limited rather than an excessive differential diagnosis. The pathologist, like the clinician and the imager, should do a major attempt to be a "sniper." This role is greatly helped by taking into account all available information including a priori likelihood and should ideally avoid very elaborate and defensive statements.

The present book is a guide for pathologists or clinicians who run into puzzling questions provoked by the findings on the liver biopsy specimen. Key disease patterns need to be recognized. The book then takes the reader on a quick tour through a broad range of findings on liver biopsy specimens and provides illustrative examples of relevant pathology. It is an addition to rather than a replacement for more traditional textbooks. The readers, pathologists or clinicians, will find in this book a very handy combination of text and images to help arrive at a diagnosis.

The authors have established themselves as a quality collaborative couple with various extensive interactions over the years and rightly gained the respect of their peers. Swan Thung brings the heritage of the Hans Popper/Mount Sinai tradition in New York City and adds years of her own experience to that. Arief Suriawinata benefitted from experiences in Mount Sinai and Memorial Sloan-Kettering and then became part of the growing gastrointestinal and liver program at Dartmouth-Hitchcock Medical Center in New Hampshire. Jointly, and by their extensive clinical and pathologic networking, they have encountered most challenges in diagnostic liver pathology worldwide. Both live in the real world of liver pathology with close interactions with their clinical and basic science colleagues.

The reader will benefit from and enjoy a wealth of experience contained in this book. May the book travel widely and be enjoyed by many.

References

1. Sherlock S, Dick R, van Leeuwen DJ. Liver biopsy today: the Royal Free Hospital Experience. *J Hepatol.* 1984;1: 75-85.
2. Van Leeuwen DJ, Balabaud C, Crawford JM, Bioulac-Sage P, Dhillon AP. A clinical and histopathological perspective on evolving noninvasive and invasive alternatives for liver biopsy. *Clin Gastroenterol Hepatol.* 2008;6:491-6.

Dirk J. van Leeuwen, MD, PhD
Professor of Medicine
Adjunct, Dartmouth Medical School
Hanover, New Hampshire
Consultant Gastroenterologist and Hepatologist
Staff Member of the Teaching Hospital
Onze Lieve Vrouwe Gasthuis
Amsterdam, The Netherlands

Preface

The knowledge and treatment of liver disorders have evolved over the years, and so have the indications for liver biopsy. Although some of the indications of liver biopsy have been obviated by the advancement of serologic testing, imaging techniques, and noninvasive methods, liver biopsy remains considered as the criterion standard in the diagnosis of liver disease by many. Therefore, considering all the effort and risk of performing liver biopsy, precise diagnosis rendered from a liver biopsy is and will continue to be of paramount importance.

This book is designed to help the practicing pathologists, hepatologists, gastroenterologists, internists, and trainees in understanding common histologic patterns and key pathologic features of frequently encountered liver disorders. It is not meant to replace the traditional exhaustive liver textbook, but rather a companion "first-base" book for the interpretation of liver specimens and, in many instances, to sufficiently serve as a guide to the "home plate" as well.

Many pathologists without special training in hepatopathology will be able to produce a differential diagnosis of two or three entities but will have difficulty in narrowing down the differential diagnosis. We hope that this book will help many pathologists to arrive at a definite conclusion and final diagnosis necessary for patient management. There-

fore, rather than elaborating each individual liver disorder at length, we discuss frequently encountered liver disorders in consideration by our clinical colleagues in a practical and concise format and concentrate on the classic rather than atypical features of these disorders. A brief discussion of associated clinical findings, prognosis, and treatment is provided. Differential diagnoses are presented in tables to provide better overview. The illustrations were selected to represent key pathologic features and demonstrate the differential features. At the end of this book, key and review articles pertaining to the topics are listed and serve as a starting point for further reading and investigation.

Pathologists and hepatologists in training will find this book very useful in understanding normal liver histology, histopathologic features of liver disorders, and special procedures in the assessment of liver specimens to guide them to arrive at the final diagnosis.

We hope that this book will be an indispensible companion in the interpretation of liver biopsy specimens and the diagnosis of liver disorders, which will ultimately benefit patients with liver disorders.

Arief A. Suriawinata, MD
Swan N. Thung, MD

Acknowledgments

We are indebted to our teachers, our pathology and clinical colleagues, residents, and fellows at The Mount Sinai Medical Center and Dartmouth-Hitchcock Medical Center for their invaluable contributions. We are grateful to Dr. Dirk van Leeuwen for the insightful comments.

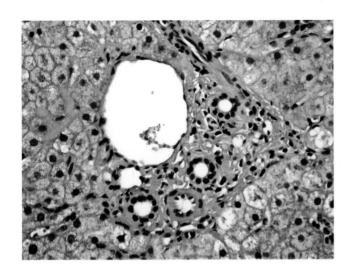

CHAPTER 1

APPROACH TO LIVER SPECIMENS, NORMAL, MINOR, AND STRUCTURAL ALTERATIONS

1.1 Approach to Liver Specimens

Liver Biopsy

A significant proportion of liver biopsies nowadays are performed for chronic viral hepatitis and fatty liver disease to assess liver damage and response to therapy, evaluate liver allograft, and diagnose space-occupying lesions. With the availability of serologic and imaging studies, biopsy of acute liver disease is rarely required, except when there is doubt on the clinical diagnosis or unclear etiology of elevation of liver enzymes.

Liver biopsy is an invasive procedure; therefore, indications and techniques should be carefully considered. The current techniques of liver biopsy include percutaneous, transjugular, open, and laparoscopic biopsies (see Table 1.1.1). Each technique has its own indication and advantages. The complication rate of liver biopsy is low but significant, which includes bleeding, intrahepatic/subcapsular hematoma, bile peritonitis, hemobilia, pneumoperitoneum, pneumothorax, sepsis, subphrenic abscess, and intrahepatic arteriovenous fistula. Severe right upper quadrant or shoulder pain can be encountered in a third of patients.

At the time of biopsy, the specimen should be immediately examined for adequacy and immersed in a fixative. A specimen size of at least 1.5 cm in total length is required to minimize sampling error, or another pass is recommended. The routine fixative for liver biopsies is 10% neutral buffered formalin. Saline should not be used. Liver biopsy performed in infants and children with jaundice requires additional handling, such as a snap-frozen section for molecular study and glutaraldehyde fixation for electron microscopy, because of the broad differential diagnosis that often includes an inherited metabolic disease. Abnormal gross morphology and color of liver biopsy specimen may indicate severe liver disease; for example, fragmented liver needle core specimen indicates cirrhosis (Figure 1.1.2), firm white needle core specimen is seen in biopsy of tumors, yellow discoloration indicates severe fatty liver, green discoloration indicates severe cholestasis, brown discoloration is seen in severe iron overload, and dark brown or black tissue can be seen in metastatic melanoma.

Initial histologic examination is best conducted without the knowledge of clinical and laboratory information. After the structure and generalized pattern of injury have been appreciated, a differential diagnosis and, eventually, a diagnosis can be rendered in combination with clinical and laboratory information.

Liver Resection

Liver resections are performed to remove focal lesions. The extent of the resections varies from small wedges to the removal of an entire lobe. Several surfaces may be covered by a hepatic capsule, whereas the exposed and often cauterized surface is the surgical margin and may be designated by the surgeon, especially when the lesion is close to a particular margin of concern (Figure 1.1.4). Once the margin is identified, the specimen is measured and weighed. A bulge in the surface of the liver or retraction of the capsule can aid in localizing the lesion.

The specimen is serially sectioned at 0.5- to 1-cm intervals, with the initial section passing through the center of the lesion to demonstrate surgical margin clearance and to measure the largest diameter of the lesion. The number of lesions, appearance, margin clearance, and gross vascular invasion are recorded. A positive margin or minimal clearance potentially leads to an additional excisional margin.

Liver Explantation

Liver explantation is performed during liver transplantation or retransplantation. Explanted liver should be evaluated for the underlying chronic liver disease, the cause of acute liver failure, and the presence of tumor. Thorough examination of the hilar region, including patency of the hepatic artery, portal vein, and bile duct, should be done before the specimen is sectioned. Lymph nodes in the hilar soft tissue should also be sampled. After hilar structures have been carefully examined and sampled, the entire liver parenchyma is sectioned using a long and sharp knife in a coronal plane at 0.5- to 1-cm intervals. Thin sectioning is necessary to avoid missing dysplastic nodules and small hepatocellular carcinoma (Figure 1.1.6). Gross characteristics of the liver parenchyma, appearance, and the number of nodules are recorded. Key samples for histologic examination and special studies should be obtained immediately.

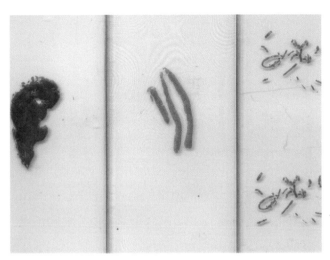

Figure 1.1.1 Different sizes of wedge biopsy, percutaneous biopsy, and transjugular biopsy specimens.

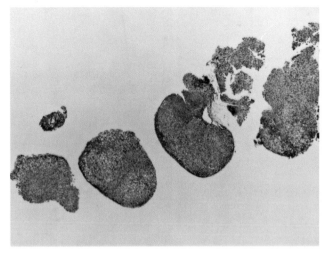

Figure 1.1.2 Fragmented needle biopsy of cirrhotic liver parenchyma (trichrome stain).

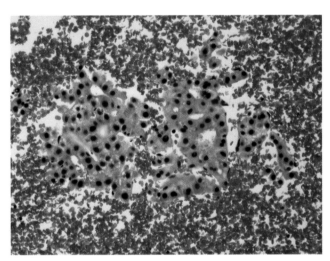

Figure 1.1.3 An imaging-guided fine-needle aspiration of hepatocellular carcinoma yielding a cord of neoplastic cells in pseudoglandular configuration, partially wrapped by flat endothelial cells.

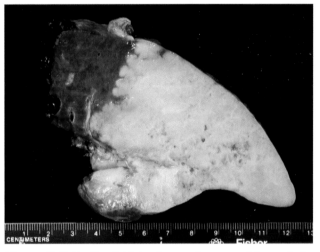

Figure 1.1.4 Partial lobectomy of a grey white and circumscribed cholangiocarcinoma. The resection margin has been inked black.

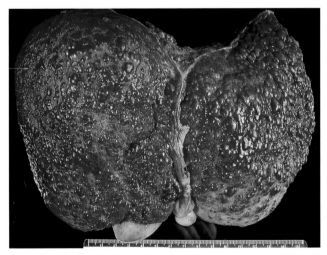

Figure 1.1.5 Explanted liver showing diffusely nodular cirrhotic liver.

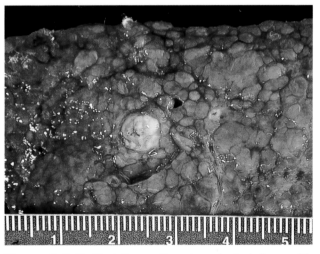

Figure 1.1.6 Serially sectioned explanted liver with subcentimeter hepatocellular carcinoma.

Table 1.1.1 Liver Biopsy Methods

Methods	Technique	Comments
Percutaneous biopsy	Suction needle (Menghini, Klatskin, Jamshidi) or cutting needle (Vim-Silverman, Tru-Cut) or spring-loaded cutting needle (ASAP gun, etc).	Most common method, provides adequate specimen for review and other studies. Complications and specimen outcome are related to the experience of the operator. Major contraindication is bleeding tendency. Relative contraindications are ascites, morbid obesity, and infection of pleural cavity.
Transjugular (transvenous) biopsy	Catheter through the internal jugular vein, right atrium, and inferior vena cava. Ability to measure hemodynamics when combined with wedged hepatic pressure and venography.	Second-line procedure for patients with coagulopathy, gross ascites, morbid obesity, or fulminant hepatic failure. Smaller and often fragmented specimens. Complications include arrhythmia and reaction to contrast material.
Laparoscopic or open abdominal biopsy	Needle or wedge biopsy. Direct visualization of the liver and peritoneal cavity.	Largest specimen. More sensitive for diagnosis of zonal chronic liver diseases and structural changes, such as primary sclerosing cholangitis, hepatoportal sclerosis, and nodular regenerative hyperplasia. Useful for initial diagnosis or staging of neoplasm. Laparoscopic bariatric surgery for obesity has increased the number of intraoperative biopsies for steatohepatitis evaluation. Risk of anesthesia and hemorrhage.
Computed tomography or ultrasound-guided biopsy	Ultrasound or computed tomography is used for visualization of hepatic lesion and anatomic structures and to avoid intersecting large vessels. <1-mm needle is usually used (fine-needle aspiration), but larger caliber similar to percutaneous biopsy can also be used.	For histologic or cytologic diagnosis of space-occupying lesion or when the patient's anatomy makes finding landmarks difficult. Cell block increases sensitivity and allows special or immunostaining. Controversial issues remain regarding dissemination of malignant cells, although these are less common than with thick-needle biopsies.

1.2 Routine and Special Stains

It is generally accepted that hematoxylin and eosin (H&E) stain is the standard stain in liver pathology. H&E stain allows accurate histologic evaluation in most liver specimens of nonneoplastic and neoplastic liver diseases. In addition to the H&E stain, special stains are frequently requested to confirm structures or findings seen or suspected on the H&E slide. Table 1.2.1 lists various special stains commonly performed in liver pathology.

Nonneoplastic Diseases

"Routine" special stain varies from one practice to another, but in most practices, routine special stains include at least a special stain for connective tissue and a special stain for iron. Other special stains are ordered as necessary after the initial histologic examination.

Special stain for connective tissue, commonly trichrome stain, identifies normal structures, such as portal triads and terminal hepatic venules, necessary for the evaluation of the lobular architecture and for the assessment of the degree of fibrosis in chronic liver diseases (Figures 1.2.1 and 1.2.2). Mature fibrous tissue and portal tract stroma are dark blue, while immature fibrous tissue is pale blue. Trichrome stain also greatly aids the identification of normal structures and portal tracts in autopsy liver with autolysis. Sirius red stain is an alternative to trichrome stain, particularly when morphometric quantification of fibrosis is desired, but it is not useful in identification of normal structures (Figure 1.2.3). Reticulin stain should be ordered when alteration of lobular architecture and hepatocyte plate thickness are suspected, such as in nodular regenerative hyperplasia and various vascular problems (Figure 1.2.4).

Special stain for iron, usually Perl's iron, is a common routine special stain for the identification of iron in the liver parenchyma (Figures 1.2.5 and 1.2.6). Copper (rhodanine) stain is ordered for the evaluation of Wilson disease and in various diseases resulting in chronic cholestasis, such as primary sclerosing cholangitis, primary biliary cirrhosis, chronic bile duct obstruction, and ductopenia (Figure 1.2.7). Mallory-Denk hyaline and copper colocalize in periportal and periseptal hepatocytes in chronic cholestasis. Bile stain (Figure 1.2.8) is usually not required for the identification of bile because bile can be readily identified with H&E stain as green-brown discoloration of the hepatocyte cytoplasm and bile plugs in bile canaliculi. Periodic acid–Schiff (PAS) with diastase reaction aids the identification of intracytoplasmic globules in α-1-antitrypsin deficiency (Figure 1.2.9) and chronic passive congestion, the identification of ceroid-laden macrophages as evidence of hepatocyte drop out and disruption of basement membrane surrounding bile ducts in primary biliary cirrhosis.

Special stains for microorganisms are ordered when infectious disease is suspected or in liver biopsy of immunocompromised patients. As an alternative to immunohistochemistry, Victoria blue stain is used to identify ground glass hepatocytes containing hepatitis B surface antigen; in addition, Victoria blue stain can be used to identify copper binding protein as well as elastic fibers in the evaluation of the maturity of fibrosis.

Neoplastic Diseases

Reticulin stain is the most common special stain ordered in the evaluation of hepatocellular adenoma, dysplastic nodules, and hepatocellular carcinoma. Other stains may be ordered but are usually unnecessary for diagnosis, such as Perl's iron to demonstrate differential iron deposition in dysplastic nodule and/or hepatocellular carcinoma and their surrounding cirrhotic nodules, and rhodanine stain to demonstrate copper deposition in some of benign hepatocellular tumors such as focal nodular hyperplasia. In general, immunohistochemistry plays a more important role in neoplastic diseases.

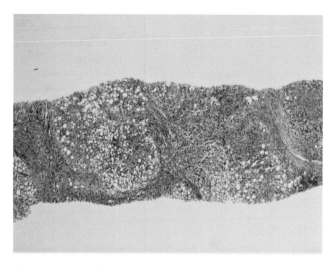

Figure 1.2.1 Trichrome stain demonstrating cirrhosis.

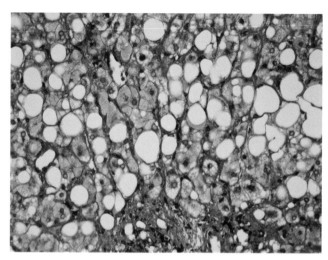

Figure 1.2.2 Trichrome stain demonstrating pericellular fibrosis.

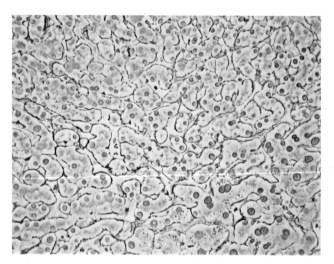

Figure 1.2.3 Reticulin stain showing 1-cell-thick to occasional 2-cell-thick normal hepatocyte cords.

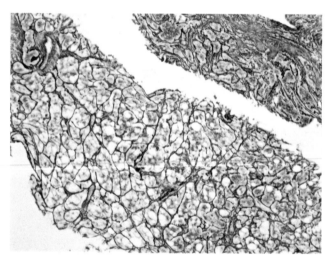

Figure 1.2.4 Reticulin stain demonstrating irregularly thickened cords of hepatocellular carcinoma.

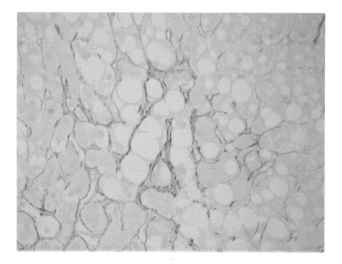

Figure 1.2.5 Sirius red stain demonstrating pericellular fibrosis in steatohepatitis.

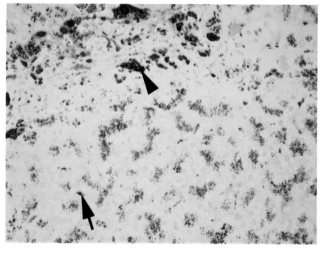

Figure 1.2.6 Perl's stain demonstrating iron deposition in hepatocytes, Kupffer cells (arrow), and portal macrophages (arrowhead) in hereditary hemochromatosis.

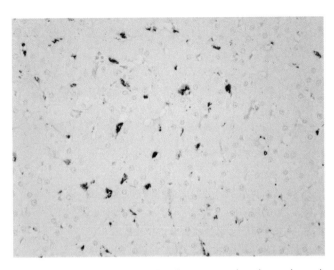

Figure 1.2.7 Perl's stain demonstrating iron deposition in Kupffer cells in secondary iron overload.

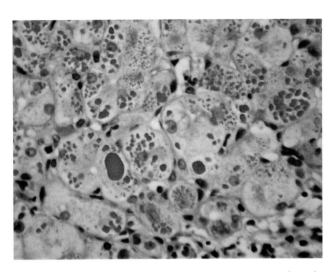

Figure 1.2.8 Eosinophilic α-1-antitrypsin cytoplasmic globules, predominantly periportal, are identified by PAS with diastase digestion.

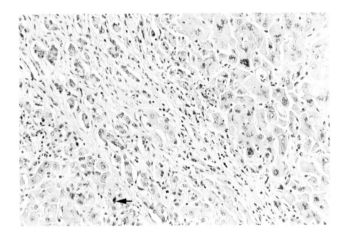

Figure 1.2.9 Rhodanine stain demonstrates orange granules of copper in the periportal hepatocytes in chronic cholestasis (cholate stasis). The green pigment is bile (arrow).

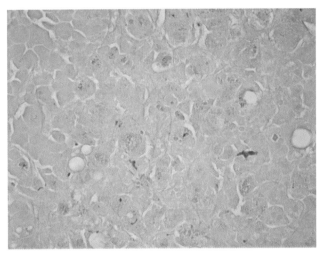

Figure 1.2.10 Hall's stain aids the identification of bile (green) in bile canaliculi and the cytoplasm of hepatocytes.

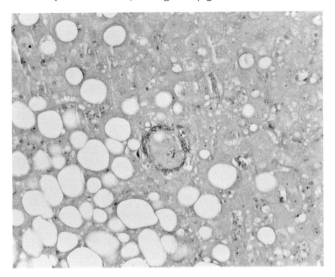

Figure 1.2.11 Phosphotungstic acid hematoxylin demonstrating purple fibrin-ring granuloma in Q fever.

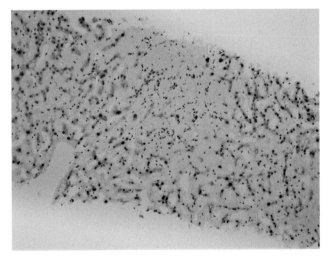

Figure 1.2.12 Congo red stain demonstrating diffuse amyloid deposition in perisinusoidal spaces, occluding the sinusoidal spaces.

Table 1.2.1 Commonly Performed Special Stains in Liver Pathology

Special Stain	Primary Use	Interpretation
Connective and muscle tissues		
Masson's trichrome	Identification of type I collagen; routine stain for fibrosis assessment or staging of chronic hepatitis	Muscle, keratin, cytoplasm, megamitochondria, Mallory-Denk bodies = red; collagen = blue
Sirius red	Idenfitication and morphometric quantitation of type I collagen; sensitive staining for fibrosis; alternative to trichrome stain	Collagen = red
Gordon and Sweets reticulin	Identification of type III collagen; evaluation of lobular architecture and hepatocyte plate thickness in dysplastic nodules, hepatocellular carcinoma, and nodular regenerative hyperplasia	Reticulin = black; collagen = rose color
Phosphotungstic acid hematoxylin	Identification of fibrin in fibrin-ring granuloma and toxemia in pregnancy	Fibrin, nuclei, cytoplasm, mitotic figures, mitochondria = purple; collagen = red
Microorganisms		
Ziehl-Neelsen	Identification of acid fast bacilli	Mycobacterium, lipofuscin, ceroid = red; background = light blue
Shikata orcein	Identification of hepatitis B surface antigen	Elastic fibers, hepatitis B surface antigen, copper-binding protein = dark brown
Victoria blue	Identification of hepatitis B surface antigen	Elastic fibers, hepatitis B surface antigen, copper-binding protein, lipofuscin, mast cell = blue; cytoplasm, nuclei = red
Groccot methenamine silver	Microorganisms	Fungi, bacteria, mucin, glycogen, melanin = black; background = green
Warthin-Starry	Spirochetes	Spirochete = black; background = yellow
Pigments and minerals		
Perl's iron	Identification, semiquantitative assessment, and distribution of iron/hemosiderin in iron overload	Iron (ferric state) = blue
Hall's	Idenfication of bilirubin in cholestatic diseases and tumor	Bilirubin = green; muscle and cytoplasm = yellow; collagen = red
Rhodanine	Identification of copper in Wilson's disease and chronic cholestasis	Copper = reddish-orange
Fontana Masson	Identification of Dubin-Johnson pigment and melanin	Dubin Johnson pigment, lipofuscin, bile, melanin = black; hepatocytes = pink/red
Glycogen		
PAS	Identification of glycogen.	Glycogen, fungi = magenta
PAS-D	Identification of intracytoplasmic globules in α-1-antitrypsin deficiency or ceroid laden macrophages as indication of hepatocellular dropout.	Glycoprotein, basement membrane, α-1-antitrypsin, atypical *Mycobacterium*, ceroid laden macrophages = magenta; glycogen = clear
Amyloid		
Congo red	Identification of amyloid in vessels, portal stroma, and perisinusoidal spaces	Amyloid = salmon pink; nuclei = blue; elastic fiber = pink
Lipids		
Oil red O	Identification of fat; requires fresh tissue and frozen section preparation	Fat = red; nuclei = blue

1.3 Immunohistochemistry

The availability of highly specific monoclonal antibodies and highly sensitive immunohistochemical staining techniques has made it possible to demonstrate many antigens in routinely processed tissue sections of nonneoplastic and neoplastic liver diseases. Table 1.3.1 lists various immunohistochemical staining commonly performed in liver pathology.

Nonneoplastic Diseases

Immunohistochemistry in nonneoplastic liver diseases is commonly performed for (1) localization of hepatotropic and nonhepatotropic viral antigens, (2) identification of biliary epithelium, and (3) identification of inclusion bodies in storage and hereditary diseases.

Immunohistochemistry for the identification of hepatitis B surface and core antigens are commonly performed in liver biopsy of serologically hepatitis B–positive patients to confirm the diagnosis (Figures 1.3.1 and 1.3.2). Various systemic nonhepatotropic virus immunohistochemical stains are available for identification and confirmation of diagnosis, particularly in immunocompromised and organ transplant patients (Figure 1.3.12). For hepatitis C virus, there is no reliable immunohistochemical stain for formalin-fixed paraffin-embedded tissue.

Cytokeratin (CK) 7 or 19 immunostain is performed for identification and counting of bile duct when bile duct loss/ ductopenia, graft-versus-host disease, or chronic allograft rejection is suspected. In addition, both CKs can be used to evaluate the degree of ductular reaction in biliary diseases and chronic viral hepatitis. CK7 staining of periportal cholestatic hepatocytes confirms long-standing cholestasis.

α-1-Antitrypsin and fibrinogen immunostains are performed to identify intracytoplasmic inclusion bodies in α-1-antitrypsin deficiency and fibrinogen storage disease, respectively.

Neoplastic Diseases

The most common use of immunohistochemistry for liver specimen is for identification, immunophenotyping, classification, and prognostication of primary or metastatic tumors to the liver. It should be noted, however, that primary or metastatic poorly/undifferentiated tumors may lose their organ-specific antigenicity; therefore, in rare instances, immunohistochemistry may fail to pinpoint organ of origin of the tumor and may require clinical correlation or further imaging studies.

For the identification of hepatocellular carcinoma, the expected staining is cytoplasmic positivity of HepPar1, TTF-1, glypican-3, CK8, and CK18, and canalicular staining for polyclonal CEA and CD10. Poorly differentiated hepatocellular carcinoma may lose some of the antigenicity to some of these antibodies, particularly in needle biopsy specimen due to limited sampling of the tumor. Positivity for CK7 or CK19 in hepatocellular carcinoma suggests cholangiocellular differentiation or mixed hepatocellular carcinoma-cholangiocarcinoma. In addition, positivity for CK19 has been suggested in hepatocellular carcinoma with aggressive behavior. Positivity for glypican-3 can be used to differentiate hepatocellular carcinoma from dysplastic nodules and cirrhotic nodules.

In benign hepatocellular tumors, serum amyloid A, C-reactive protein, glutamine synthetase, β-catenin, CK7, and Ki67 play an important role in differentiating these lesions. Focal nodular hyperplasia shows positivity for CK7 in the ductules and map-like staining pattern for glutamine synthetase. Inflammatory hepatocellular adenoma shows positive staining for serum amyloid A and C-reactive protein and occasional CK7 staining in ductular structures. Conventional hepatocellular adenoma shows diffuse or patchy (not map-like) positivity for glutamine synthetase, and it is negative for CK7 and serum amyloid A. In addition, higher rate of Ki67, diffuse strong positivity for glutamine synthetase, and nuclear positivity for β-catenin are seen in hepatocellular adenoma with high risk of transformation to well-differentiated hepatocellular carcinoma.

Workup for metastatic tumors involves various antibodies, including establishing a line of differentiation (epithelial, stromal, or melanoma) and organ of origin. For epithelial tumor or adenocarcinoma, CK7 and CK20 immunostaining profile and additional organ-specific antibodies (TTF-1, CDX-2, etc.) are required.

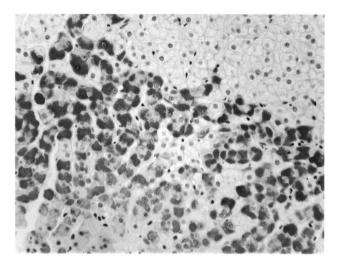

Figure 1.3.1 Hepatitis B surface antigen immunostain in chronic hepatitis B demonstrating hepatitis B surface antigen reactivity in the cytoplasm of ground glass hepatocytes. Notice the lack of staining of the nuclei.

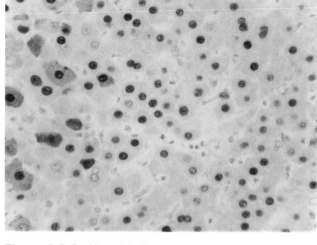

Figure 1.3.2 Hepatitis B core antigen (HBcAg) immunostain in chronic hepatitis B demonstrating nuclear HBcAg with occasional cytoplasmic HBcAg reactivity. The HBcAg staining correlates with active viral replication.

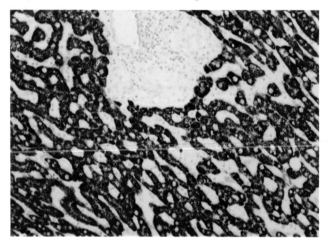

Figure 1.3.3 HepPar1 immunostain demonstrating intense granular staining of the cytoplasm of normal hepatocytes.

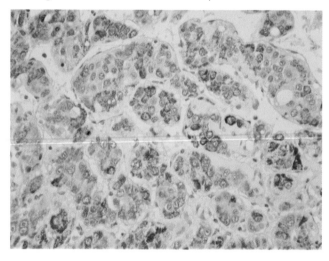

Figure 1.3.4 HepPar1 immunostain showing patchy cytoplasmic positivity in hepatocellular carcinoma.

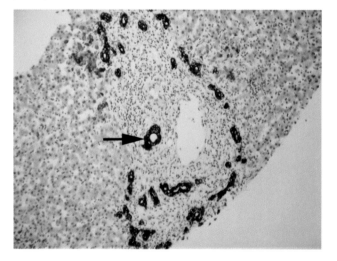

Figure 1.3.5 Bile duct (arrow), bile ductules, and ductular hepatocytes are reactive for cytokeratin 7.

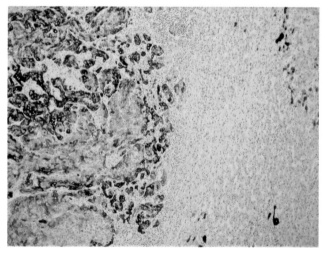

Figure 1.3.6 Cytokeratin 7 immunostain showing positive staining of cholangiocarcinoma (predominantly in the left field) and bile ductules (scattered in the right field), whereas hepatocytes in the right field are negative.

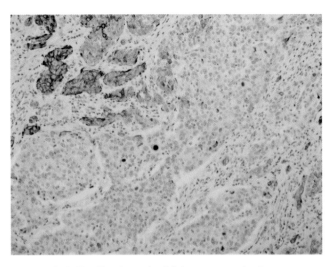

Figure 1.3.7 Cytokeratin 19 immunostain demonstrating cholangiocellular differentiation in mixed hepatocellular carcinoma—cholangiocarcinoma.

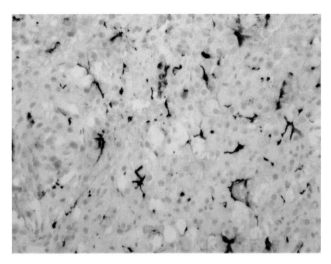

Figure 1.3.8 Polyclonal carcinoembryonic antigen immunostain demonstrating canalicular differentiation in hepatocellular carcinoma.

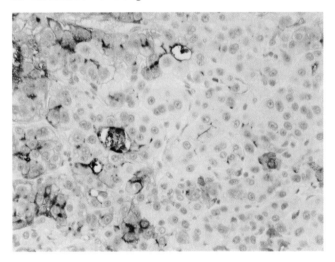

Figure 1.3.9 CD10 immunostain demonstrating canalicular differentiation in hepatocellular carcinoma.

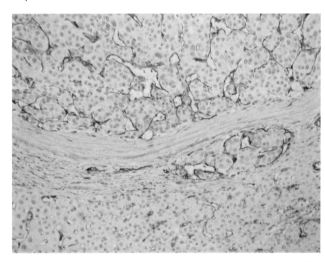

Figure 1.3.10 CD31 immunostain showing positive staining of endothelial cells, wrapping around thick cords of hepatocellular carcinoma in the upper field. The cirrhotic nodule is in the lower field.

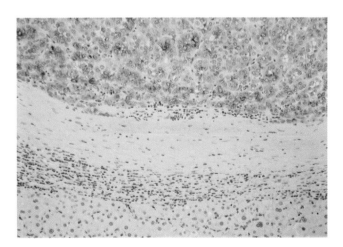

Figure 1.3.11 Glypican-3 immunostain showing cytoplasmic and membranous reactivity of hepatocellular carcinoma in the upper field and negative staining in the cirrhotic nodule in the lower field.

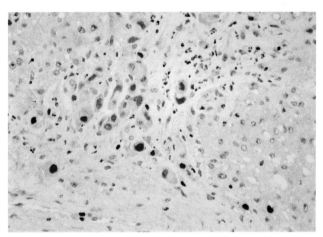

Figure 1.3.12 Immunohistochemical stain for cytomegalovirus showing nuclear and cytoplasmic positivity in CMV hepatitis, colocalizing with viral cytopathic changes in the H&E stain.

Table 1.3.1 Commonly Performed Immmunohistochemistry in Liver Pathology

Immunohistochemical Stains	Utility and Interpretation
Detection of viral antigens	
HBsAg and HBcAg	Visual aid to idenfication of HBsAg-positive ground glass hepatocytes and confirmation of hepatitis B infection. HBcAg provides status of HBV replication, particularly in combined hepatitis viral infections.
HDV	Confirmation of HDV coinfection or superinfection in HBV-infected patients.
Nonhepatotropic viruses	Identification of nonhepatotropic viruses (cytomegalovirus, herpes simplex, EBV, adenovirus, etc).
Hepatitis C virus	No reliable immunohistochemical stain currently available.
Identification and classification of tumors	
Hepatocyte paraffin 1	Positive in 90% well and moderately differentiated HCC, but often negative in poorly differentiated HCC.
α-fetoprotein	Positive in 40% HCC, in all hepatoblastomas and fetal livers. Hepatocytes in cirrhotic nodules may occasionally show focal positive staining.
Polyclonal CEA	Bile canalicular staining or canalicular differentiation in HCC. Cytoplasmic and membranous staining in adenocarcinoma.
Glypican-3	Positive in 80% hepatocellular carcinoma and focally in dysplastic nodules.
Serum amyloid A	Positive in inflammatory hepatocellular adenoma.
CD10, villin	Bile canalicular staining or canalicular differentiation in HCC.
Monoclonal CEA	Negative in HCC. Positive in 60% adenocarcinoma, cytoplasmic, and membranous staining.
MOC-31	Negative in HCC. Positive in 80% adenocarcinoma.
Cytokeratins	Coordinate CK7/CK20 staining are commonly used in the evaluation of metastatic carcinomas, both are negative in HCC. Hepatocytes are positive for CK8 and CK18. CK7 and CK19 are positive in the presence of cholangiocellular differentiation in HCC and cholangiocarcinoma.
NCAM (CD56)	Positive in bile ductules and cholangiolocarcinoma, but negative or focally positive in bile duct and cholangiocarcinoma
Thyroid transcription factor-1	Cytoplasmic staining indicates hepatocellular differentiation. Nuclear staining indicates pulmonary adenocarcinoma or thyroid origin tumors. Positive in pulmonary small cell neuroendocrine carcinoma, and to less extent in its extrapulmonary counterpart.
Epithelial membrane antigen	Negative in HCC. Positive in adenocarcinoma.
Factor VIII-related antigen, CD31 and CD34	Vascular tumors or endothelial cells of HCC. Sinusoidal endothelial cells are generally negative in normal liver except in the immediate periportal region and chronic liver diseases.
P63	Positive in squamous cell carcinoma, nuclear staining.
Organ-specific antigens	TTF-1 (lung or thyroid), GCDFP or breast-2 (breast), prostate-specific antigen, estrogen and progesterone receptors (breast or gynecologic tract), renal cell carcinoma, CDX-2 (intestinal differentiation).
Prognostication of tumors	
Ki67 or PCNA	Differentiating HCC from high-grade dysplastic nodule or hepatocellular adenoma.
CK19	HCC with aggressive behavior.
Beta catenin	Nuclear positivity for beta catenin is seen in hepatocellular adenoma with high risk of transformation to HCC.

Table 1.3.1 *(continued)*

Immunohistochemical Stains	Utility and Interpretation
Identification of bile duct epithelium	
Cytokeratins 7 or 19	Identification of bile ducts and ductules in the evaluation of ductopenia or chronic rejection. Confirming the degree of ductular reaction in biliary diseases and chronic viral hepatitis.
Storage and hereditary diseases	
α-1-Antitrypsin	Predominantly periportal intracytoplasmic globules in α-1-antitrypsin deficiency
Fibrinogen	Intracytoplasmic fibrinogen deposition in fibrinogen storage disease
Miscellaneous	
Leukemia/leukemia phenotyping	Differentiating and/or confirming PTLD from EBV hepatitis or acute rejection
Cytokeratins 8, 18, and 19	Embryonal hepatocytes, expression of CK19 disappears by 10th week of gestation
Synaptophysin, glial fibrillary acidic protein, and neural cell adhesion molecule	Neural/neuroectodermal differentiation markers can be used to identify resting hepatic stellate cells
Ubiquitin, cytokeratins 8 and 18, p62	Idenfitication of Mallory-Denk hyalins
Vimentin, desmin, and smooth muscle actin	Myofibroblastic differentiation in activated hepatic stellate cells (including vitamin A toxicity)
HMB45, MART1	Positive in angiomyolipoma and melanoma

HBsAg indicates hepatitis B surface antigen; HBcAg, hepatitis B core antigen; HDV, hepatitis delta virus; HCC, hepatocellular carcinomas;

HBV, hepatitis B virus; PCNA, proliferating cell nuclear antigen; PTLD, posttransplant lymphoproliferative disease; EBV, Epstein-Barr virus.

1.4　Molecular Studies and Electron Microscopy

Molecular Studies

Much of the routine molecular diagnostic applications associated with liver disease are geared toward the assessment of hepatitis B and C. Molecular technologies have been developed for the qualitative and quantitative detection and genotyping of these viruses, providing prognostic indicator and guidance of therapeutic options. With regard to neoplastic diseases of the liver, molecular assays are currently used in investigational studies to understand the pathogenesis of benign hepatocellular tumors, preneoplastic nodules, hepatocellular carcinoma, and cholangiocarcinoma, which can provide better surveillance, diagnosis, treatment, and prognostication of these lesions.

In situ hybridization employs radioactive/fluorescent/ antigen-labeled complementary DNA or RNA sequences to localize a specific DNA or RNA sequence in tissue. In situ hybridization has been applied to liver tissue for the identification of hepatitis A, B, C, and D viruses; cytomegalovirus; and Epstein-Barr virus. In situ hybridization can be used to identify albumin messenger RNA, which is highly specific for normal hepatocytes and hepatocellular tumors.

Polymerase chain reaction is a technique used to amplify exponentially a single or few copies of DNA sequence, employing DNA polymerase and generating thousands to millions of copies of the particular DNA sequence. Reverse transcription–polymerase chain reaction allows the identification of RNA. Currently, these techniques are the most sensitive and specific method to demonstrate hepatitis B virus DNA, hepatitis C virus RNA, and their genotypes in the blood and liver tissue. In addition, PCR can be used to identify infectious organisms or specific genetic mutations.

Microarray analysis provides an arrayed series of thousands of DNA sequences. Each may contain a specific DNA sequence, in which relative abundance is determined by chemiluminescence-labeled targets. It can be used to measure changes in expression levels, to detect single nucleotide polymorphisms, and for comparative studies in neoplastic and nonneoplastic liver diseases.

Electron Microscopy

Electron microscopy has a limited but well-defined role in investigating (1) hereditary and metabolic liver diseases, (2) viral infection not otherwise identified by light microscopy or serology, (3) tumors of unknown histogenesis, (4) certain drug-induced liver injuries, and (5) diseases of unclear etiology. Tissue obtained for electron microscopic study should be fixed in 3% glutaraldehyde.

Table 1.4.1　Molecular Studies in Liver Pathology

In situ hybridization

Detection of hepatotropic and nonhepatotropic viruses

Detection of albumin messenger RNA in hepatocellular tumors

Polymerase chain reaction

Quantification of hepatitis B virus DNA and hepatitis C virus RNA

Genotyping of hepatitis B and C virus

Detection of infectious agents (virus, bacteria, parasite)

Detection of genetic mutations (hereditary hemochromatosis, progressive familial intrahepatic cholestasis)

Microarray analysis

Gene expression profile

Comparative genomic hybridization

Detection of single nucleotide polymorphism

Table 1.4.2 Electron Microscopy Findings in Liver Pathology

Indication	Findings
Detection of viral infection	
Hepatitis B virus	Intranuclear core virus particle, dilated smooth endoplasmic reticulum containing HBsAg reactive filaments
Suspected virus with no serologic test or culture	Intranuclear or intracytoplasmic virions
Evaluation of genetic and metabolic disease	
Glycogenoses	Glycogen pools displacing organelles to the periphery of cells. Lipid droplets.
Glycogenosis type II (Pompe disease)	Enlarged lysosomes containing glycogen, cytoplasmic glycogen rosettes
Glycogenosis type IV (Anderson disease)	Undulating, random, delicate, nonmembrane bound fibrillar inclusions
Myoclonus epilepsy (Lafora disease)	Lafora inclusions (fibrillar and granular non-membrane bound material)
Hereditary fructose intolerance	Concentric and irregularly disposed membranous arrays and rarefaction of hyaloplasm
Mucopolysaccharidosis	Vacuolated lysosomes containing dense mucopolysaccharide material in hepatocytes and Kupffer cells
Cystinosis	Spaces created by cystine crystals in lysosomes of Kupffer cells
Fibrinogen storage disease	Densely packed tubular structures in fingerprint-like pattern in rough endoplasmic reticulum
Wolman diseases	Cholesterol crystals in lysosomes of Kupffer cells and cytoplasm of hepatocytes
Cholesterol ester storage disease	Triglyceride droplets in cytoplasm of hepatocytes
Gangliosidosis	Granulofibrillar material in Kupffer cells or membrane-bound inclusions in Kupffer cells and hepatocytes
Galactosidase deficiency (Fabry disease)	Dense and laminated inclusions in hepatocytes and Kupffer cells
Ceramidase deficiency (Farber disease)	Recti/curvilinear cytoplasmic inlcusion in macrophages, dense bodies and clear vacuoles in hepatocytes
Glycosylceramide lipidosis (Gaucher disease)	Cytoplasmic tubular bodies (dense ring in cross section) in macrophages
Sphingomyelin lipidosis (Niemann-Pick disease)	Lamellar lipid inclusions in lysosomes of hepatocytes and Kupffer cells
Mitochondrial disorders	Pleomorphic mitochondria with granular matrix and loss of cristae
Dubin-Johnson syndrome	Complex dense bodies
α-1-Antitrypsin deficiency	Finely granular material in the cisternae of dilated endoplasmic reticulum of hepatocytes
Wilson disease	Variation of mitochondria, vacuolation, deposition of crystalline material
Diagnosis of tumor of uncertain histogenesis	
Carcinoma	Intercellular bridges, microvilli
Sarcoma	Intermediate filaments: vimentin, actin
Neuroendocrine tumor	Neurosecretory granules
Melanoma	Melanosomes, premelanosomes
Evaluation of drug-related changes	
Phospholipidosis	Enlarged lysosome containing lamellar and reticular inclusions resembling myelin
Reye syndrome	Abnormal, swollen mitochondria
Hypervitaminosis A	Multivesicular hepatic stellate cells (Ito cells) with fat droplets

1.5   Normal Liver

Histologic examination of liver biopsies should conform to a specific routine, which includes evaluation of normal structures of the liver (lobular architecture, portal triads, limiting plate, hepatocytes, sinusoidal cells, and terminal hepatic venules) and their deviation; therefore, basic knowledge of the normal structures of the liver is important. An initial low-magnification examination of the liver parenchyma should give the overall impression of the architecture and the presence or absence of focal changes, which is then followed by a higher-magnification examination of each of the structures in the liver.

Hepatic Parenchyma

The hepatocytes are arranged in functional units referred to as either the lobule of Kiernan or the acinus of Rappaport. A hepatic lobule of Kiernan consists of a central venule with cords of hepatocytes radiating out toward several portal tracts, and zonal changes in the lobules are described as being centrilobular, midzonal, or periportal (Figures 1.5.1 and 1.5.2). A hepatic acinus of Rappaport consists of a portal tract as the axis that contains portal veins and hepatic arterioles, with blood flowing through the acinar sinusoids into several terminal hepatic venules, and the changes in the acini are described as being in zones 1, 2, and 3, corresponding to progressive decrease in tissue oxygenation.

Hepatocytes are polygonal epithelial cells with one or more centrally located round nuclei and are arranged in 1-cell-thick plates (Figure 1.5.3). The number of binucleate and polyploid hepatocytes increases with age. These changes are more prominent in the midzonal region, and their significance is unknown (Figure 1.5.4). Rare acidophilic or apoptotic bodies or mitoses may indicate physiologic turnover of hepatocytes in otherwise apparently normal liver parenchyma. The presence of 2-cell-thick plates and rosette formation in adults indicates hepatocyte regeneration.

The cytoplasm of normal hepatocytes contains a variable amount of glycogen and is often irregular in distribution, following diurnal and diet-related variations. Cytoplasmic glycogen imparts a fine, reticulated, foamy appearance to the cytoplasm. An irregular distribution pattern may be found normally in biopsies and is not of diagnostic significance. Scattered periportal glycogenated nuclei are normal in adolescents and young adults (Figure 1.5.5), whereas excessive glycogenated nuclei in adults are often seen in patients with glucose intolerance, diabetes mellitus, and Wilson disease.

Sinusoidal lining cells consist of specialized fenestrated endothelial cells and macrophages (Kupffer cells), which are usually inconspicuous in normal liver parenchyma.

Occasional lymphocytes and rare neutrophils may be identified in the sinusoids. Collections of neutrophils without clinical importance, termed *surgical hepatitis*, are often found in surgical biopsy or resection specimens due to exposure of the liver to free air. In between the sinusoidal lining cells and hepatocytes lies the space of Disse, containing hepatic stellate cells (Ito or fat-storing cells) and pit cells (natural killer lymphocytes). Hepatic stellate cells are modified resting fibroblasts that can store lipid and vitamin A and play a significant role in fibrogenesis (Figure 1.5.9) Elastic fibers and basement membrane material are absent from normal sinusoids.

Blood in the sinusoids drains into the terminal hepatic venule, which has a very thin wall and is in direct contact to the hepatocytes. Thickening of the terminal hepatic venule wall is often part of pericellular fibrosis in steatohepatitis, central hyalin sclerosis in alcoholic liver disease, or chronic passive congestion in congestive heart failure.

In older individuals, particularly those older than 60 years, there is more variation in the size of hepatocytes and the number of their nuclei (polyploidy) and an increase in lipofuscin pigment deposition. There may be apparent dilatation of sinusoids because of hepatocyte atrophy. These changes are accompanied by alterations in the metabolic function of the liver, including the metabolism of various toxins and drugs.

Portal Tracts

The portal tracts contain a bile duct, several bile ductules, a hepatic artery, a portal vein, and lymphatic channels (Figure 1.5.6). Bile ducts are lined by cuboidal or low columnar cholangiocytes. A bile duct is always accompanied by a hepatic artery of the same caliber. Larger bile ducts have more periductal fibrous tissues than smaller ones (Figure 1.5.7). Bile ductules are found at the periphery of the portal tracts, lined by cuboidal cholangiocytes. The absence of the portal vein may be encountered in up to 30% of portal tracts, whereas the absence of the bile duct and the hepatic artery does not exceed 10% of portal tracts. Portal tracts almost always contain a paired bile duct and hepatic artery of approximately equal diameter. Lymphatic channels are inconspicuous in a normal liver. Large portal tracts are often seen in the subcapsular parenchyma in liver biopsies (Figure 1.5.10).

In aged individuals, the portal tracts may contain denser collagen, a mild increase in chronic inflammatory cells, atrophic bile ducts, and thickened hepatic arteries even in normotensive individuals (Figure 1.5.8). Obliteration of the subcapsular portal vein is common in aged individuals.

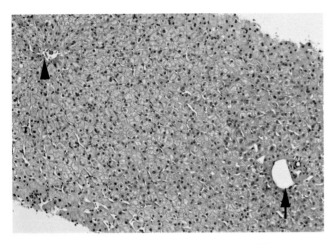

Figure 1.5.1 Low magnification of normal liver parenchyma with preserved lobular architecture, containing a portal tract (arrow) and a central or terminal hepatic venule (arrowhead).

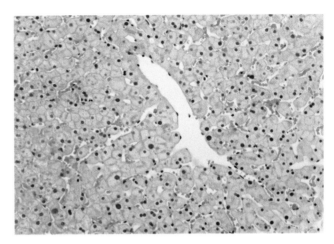

Figure 1.5.2 Normal centrilobular area demonstrating cords of hepatocytes radiating out from the terminal hepatic venule. Centrilobular hepatocytes with brown discoloration due to a normal amount of the lipofuscin pigment. Sinusoids contain red blood cells.

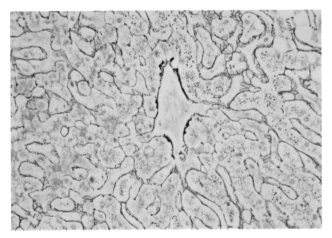

Figure 1.5.3 Reticulin fibers lined 1-cell-thick cords of hepatocytes in normal liver parenchyma.

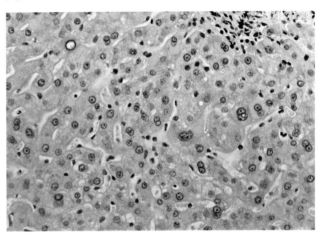

Figure 1.5.4 Binucleate and polyploid hepatocytes are often found in the midzonal region at an increasing number in older individuals.

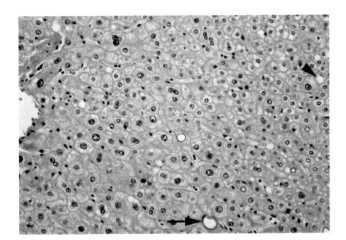

Figure 1.5.5 A small amount of macrovesicular fat droplets (in <5% of hepatocytes, arrowhead) can be encountered in an otherwise normal liver. Occasional hepatocytes with glycogenated nuclei (arrow) in periportal location are normal in adolescents and young adults.

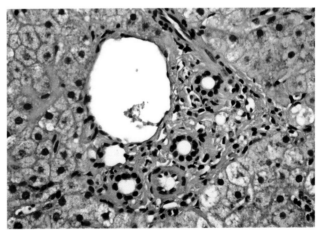

Figure 1.5.6 Normal portal tract containing a portal vein, a hepatic artery, and a bile duct. In most portal tracts, a hepatic artery accompanies a bile duct at approximately the same caliber. A tortuous bile duct may be cut across at several points producing the impression of multiplicity in this microphotograph.

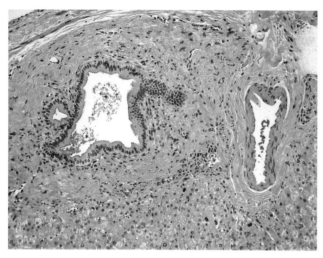

Figure 1.5.7 A larger bile duct has more periductal connective tissues compared with a small bile duct.

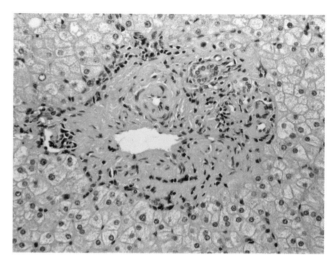

Figure 1.5.8 In aged individuals, the portal tract shows an increase in fibrous stroma and thickening of the hepatic artery.

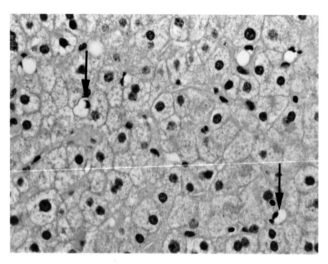

Figure 1.5.9 Hepatic stellate cells (Ito cells) containing fat vacuoles with "tent"-like nuclei (arrows).

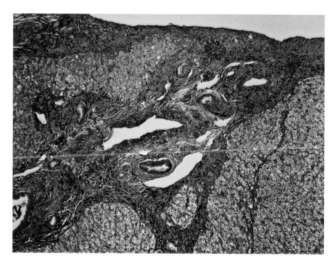

Figure 1.5.10 Subcapsular large portal tracts are often encountered in a normal liver.

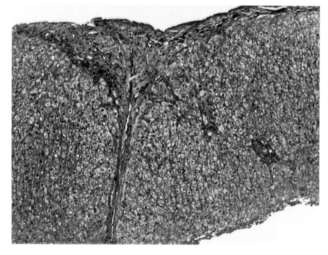

Figure 1.5.11 Subcapsular fibrous septum as part of the normal liver framework in superficial biopsy, mimicking bridging fibrosis in chronic liver disease.

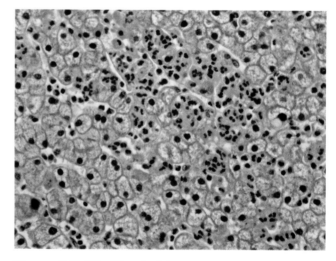

Figure 1.5.12 "Surgical hepatitis" represents collections of neutrophils, resembling microabscesses, as a result of exposure of liver to free air in open liver biopsy.

1.6 Hepatocyte Degeneration, Death, and Regeneration

Normal liver structure and function depends on the balance between hepatocyte death and regeneration. A limited minor hepatocyte injury results in immediate regeneration of the hepatocytes without significant or prolonged effect in the liver structure and function, whereas a severe acute hepatocyte injury may exceed the regenerative capacity of the hepatocytes and results in parenchymal collapse and liver failure.

Hepatocyte Degeneration and Death

Two types of hepatocyte death can be distinguished by morphologic features: (1) apoptosis and (2) cytolytic necrosis. It is likely, however, that these are two ends of a spectrum with possible intermediate forms.

Apoptosis involves shrinkage, nuclear disassembly and fragmentation of the cell into discrete acidophilic bodies with intact plasma membranes, which are then rapidly phagocytosed by neighboring Kupffer cells (Figure 1.6.2).

In cytolytic necrosis, the process begins with ballooning degeneration where hepatocytes become swollen, rounded, and pale staining as a result mainly from dilation of the endoplasmic reticulum, which is the consequence of mitochondrial dysfunction and ATP depletion, leading to the loss of ion homeostasis and plasma membrane integrity. The cytoplasm is partially rarefied, particularly along the cellular periphery, and the cytoplasmic cytoskeleton clumps around the nucleus; cell membranes are frequently indistinct (Figure 1.6.1). Ballooned hepatocytes undergo lytic necrosis, which is not visible, but the occurrence can be inferred to small foci of stromal collapse that are accompanied by collections of lymphocytes and Kupffer cells (Figure 1.6.4), referred to as spotty necrosis. The degree of ballooning degeneration varies across the lobule in hepatocellular injury, although classically, the centrilobular region is the most severely affected.

Hepatocyte Regeneration

The liver is the only human organ that is capable of natural regeneration. Regeneration may be rapid as seen after partial hepatectomy. This is predominantly due to the hepatocytes reentering the cell cycle: quiescent cells stimulated by mediators, including cytokines, move into a primed state (G0 to G1) when growth factors can stimulate DNA synthesis and cellular replication.

In the event of injury, regeneration is observed predominantly in the periportal hepatocytes in mild injury or throughout the hepatic parenchyma in severe injury. It is manifested by mitoses, multinucleation, and crowding of the periportal cell plates by small, uniform, clear, or basophilic hepatocytes (Figure 1.6.5). Liver cell plates in the periportal region become irregularly thickened, and occasional hepatocellular rosettes may appear. Nuclear displacement to the sinusoidal pole with hyperchromasia is a cytologic indication of regenerative activity. All of these changes impart a darkened periportal region under low magnification, which is often the only remarkable change in mild acute hepatitis or in residual hepatitis as a reaction to recent injury. In severe hepatocellular injury or hepatitis, the feature of regeneration may be overwhelmed by the amount of ballooning degeneration, cytolytic necrosis, apoptosis, bridging necrosis, and inflammatory infiltrate.

The degree of hepatocyte regeneration often correlates with the degree of necroinflammatory activity in chronic hepatitis, particularly when interface hepatitis is the predominant process. Similarly, hepatocyte regeneration occurs in the periphery or periseptal region of cirrhotic nodules when the necroinflammatory activity persists, resulting in regenerative nodules in cirrhosis.

If hepatocytes are extensively damaged, such as in massive hepatic necrosis, the conventional hepatocyte regeneration is impaired. Hepatocytes may be derived from bipotential stem cells, so-called oval cells, which are thought to rest in the canals of Hering. These cells can differentiate into either hepatocytes or cholangiocytes.

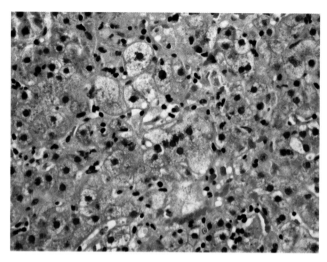

Figure 1.6.1 Hepatocytes are swollen with pale and rarefied cytoplasm in ballooning degeneration.

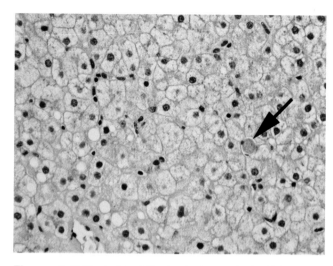

Figure 1.6.2 Acidophilic body (arrow) signifying apoptotic hepatocyte, found in an otherwise normal liver or in abundance in acute hepatocellular injury.

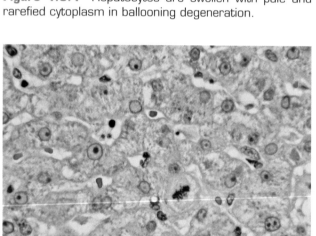

Figure 1.6.3 Mitosis signifying hepatocellular regeneration. It is rarely encountered in an otherwise normal liver as a physiological turnover.

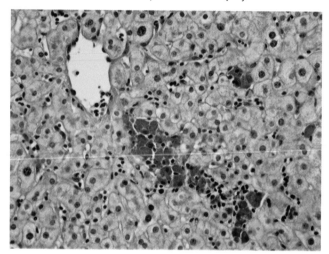

Figure 1.6.4 The PAS reaction after diastase demonstrates clusters of macrophages, engulfing hepatocellular debris after an episode of hepatocellular injury.

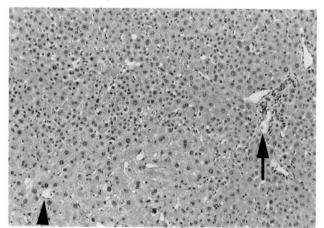

Figure 1.6.5 Hepatocytes of different sizes are evident in resolving acute hepatocellular injury. The smaller regenerative hepatocytes are in the periportal region (portal tract, arrow), whereas the larger mature hepatocytes are in the centrilobular region (central venule, arrowhead).

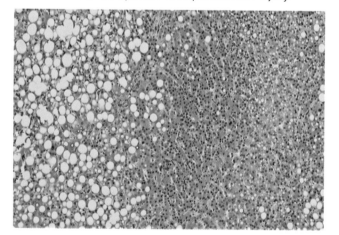

Figure 1.6.6 Smaller regenerative nonsteatotic hepatocytes are noted in this biopsy of a patient with acute hepatocellular injury superimposed on fatty liver disease.

1.7 Nonspecific Reactive Hepatitis, Mild Acute Hepatitis, and Residual Hepatitis

Hepatocellular injury may cause subtle histopathologic changes. These mild changes include mild acute hepatitis, residual hepatitis, and nonspecific reactive hepatitis. The elevation of liver enzyme activities in these conditions can be clinically significant, prompting liver biopsy.

Mild Acute Hepatitis

Mild acute hepatitis is a mild diffuse hepatocellular injury due to hepatitis viruses, drugs, or other causes, resulting in gastrointestinal and influenza-like symptoms, such as malaise, anorexia, nausea, fever, and right upper quadrant discomfort. Aminotransferase and other liver enzyme activities are elevated. The disease usually resolves in a few months. Mild acute hepatitis is characterized by subtle but diffuse changes (Figures 1.7.1 and 1.7.2). These include panlobular disarray with degeneration and regeneration of the hepatocytes, accompanied by activation of sinusoidal lining cells and diffuse infiltration of sinusoids and portal tracts by inflammatory cells, primarily lymphocytes and macrophages and some plasma cells. Cholestasis or bridging necrosis is not seen in mild acute hepatitis.

Mild acute hepatitis requires no specific treatment. The prognosis of mild acute hepatitis depends on the causative agent and its potential in progression to chronicity.

Residual Hepatitis

The term *residual* or *prolonged hepatitis* is used to describe changes in liver biopsies taken late in the course of acute hepatitis with residual abnormalities in liver enzyme activities. At the late stage of acute hepatitis, diffuse hepatocellular damage and inflammation have subsided, except for mild pleomorphism of the hepatocytes, irregular cell plates, and a few foci of lobular necrosis and mild inflammation, predominantly in the centrilobular areas (Figure 1.7.3). Clusters of periodic acid–Schiff diastase–resistant macrophages are observed predominantly in the centrilobular area and portal tracts (Figure 1.7.4). These macrophages contain debris of necrotic or apoptotic hepatocyte or ceroid pigment and may be iron-positive. Focal reticulin fiber condensation may be seen as a result of hepatocyte loss. The portal tracts may be expanded with mild lymphocytic infiltrate and mild fibrosis or with thin fibrous septa.

Because most of hepatocellular injury has occurred, the prognosis of residual hepatitis is good and does not require further treatment when the cause of injury has been identified.

Nonspecific Reactive Hepatitis

Nonspecific reactive hepatitis is a mesenchymal tissue reaction in the liver in response to systemic or extrahepatic diseases or unknown causes. The symptoms are nondescript or related to the extrahepatic diseases, which include extrahepatic biliary diseases, gastrointestinal diseases, neoplastic diseases, acquired immunodeficiency syndrome, and febrile conditions.

Nonspecific reactive hepatitis is characterized predominantly by activation of sinusoidal lining cells (Figure 1.7.6). Fat-storing cells (Ito cells) are occasionally prominent. Portal tracts are slightly expanded by mild lymphocytic infiltrate and mild fibrosis, but the limiting plate is intact. There is no direct or diffuse hepatocellular injury, although rare spotty necrosis, mild inflammation, focal macrovesicular steatosis, and slight pleomorphism of the hepatocytes may be present. The underlying systemic disease determines the prognosis and treatment of nonspecific reactive hepatitis.

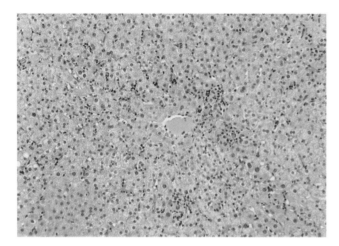

Figure 1.7.1 Mild acute hepatitis is characterized by mild lymphocytic infiltrates in the sinusoids, often predominantly in the centrilobular region.

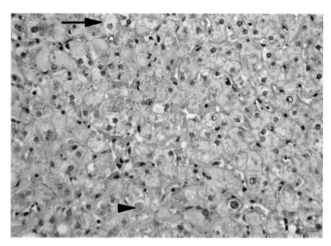

Figure 1.7.2 Subtle hepatocellular changes, such as rare ballooning degeneration (arrow) and acidophilic body (arrowhead), can be the only findings in mild acute hepatitis.

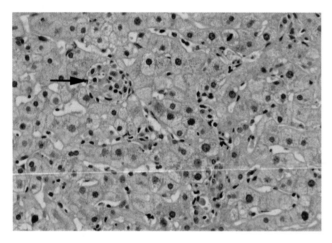

Figure 1.7.3 Clusters of hypertrophic Kupffer cells and macrophages (arrow) are often the only histopathologic changes in mild acute hepatitis or residual hepatitis.

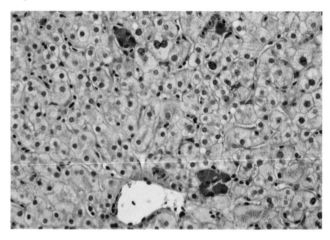

Figure 1.7.4 The PAS reaction after diastase demonstrates clusters of hypertrophic Kupffer cells and macrophages as evidence of previous hepatocellular dropout.

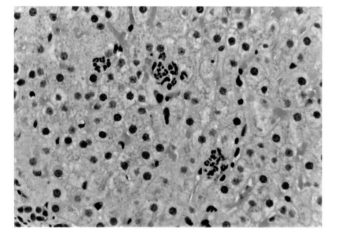

Figure 1.7.5 Although the most common inflammatory infiltrate is lymphocytic, on rare occasions, neutrophilic infiltrate can be encountered in mild acute hepatitis or mild drug-induced injury.

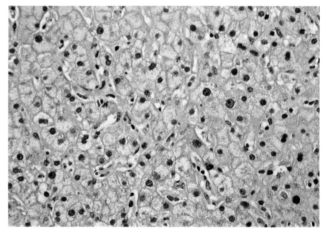

Figure 1.7.6 Nonspecific reactive hepatitis with hypertrophic sinusoidal lining cells.

Table 1.7.1   Differential Diagnoses of Nonspecific Reactive Hepatitis, Mild Acute Hepatitis, and Residual Hepatitis

Histologic Features	Nonspecific Reactive Hepatitis	Mild Acute Hepatitis	Residual Hepatitis	Large Duct Obstruction	Sepsis
Sinusoidal lining cell activation	++	+	−	+	+
Lobular inflammation	+/−	+	−	−	+
Hepatocyte necrosis	+/− (rare)	+	+/−	+/− (rare)	++ (in septic shock)
PAS-D–positive macrophages in clusters	−	+	++	−	+/−
Portal inflammation	+/−	+	+/−	+ (neutro-phils)	+ (neutrophils)
Portal edema	−	−	−	++	+/−
Ectatic bile duct	−	−	−	+	−
Periductal edema	−	−	−	+	−
Ductular reaction	−	−	−	++	+
Hepatocellular cholestasis	−	−	+/−	++	+
Canalicular cholestasis	−	−	+/−	++	+
Ductular cholestasis (bile casts)	−	−	−	−	++
Bile infarct/lakes	−	−	−	+/−	+/−

++, indicates almost always present; +, usually present; +/−, occasionally present; − usually absent.

1.8 Portal and Vascular Problems

The liver has 2 afferent vessels: the hepatic artery and the portal vein. A compromise, abnormality, or obstruction of the vasculature may produce clinically silent changes, but, if severe, it may lead to portal hypertension and varices, generally without ascites or liver failure. The changes in the liver parenchyma may be subtle, requiring the understanding of normal and minor structural alteration of liver parenchyma. The most important of these are portal vein thrombosis, hepatoportal sclerosis, and nodular regenerative hyperplasia.

Nodular Regenerative Hyperplasia

Nodular regenerative hyperplasia is a diffuse nodular regeneration of the hepatocytes, associated with other disorders such as autoimmune diseases (rheumatoid arthritis, systemic sclerosis, systemic lupus erythematosus), chronic venous congestion, hematologic malignancies, endocrine or metabolic disorders, or hepatotoxic drugs. In most cases, the cause is obliteration of small portal veins, and the hepatic circulation is replaced by arterial flow.

Nodular regenerative hyperplasia occurs in both sexes at any age, but most frequently between the ages of 40 and 70 years. Many patients are asymptomatic, but they may develop portal hypertension as in cirrhosis and rarely hepatic failure or ascites or rupture of liver with massive hemorrhage.

The liver parenchyma shows widely scattered parenchymal nodules varying in diameter from 0.1 to 0.4 cm. The capsular surface of the liver often reveals minimal shallow irregularities that may be mistaken for cirrhosis. The nodules either replace almost the entire parenchyma or are confined to one portion of the liver. The nodules in nodular regenerative hyperplasia are not surrounded by fibrous septa; therefore, they are ill defined and soft, distinct from those found in cirrhosis. Irregular areas of congestion may be present, resulting in a mottled appearance of the cut surface of the liver. The nodules consist of hyperplastic hepatocytes arranged in plates more than 1-cell-layer thick, particularly adjacent or surrounding the portal tracts. The surrounding centrilobular parenchyma is compressed and atrophic, and the sinusoids are congested (the so-called linear congestion) (Figure 1.8.1). Reticulin stain shows condensation of the reticulin framework around the expanding nodules and the irregular thickened hepatocyte plates within the nodules, but dense septa as in cirrhosis are not seen (Figure 1.8.2). There is little, if any, pericellular fibrosis. The hyperplastic hepatocytes are slightly larger and more variable than normal and are arranged in 2-cell-thick plates with occasional binucleation. Obliteration of small portal veins is often seen.

The diagnosis is often difficult in needle biopsy specimen and may require an open liver biopsy. Alternating areas of hyperplastic hepatocytes and atrophic hepatocytes with linear congestion on needle biopsy should lead to a reticulin stain to rule out nodular regenerative hyperplasia.

The prognosis of nodular regenerative hyperplasia is determined by its complications, particularly portal hypertension.

Hepatoportal Sclerosis

Hepatoportal sclerosis, also known as idiopathic portal hypertension, noncirrhotic portal hypertension, or obliterative portal venopathy, denotes a condition consisting of portal hypertension, splenomegaly, and anemia secondary to hypersplenism in a noncirrhotic patient with dense portal tract fibrosis and obliteration of portal veins. One of the known causes of hepatoportal sclerosis is chronic exposure to copper, arsenic, and vinyl chloride. Per definition, parasitic infection, myeloproliferative disease, and portal thrombosis should be excluded.

The liver is usually mildly atrophic with a wrinkled capsule (Figures 1.8.3 and 1.8.4). Portal tracts are fibrotic with either fibrous obliteration of larger portal veins or numerous dilated small portal vein branches (Figure 1.8.5). Fibrin thrombi and recanalization of portal veins can be seen. Bile ducts may show periductal fibrosis. The centrilobular hepatocytes become atrophic, causing dilatation of sinusoids and reverse lobulation. On occasion, portal-to-portal bridging fibrosis may occur.

Portal Vein Thrombosis

Portal vein thrombosis frequently occurs in patients with cirrhosis. In the absence of cirrhosis, thrombosis in a large portal vein occurs as a result of a tumor in the hepatic hilum or pancreas, traumatic injury, and hypercoagulable states, whereas thrombosis in a small portal vein occurs as a result of local inflammation and injury, such as in primary biliary cirrhosis, primary sclerosing cholangitis, sarcoidosis, polyarteritis nodosa, schistosomiasis, and toxic injury (cyclophosphamide, azathioprine, arsenic).

Thrombosis of a large portal vein can be detected by imaging studies, but thrombosis of a small portal vein requires a liver biopsy to diagnose the underlying liver disease that causes portal hypertension. The portal vein is occluded and replaced by small recanalization vascular channels (Figure 1.8.6). Portal vein thrombosis causes hepatocyte atrophy, particularly in the centrilobular area, resulting in sinusoidal dilatation and eventually lobar atrophy.

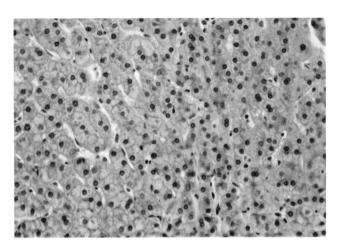

Figure 1.8.1 Linear compression of cords of hepatocytes in the centrilobular region is a characteristic of nodular regenerative hyperplasia.

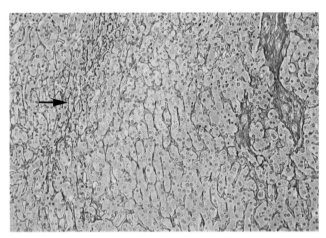

Figure 1.8.2 In nodular regenerative hyperplasia, reticulin fibers outline the thicker cords on either side and the atrophic, compressed cords of hepatocytes in between (arrow) (reticulin stain).

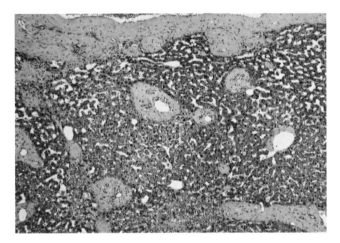

Figure 1.8.3 Atrophic liver parenchyma with rounded fibrotic portal tracts, fibrous obliteration of portal veins, and sinusoidal dilatation in hepatoportal sclerosis (trichrome stain).

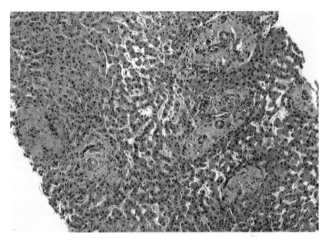

Figure 1.8.4 Patients with hepatoportal sclerosis often present with clinical portal hypertension but with non-cirrhotic liver parenchyma on biopsy. There is no bridging fibrosis or regenerative nodule.

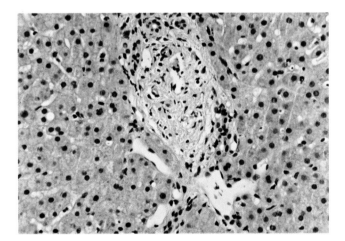

Figure 1.8.5 Engorged periportal sinusoids or herniation of small portal vein branches to the periportal liver parenchyma is often seen in hepatoportal sclerosis.

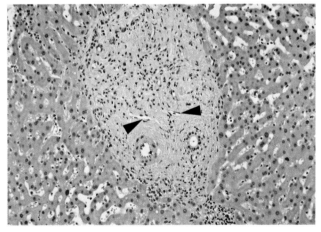

Figure 1.8.6 Portal vein thrombosis leaving narrow residual lumen (arrowheads).

Table 1.8.1 Differential Diagnoses of Vascular and Portal Problem

Histologic Features	Portal Vein Thrombosis	Hepatoportal Sclerosis	Nodular Regenerative Hyperplasia	Cirrhosis
Bridging fibrous bands/septa	–	–	–	++
Nodule formation	–	–	+	++
Hepatocyte hyperplasia	–	–	++	+
Compression of hepatocytes	–	–	++	–
Hepatocyte atrophy	++	++	+	–
Sinusoidal dilatation	++	++	+/–	–
Herniation of portal vein branches	–	+	–	–
Portal fibrosis	+/–	+	–	++
Portal vein obliteration	+	++	+/–	+/–
Portal vein recanalization	+	–	–	–

++ indicates almost always present; +, usually present; +/–, occasionally present; –, usually absent.

1.9   Brown Pigments in the Liver

There are several pigments that can cause brown discoloration of the liver parenchyma. In normal condition, the only brown pigment that can be encountered is lipofuscin. Bile, iron, and copper are seen in hepatocytes in pathologic conditions. There are other rare brown pigments that can be seen in portal macrophages and Kupffer cells, such as talc pigments in intravenous drug abuser and parasite-associated pigments in malaria and schistosomiasis.

Lipofuscin

Lipofuscin pigment appears as a brown pigment in the pericanalicular cytoplasm of centrilobular hepatocytes (Figures 1.9.1 and 1.9.2). Often, it is accompanied by variation in the size of the hepatocytes and their nuclei, with increased polyploidy, particularly in older individuals. An increase in the lipofuscin pigment occurs in atrophic liver, old age, starvation, chronic wasting diseases, and malignancies. It has no functional or clinical significance. Atrophy of the liver presents as small dark brown liver without other abnormalities.

Lipofuscin is produced by lysosomal oxidation of lipids. Under the electron microscope, lipofuscin granules appear as secondary lysosomes in the pericanalicular location that contains irregular and lobulated electron-dense granules, lipid droplets, and a heterogenous matrix.

Dubin-Johnson Pigment

Dubin-Johnson syndrome is an autosomal recessive familial disorder of bilirubin metabolism characterized by chronic or intermittent benign jaundice due to defect in hepatocellular excretion of organic anions into the bile, and may be exacerbated during pregnancy or after taking oral contraceptives. Dubin-Johnson syndrome has an excellent prognosis, long-term sequelae do not occur, and treatment is not necessary.

Dubin-Johnson syndrome results in black to dark green discoloration of the liver that can be recognized macroscopically even on a needle biopsy specimen. Otherwise, the liver is grossly normal. Abundant dark brown coarse pigment in the pericanalicular cytoplasm of centrilobular hepatocytes is noted. In contrast to lipofuscin, the granules are darker and more variable in size and extend into the midlobular and periportal hepatocytes. An electron microscope demonstrates distinctive oval or irregularly shaped, pleomorphic electron-dense lysosomes, frequently associated with lipid droplets, in a finely granular background, and lack the typical lobulation of lipofuscin granules. Other liver abnormalities and particularly cholestasis are not seen.

Hemosiderin

In the early stages, hereditary hemochromatosis and secondary iron overload result in a distinct pattern of hemosiderin deposition, but as the disease progresses, the histologic distinction between them becomes less clear.

Hereditary hemochromatosis causes preferential hemosiderin deposition in periportal hepatocytes of homozygotic patients in the early stages and heterozygotic patients throughout life. Kupffer cells do not contain excess iron, and other liver abnormalities are not observed. With increasing age, continued iron deposition in hepatocytes leads to hepatocellular damage and fibrosis that are directly related to the iron content of the liver. Iron is deposited in all hepatocytes throughout the hepatic lobules, as well as in Kupffer cells, portal macrophages, and bile ducts and ductules (Figures 1.2.6 and 1.9.4). Iron in bile ducts and ductules is typical but not pathognomonic for hereditary hemochromatosis.

Secondary iron overload results in hemosiderin deposition primarily in Kupffer cells, distributed evenly throughout the liver lobules and only in severe cases in hepatocytes, a histologic pattern quite different from hereditary hemochromatosis. Fibrosis or cirrhosis is usually absent. Severe secondary iron overload, such as in sideroblastic anemias and thallasemia major, can mimic to a large degree hereditary hemochromatosis with fibrosis and cirrhosis, but there is more iron in clustered macrophages and Kupffer cells (Figures 1.2.7 and 1.9.3). Other conditions associated with iron overload are alcoholic liver disease, transfusion, and porphyria cutanea tarda. Secondary iron overload from excessive ingestion or peripheral hemolysis (such as caused by ribavirin) results in primarily hepatocyte deposition.

Copper-Associated Protein

Copper-associated protein is usually found in periportal hepatocytes or, in cirrhosis, in hepatocytes at the periphery of nodules. Copper itself is also demonstrable in the same location. Increase in copper deposition is seen in chronic cholestasis (cholate stasis) and Wilson disease (Figure 1.2.9). In Wilson disease, copper-associated protein is distributed throughout the lobule or the cirrhotic nodule, in contrast to the periportal or periseptal deposition in chronic cholestasis.

Bile

In normal condition, bile in liver parenchyma is invisible. Bile can be visualized only in pathologic conditions, referred generally as cholestasis. Bile can accumulate in the cytoplasm of hepatocytes, canalicular spaces, Kupffer cells, bile ducts, and ductules (Figure 1.9.5). Accumulation in the cytoplasm of hepatocytes is called hepatocytic or parenchymal cholestasis, in canalicular spaces is called canalicular cholestasis, and in bile ductules is called ductular cholestasis. Bile can also be encountered in dilated bile canaliculi of hepatocellular carcinoma and also in bile duct hamartoma.

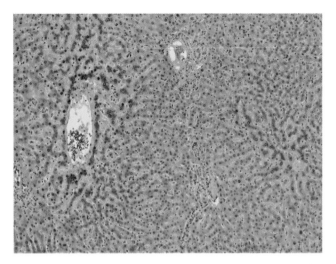

Figure 1.9.1 Lipofuscin pigments causing brown discoloration of the centrilobular liver parenchyma.

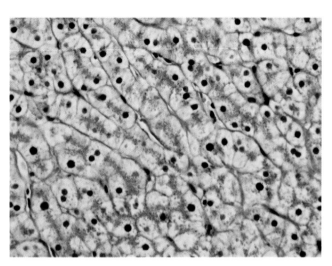

Figure 1.9.2 Lipofuscin pigments located in the pericanalicular cytoplasm of centrilobular hepatocytes (PAS-D stain).

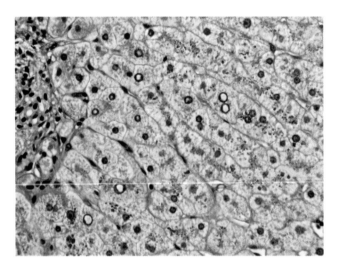

Figure 1.9.3 Hemosiderin pigment in a patient with alcoholic liver disease and negative for *HFE* gene mutation.

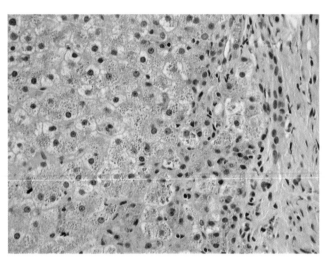

Figure 1.9.4 Hemosiderin pigment in untreated hereditary hemochromatosis with cirrhosis is deposited in all hepatocytes throughout the hepatic lobules.

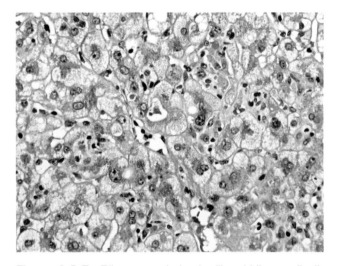

Figure 1.9.5 Bile accumulating in dilated bile canaliculi.

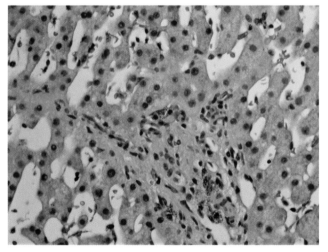

Figure 1.9.6 Dark brown pigment in portal macrophages and Kupffer cells in schistosomiasis.

Table 1.9.1   Differential Diagnoses of Brown Pigments in the Liver

Characteristics	Lipofuscin	Dubin-Johnson Pigment	Hemosiderin	Copper-Associated Protein/Copper	Bile
Color	Golden brown	Dark brown to black	Dark brown, refractile	Pink-brown	Yellow to green-brown
Cellular distribution	Centrilobular hepatocytes, Kupffer cells	Centrilobular to periportal hepatocytes	Periportal hepatocytes, Kupffer cells, portal macrophages, cholangiocytes	Periportal hepatocytes	Hepatocytes, Kupffer cells
Location	Cytoplasmic, pericanalicular	Cytoplasmic, pericanalicular	Pericanalicular to diffuse cytoplasmic	Diffuse cytoplasmic	Cytoplasmic and intracanalicular
Relative size	Fine	Coarse	Fine to coarse	Fine	Small to large plugs
Bile stain	−	−	−	−	+
Perl's iron stain	−	−	+	−	−
Acid fast	+	+	−	−	−
PAS-D	+	+	−	−	+/−
Orcein/Victoria blue/Rhoda-nine	−	−	−	+	−
Fontana Masson	+	+	−	−	+

− indicates negative staining; +, positive staining; +/−, weak positive staining.

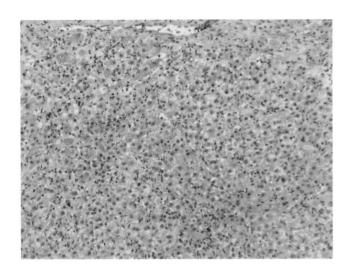

ACUTE LIVER DISEASES

2.1 Acute Hepatitis

Acute hepatitis is a diffuse hepatocellular injury that occurs no longer than 6 months. Common causes of acute hepatitis are hepatotropic viral infection and drug-induced injury, but the term *acute hepatitis* can also be used for general hepatocellular injury due to other causes that occurs for less than 6 months with characteristic changes, including panlobular disarray and diffuse lobular inflammation accompanied by marked hepatocellular degeneration and regeneration.

Acute hepatitis may be asymptomatic or may present with a fairly well-defined onset of symptoms, influenza-like or gastrointestinal symptoms, including anorexia, nausea, vomiting, mild fever, right upper quadrant discomfort, and profound malaise. The liver is palpable and tender. Jaundice may or may not develop later in the course. Serum aminotransferase activities are markedly elevated.

Pathologic Features

The major histologic changes in acute hepatitis are located in the parenchyma. The architecture shows panlobular disarray, markedly increased cellularity, and pleomorphism of the hepatocytes caused by a combination of diffuse hepatocellular degeneration, hepatocellular regeneration, and inflammation (Figure 2.1.1). Degeneration of the hepatocytes, accompanied by formation of acidophilic or apoptotic bodies and ballooning degeneration leading to lytic necrosis, is scattered throughout the lobules (Figure 2.1.2). Regeneration is reflected by occasional mitoses, clusters of small hepatocytes, and binucleation or multinucleation of hepatocytes. The combination of degeneration and regeneration results in marked variation in the size, shape, and staining qualities of hepatocytes. There is diffuse lobular inflammation with lymphocytes, few plasma cells, and activation of sinusoidal lining cells, particularly Kupffer cells (Figures 2.1.5 and 2.1.6).

The portal tracts are infiltrated by lymphocytes and macrophages and a few scattered plasma cells, eosinophils, and neutrophils. The portal tracts may be expanded by inflammatory infiltrate, and the inflammation may spill over to the adjacent parenchyma, but true interface hepatitis as seen in chronic hepatitis is absent.

Severe acute hepatitis may be complicated by bridging necrosis and collapse of the parenchyma, which connects the portal tract to the central hepatic venule or central to central hepatic venules and is easily mistaken for fibrous septa of chronic hepatitis. The bandlike parenchymal collapse consists of inflammatory cells, blood-filled sinusoids, macrophages, and condensation of reticulin fibers, but minimal fibrous tissue and elastic fibers.

Differential Diagnosis

Acute hepatitis may be indistinguishable from chronic hepatitis. Therefore, the clinical history of the duration of the disease and serologic findings are very important. Features of chronic hepatitis, such as dense portal lymphocytic infiltrate, portal fibrosis, fibrous septa, and pericellular fibrosis, are not seen in acute hepatitis. If there is suggestion of fibrosis in a case of acute hepatitis, a chronic hepatitis with severe activity or chronic hepatitis superimposed by acute hepatitis should be suspected. Other differential diagnoses of acute hepatitis include autoimmune hepatitis, and alcoholic hepatitis (see Table 2.1.1).

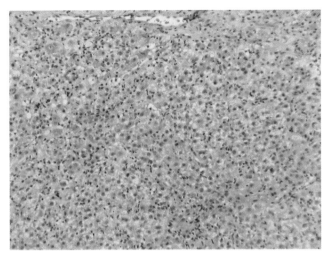

Figure 2.1.1   Diffuse panlobular necroinflammatory activity in acute hepatitis.

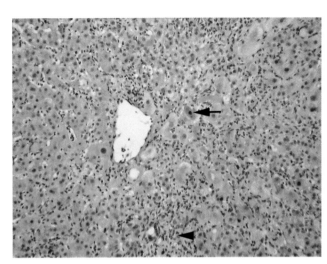

Figure 2.1.2   Diffuse lobular necroinflammatory activity, numerous apoptotic/acidophilic bodies (arrow), focal necrosis (arrowhead), and central venulitis in acute hepatitis.

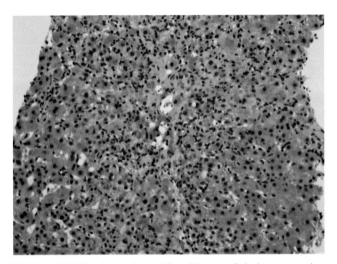

Figure 2.1.3   Acute hepatitis with centrilobular necrosis.

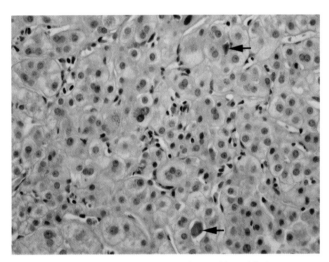

Figure 2.1.4   Resolving acute hepatitis with hepatocanalicular cholestasis (arrows).

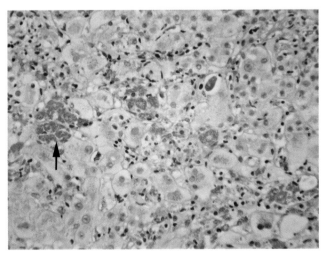

Figure 2.1.5   Numerous clusters of Kupffer cells and macrophages (arrow) in acute hepatitis demonstrated by periodic acid–Schiff with diastase stain.

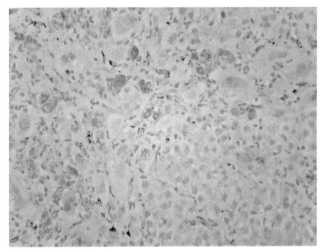

Figure 2.1.6   Accumulation of iron in Kupffer cells and macrophages seen in acute hepatitis.

Table 2.1.1 Differential Diagnoses of Acute Hepatitis

Histologic Features	Acute Hepatitis	Chronic Hepatitis	Autoimmune Hepatitis	Alcoholic Hepatitis
Inflammatory infiltrate	Predominantly lymphocytes with scattered plasma cells	Predominantly lymphocytes with scattered plasma cells	Abundant plasma cells in clusters	Neutrophils, rare lymphocytes
Portal inflammation	+	++	++	+/−
Portal fibrosis	−	++	+	+
Fibrous septa	−	+/−	+	+
Bridging fibrosis	−	+/−	+/−	+/−
Pericellular fibrosis	−	+/− (periportal)	−	++
Central hyalin sclerosis	−	−	−	+
Interface hepatitis	+/−	+	++	−
Lobular inflammation	++	+	++	+
Lobular dissaray	++	−	++	+
Hepatocyte regeneration	++	−	++	−
Ballooning degeneration	+	−	+	++
Hepatocyte necroses	++	+	++	+
Bridging necrosis	+/−	−	+	−
Acidophilic bodies	++	+/−	++	+
Mallory-Denk bodies	−	−	−	++
Centrilobular cholestasis	+/−	−	−	+/−

++ indicates almost always present; +, usually present; +/−, occasionally present; − usually absent.

2.2 Acute Hepatotropic Viral Hepatitis

Acute hepatotropic viral hepatitis, often referred simply as acute viral hepatitis, is an acute diffuse hepatocellular damage caused by hepatotropic viruses that infect the liver as the primary target organ, including hepatitis A, B, C, D, and E (see Table 2.2.1).

Acute hepatotropic viral hepatitis may be symptomatic or asymptomatic. Symptomatic infection is seen in cases of hepatitis A, B, and E and superinfection or coinfection of hepatitis B by hepatitis D (delta) virus, whereas asymptomatic infection is usually seen in hepatitis C. Symptomatic acute hepatotropic viral hepatitis is preceded by a prodromal phase that often lasts from a few days to several weeks with nonspecific symptoms, including nausea, vomiting, myalgia, and anorexia. Serologic tests for these viruses are usually diagnostic; therefore, liver biopsy is rarely needed.

The majority of acute hepatotropic viral hepatitis tends to lead to spontaneous recovery, and no specific treatment is needed. Hepatitis B and C, however, can become chronic.

Pathologic Features

Acute hepatotropic viral hepatitis produces a similar morphologic feature, characterized by diffuse hepatocellular damage, regeneration, and inflammation (Figures 2.2.1 and 2.2.2). These result in the low-magnification appearance of panlobular disarray, hypercellularity, and hepatocellular pleomorphism. All hepatocytes vary in size, shape, and staining qualities. Acidophilic or apoptotic bodies and ballooning degeneration leading to lytic necrosis are seen throughout the lobule. Regeneration is reflected in mitoses, formation of clusters of small regenerating hepatocytes, and binucleation of hepatocytes. Bridging necrosis and multilobular necrosis develop in more severe cases. The lobules and portal tracts are diffusely infiltrated by predominantly lymphocytes and macrophages, with occasional plasma cells, eosinophils, or neutrophils. The extent and intensity may vary from one case to another, depending on the severity, course of the infection, degree of host response, and virus involved. Centrilobular hepatocellular or canalicular cholestasis is usually mild and appears late in the course of acute viral hepatitis (Figure 2.2.3). Steatosis is absent or, if present, is mild. Interface hepatitis is usually not observed. Fibrosis of portal tracts and ductular reaction are absent.

In addition to the common features of acute hepatitis, acute hepatitis A often shows periportal hepatocellular injury (interface hepatitis), abundant plasma cells, and canalicular cholestasis (Figure 2.2.5), and acute hepatitis C may show sinusoidal lymphocytic infiltrate similar to mononucleosis, portal lymphocytic aggregates, and mild steatosis (Figure 2.2.6).

Immunohistochemistry is generally not useful in an episode of acute hepatotropic viral hepatitis, except for hepatitis D, because viral antigens are transiently expressed during incubation and early symptomatic periods. Similar to hepatitis D virus, hepatitis B antigens are difficult to detect during active disease. Currently, there is no reliable immunohistochemical stain for hepatitis C virus infection.

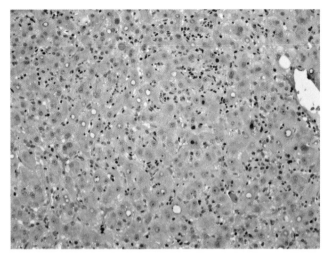

Figure 2.2.1 Acute viral hepatitis with diffuse lobular necroinflammatory activity.

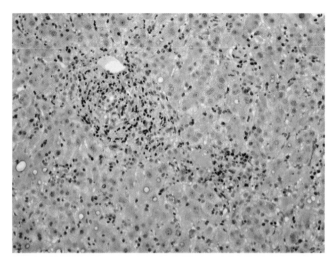

Figure 2.2.2 The inflammatory infiltrate in the portal tract is the same as in hepatic parenchyma in acute viral hepatitis.

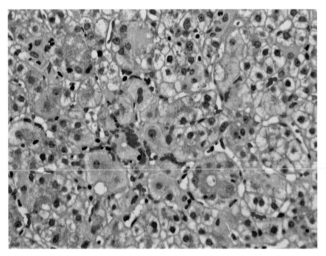

Figure 2.2.3 Hepatocanalicular cholestasis in acute viral hepatitis A.

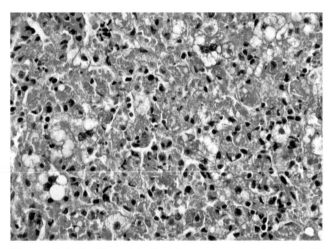

Figure 2.2.4 Hepatitis B with severe acute hepatitis D superinfection resulting in extensive necrosis.

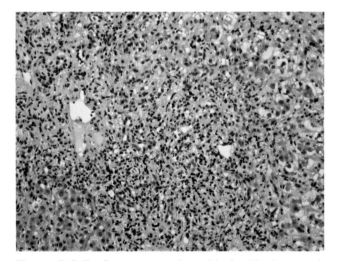

Figure 2.2.5 Severe acute hepatitis A with plasmacellular infiltrate.

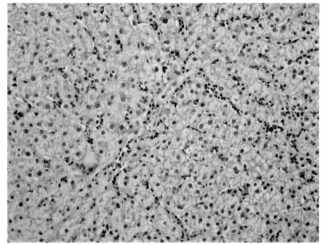

Figure 2.2.6 Acute hepatitis C with mononucleosis-like sinusoidal lymphocytic infiltrate.

Table 2.2.1   Acute (Hepatotropic) Viral Hepatitis

| | Acute Hepatitis | | | | |
	A	B	C	D	E
Virus type	RNA, picornavirus	DNA, hepadnavirus	RNA, flavivirus	RNA, defective virus	RNA, calicivirus
Transmission	Fecal-oral	Parenteral, perinatal, sexual	Parenteral, sporadic, rarely sexual	Parenteral	Fecal-oral
Chronic infection	0%	~10%	60%-80%	~5% coinfection; ~70% super-infection on hepatitis B	0%
Fulminant acute hepatitis incidence	0.30%	1%	0%	20%	2%; but 20% in pregnant woman
Common histologic pattern	Acute hepatitis with abundant plasma cells, periportal inflammation, and canalicular cholestasis	Typical acute hepatitis	Mild acute hepatitis with sinusoidal lymphocytes, occasional steatosis, portal lymphocytic aggregates	Typical acute hepatitis, more severe than hepatitis B alone	Typical acute hepatitis, cholestasis

2.3 Acute Nonhepatotropic Viral Hepatitis

Nonhepatotropic viruses infect primarily other organs and tissues and involve the liver as part of a disseminated infection, particularly in immunocompromised patients, such as those with acquired immunodeficiency syndrome, immunosuppressive therapy, malignancy, organ transplants, and neonates.

Signs and symptoms related to other organs often predominate, for example, pharyngitis and lymphadenopathy in infectious mononucleosis and cytomegalovirus infection, or mucocutaneous lesions in herpes simplex, varicella-zoster, measles, and rubella virus infection. Fever, jaundice, and fulminant hepatitis may occur. Serologic tests are crucial for confirming the diagnosis. Exotic viruses are important in tropical and developing countries and for travelers, including various viral hemorrhagic fevers (dengue fever, yellow fever, Lassa fever, Marburg fever, Ebola fever, Crimean-Congo fever).

Pathologic Features

Nonhepatotropic viruses, such as herpes simplex, varicella-zoster, and adenovirus, may lead to numerous, grossly visible, mottled, small foci of parenchymal necrosis surrounded by hemorrhagic rings.

The morphologic findings of diffuse hepatocellular damage such as those seen in acute hepatotropic viral hepatitis are absent, and the hepatocytes generally appear normal. In most instances, there are mild nonspecific alterations with focal "punched out" coagulative hepatocyte necroses and neu-trophilic infiltration, which can be extensive and prominent in severe cases. In addition, some hepatocytes may show predominantly microvesicular steatosis. Viral inclusions may be detectable. Cholestasis is absent. In infectious mononucleosis, the sinusoidal lining cells become prominent, and there is increase of mononuclear inflammatory infiltrate in the sinusoids, but without direct contact with hepatocytes. Additional features of specific viruses are listed in Table 2.3.1.

Except for viral hemorrhagic fevers, hepatic necrosis in nonhepatotropic viral infection is generally nonzonal and may become confluent leading to massive hepatic necrosis. Multinucleation and scattered mitoses of the hepatocytes are often present. Giant cell transformation of the hepatocytes may be seen in adults or more often in infants.

Immunohistochemical stains for specific viruses can be used to confirm the histologic findings or to search for viral inclusions that are not readily identified on hematoxylin-eosin–stained slides.

Differential Diagnosis

The differential diagnosis of various nonhepatotropic viral hepatitis depends on the circumstances of the immunocompromised patients, for example, graft-versus-host disease in bone marrow transplantation or acute cellular rejection in liver transplantation. Acute hepatotropic viral hepatitis (usually either hepatitis A, E, B, or delta virus) enters the differential diagnosis in tropical countries and for travelers returning from those countries.

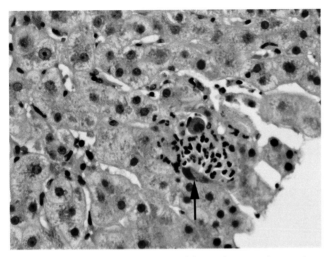

Figure 2.3.1 Microabscess with nuclear and cytoplasmic cytomegalovirus inclusion (arrow).

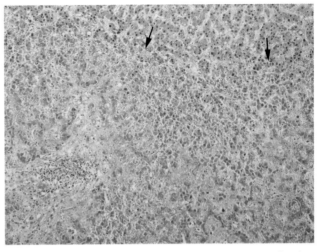

Figure 2.3.2 Coagulative necrosis in herpes simplex hepatitis (arrows).

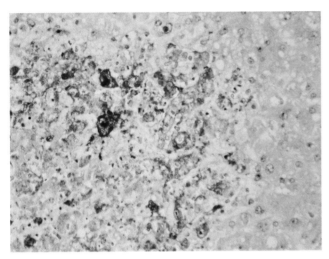

Figure 2.3.3 Herpes simplex virus 1 immunostain shows positive staining in area of coagulative necrosis.

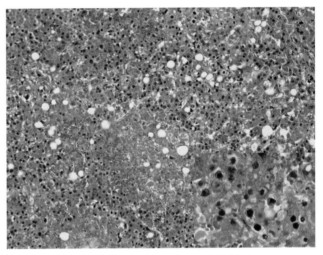

Figure 2.3.4 Hemorrhagic necrosis with hepatocytes containing intranuclear "blueberry-like" adenovirus inclusions (see inset) in the periphery of necrotic areas.

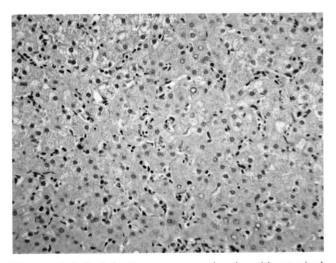

Figure 2.3.5 Infectious mononucleosis with atypical lymphocytes in the sinusoids.

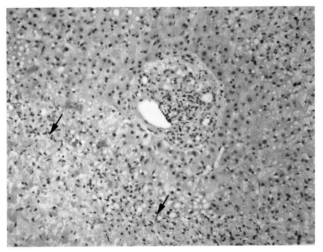

Figure 2.3.6 Midzonal necrosis (arrows) in dengue hemorrhagic fever.

Table 2.3.1 Acute Nonhepatotropic Viral Hepatitis

Common Virus Type	Pathologic Features	Viral Inclusion/Cytopathic Effect Observed
Infectious mononucleosis (Epstein-Barr virus)	Large atypical lymphocytes in the sinusoids "string of beads" and portal tracts. Increased mitoses of the hepatocytes. Rare noncaseating granulomas or fibrin ring granuloma.	No direct cytopathic effect to hepatocytes
Cytomegalovirus	Focal necroses with neutrophils forming "microabscess", with or without viral inclusion. Increased mitoses of the hepatocytes. Rare noncaseating granulomas or fibrin ring granuloma. May cause sclerosing cholangitis in immunocompromised patients. Cholestasis, giant cell transformation, and extramedullary hematopoiesis in neonates.	Cytomegalic cells with basophilic intranuclear and cytoplasmic inclusions in hepatocytes, bile duct epithelium, and Kupffer or endothelial cells
Herpes simplex/ varicella-zoster	Extensive foci of coagulative necrosis with or without intranuclear inclusion in hepatocytes at the periphery of the lesion.	Purple intranuclear inclusions with clear surrounding halo
Adenovirus	Patchy areas of necrosis with viral inclusions and inflammatory infiltrate limited to necrotic areas.	Basophilic "blueberry" intranuclear inclusions
Coxsackie virus	Microabscess and small or multilobular hemorrhagic necroses in neonates, similar to HSV infection. Centrilobular cholestasis with ballooning degeneration and lymphocytic and neutrophilic infiltrate in sinusoids and portal tracts in adults.	No cytopathic effect observed
Dengue fever	Midzonal or perivenular necroses with scant inflammation. Steatosis.	No cytopathic effect observed
Yellow fever	Midzonal focal necroses with acidophilic bodies (Councilman bodies) and small droplet fat.	Eosinophilic intranuclear inclusion (Torres bodies)
Rubella	Giant hepatocyte cells in neonatal hepatitis. Paucity of bile ducts.	No cytopathic effect observed
Measles (rubeola)	Steatosis, nonspecific portal inflammation and focal hepatocyte necroses.	Viral inclusion is rare

2.4 Acute Hepatitis With Massive Hepatic Necrosis

Acute hepatitis with massive hepatic necrosis presents with signs, symptoms, and biochemical test results of acute hepatitis with jaundice, coagulopathy, and slow or rapid progression to hepatic encephalopathy. As the disease progresses to hepatic failure, the initially enlarged liver may decrease in size, the markedly elevated serum aminotransferase activities may decline, and prothrombin time rises owing to hepatic parenchymal loss. Acute viral hepatitis, drug-induced injury, and toxins account for the most cases. In fulminant hepatic failure from acute hepatitis A, B, D, or E, viral serologic markers for hepatitis viruses are helpful for the diagnosis.

The prognosis of acute hepatitis with massive hepatic necrosis is poor, depending on the cause, age of the patient, and extent of necrosis and encephalopathy. Liver transplantation is a lifesaving treatment.

Pathologic Features

The liver becomes small, shrunken, and soft, with wrinkled capsule and spleen-like cut surface. Islands of surviving or regenerating hepatocytes are yellow-brown, forming bulging nodules, and surrounded by sunken dark-red areas of parenchymal collapse.

Acute hepatitis with massive hepatic necrosis is characterized by loss of almost all or all of the hepatocytes resulting in collapse of the reticulin framework and approximation of the portal tracts (Figure 2.4.2). Surviving hepatocytes can be identified in the lobules or at the periportal location, exhibiting ballooning and eosinophilic degeneration, cholestasis, enlargement with binucleation or multinucleation, or containing small droplets of fat. The sinusoids are filled with red blood cells, lymphocytes, and enlarged pigment-laden macrophages. Ductular hepatocyte formation or ductular reaction as an attempt of bipotential progenitor cells to replace hepatocytes loss is often seen in massive hepatic necrosis (Figure 2.4.4).

Differential Diagnosis

The differential diagnoses of acute hepatitis with massive hepatic necrosis are toxic necrosis, shock liver, and autoimmune hepatitis (see Table 2.4.1). Toxic necrosis is caused by predictable or direct hepatotoxins and drugs, such as carbon tetrachloride, mushroom poisoning, and acetaminophen. Suicidal or accidental overdoses of acetaminophen or lower doses of acetaminophen in alcoholic patients may lead to nausea and vomiting, followed by jaundice, hepatic encephalopathy, and coma. The laboratory findings of toxic necrosis are similar to acute hepatitis with massive hepatic necrosis. Toxic necrosis involves the centrilobular and midzonal areas with eosinophilic necrosis in the early stage, which is subsequently removed by macrophages, resulting in centrilobular collapse containing numerous brown pigment–laden Kupffer cells.

Shock liver develops in patients with heart failure or shock after trauma, surgery, burns, hemorrhage, or sepsis. Although aminotransferase activities are markedly elevated and prothrombin time rises, shock liver does not cause hepatic failure. Shock liver shows centrilobular ischemic coagulative necrosis, which is surrounded by a scanty neutrophilic infiltrate after a day or two and later by macrophages (Figure 2.4.5). The uninvolved parenchyma and portal tracts are not inflamed. In patients with acute heart failure, the centrilobular areas show sinusoidal dilatation, congestion, and hemorrhage that may obscure necrotic hepatocytes.

Autoimmune hepatitis is usually insidious but may be acute with features of massive hepatic necrosis, accompanied by hypergammaglobulinemia and high titers of autoantibodies (antinuclear, anti–smooth muscle, or anti–liver kidney microsomal antibody). Plasma cells are abundant, and eosinophils are always present (Figure 2.4.6).

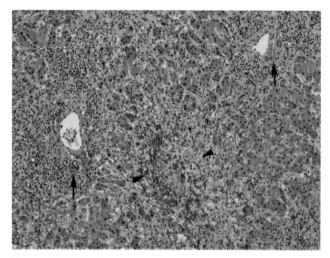

Figure 2.4.1 Acute hepatitis with submassive necrosis (arrowheads). The portal tracts are inflamed (arrows), and periportal hepatocytes are preserved.

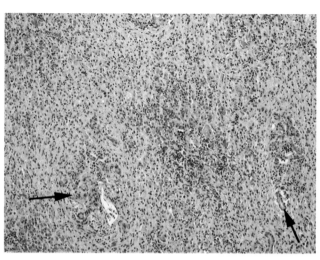

Figure 2.4.2 Acute hepatitis with massive necrosis. The portal tracts (arrows) are closer one to another because of parenchymal collapse.

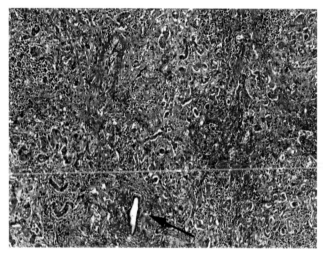

Figure 2.4.3 Portal tract (arrow) surrounded by inflammatory cells and ductular reaction in massive hepatic necrosis. The mature fibrous stroma of portal tract is more intensely blue than the collapse area (trichrome stain).

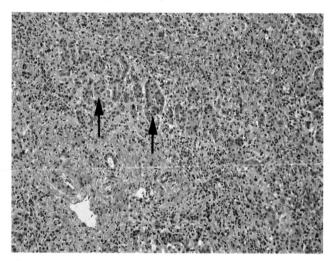

Figure 2.4.4 Ductular reaction (ductular hepatocytes, arrows) in massive hepatic necrosis.

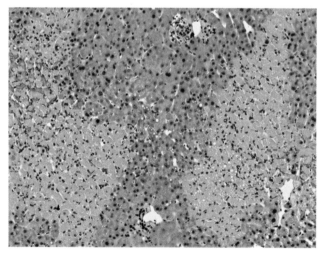

Figure 2.4.5 Shock liver with centrilobular coagulative necrosis and neutrophilic infiltrate. Periportal parenchyma and portal tracts are not involved.

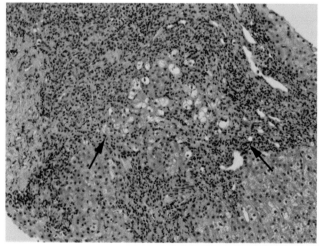

Figure 2.4.6 Autoimmune hepatitis with abundant plasma cells and severe interface hepatitis (arrows).

Table 2.4.1 Differential Diagnoses of Acute Hepatitis With Massive Hepatic Necrosis

Features	Acute Hepatitis With Massive Hepatic Necrosis	Toxic Necrosis	Shock Liver	Autoimmune Hepatitis
Hepatic failure	++	++	+	+/–
Inflammatory infiltrate	++ (predominantly lymphocytes, except for hepatitis A with plasma cells)	–	–	++ (predominantly plasma cells)
Centrilobular coagulative/ ischemic necrosis	–	+	+	+/–
Centrilobular hemorrhage	–	–	+	+/–
Steatosis (periportal or periphery of necrotic areas)	–	++	+	–
Phlebitis	+	–	–	–
Ductular reaction	++	–	–	+/–
Portal fibrosis	–	–	–	+
Portal inflammation	+	+/–	–	++

++ indicates almost always present; +, usually present; +/–, occasionally present; –, usually absent.

2.5 Granulomatous Inflammation

Granuloma is a nodular collection of macrophages, accompanied by lymphocytes and plasma cells and occasionally with giant cell formation, neutrophils, or eosinophils. Hepatic granulomas are often asymptomatic and are commonly part of systemic diseases, particularly sarcoidosis; infectious diseases (tuberculosis, schistosomiasis, bacterial and fungal infections); immunologic disorders (primary biliary cirrhosis, polyarteritis nodosa); and drug-induced injury. Therefore, the importance of granulomatous inflammation lies in the opportunity to diagnose the underlying disease.

When granulomatous inflammation is associated with hepatocellular injury, the process is referred to as granulomatous hepatitis and is often associated with drug-induced injury or infectious diseases. Small granulomas can also occur as a nonspecific reaction of macrophage or Kupffer cell to hepatocellular dropout in various acute or chronic liver diseases, including chronic hepatitis C.

In some instances, the histologic features of the granulomas may be characteristic of a specific disease or provide guidance to additional tests (see Table 2.5.1 for different types of granulomas). Both tuberculosis and sarcoidosis are among the most common causes of hepatic granulomatous diseases.

Sarcoid granulomas in the liver are seen in most cases of sarcoidosis (up to 90%). They are located in the portal tracts and to a less extent in the lobules (Figure 2.5.1). They are multiple, large nonnecrotizing granulomas, with multinucleated giant cells and rare eosinophils, containing Schaumann bodies, asteroid bodies, or calcium oxalate crystals. They often coalesce to form conglomerates of several granulomas. The granulomas usually undergo fibrosis with formation of concentric layers of dense hyalinized collagen and eventually become nodular fibrous scar. Different stages of evolution of granulomas can be seen in the same liver. Special stains show collagen deposition and abundant reticulin fibers but are negative for microorganisms. Isolated multinucleated giant cells may be found in the hepatic sinusoids of patients with sarcoidosis, even in the absence of hepatic granulomas. Rare complications of hepatic sarcoidosis include primary biliary cirrhosis-like cholestatic syndrome with bile duct loss, biliary fibrosis, and cirrhosis.

Tuberculous granulomas in the liver can be seen in more than 25% of patients with tuberculosis. The granulomas are located in the portal tracts and lobules, and all are in the same stage of development (Figure 2.5.2). Multinucleated Langhans giant cells and caseating necrosis may be absent, especially in small granulomas. The remaining liver parenchyma shows nonspecific changes, including activation of sinusoidal lining cells, sinusoidal dilatation, lymphocytic infiltrate, and scattered hepatocellular necroses. Special stains for acid-fast bacilli are positive in a small percentage of cases, but cultures or polymerase chain reaction test is usually positive. Reticulin stain demonstrated destruction of reticulin fibers within the granulomas. In AIDS or severely immunocompromised patients, granulomas are poorly formed or can be entirely absent. In patients with *Mycobacterium avium-intracellulare*, clusters of macrophages are seen filled with the organisms that are positive for periodic acid–Schiff with diastase digestion.

Drug-induced injury may result in granuloma formation and may be accompanied by acute hepatitis or cholestatic hepatitis. The granulomas are located in the portal tracts or hepatic lobules and may contain eosinophils and rarely giant cells (Figures 2.5.3 and 2.5.4). The more common drugs that cause granuloma are allopurinol, sulfonamides, phenytoin, carbamazepine, quinine, thiabendazole, and phenylbutazone.

Hodgkin and non-Hodgkin lymphomas can cause nonspecific granulomatous reaction in the liver. The possibility of a lymphoma should be considered in patients with fever of unknown origin, nonspecific symptoms, and liver biopsy with nonspecific atypical lymphocytic infiltrate.

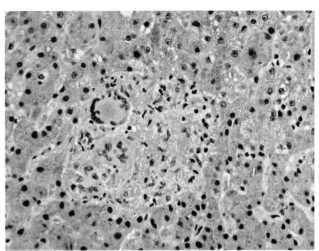

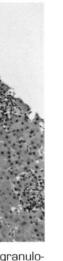

Figure 2.5.1   Multiple well-formed epithelioid granulomas with giant cells in sarcoidosis.

Figure 2.5.2   Tuberculous granuloma with multinucleated Langhans giant cells and caseous necrosis.

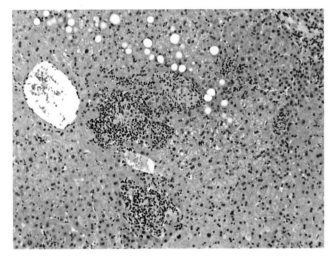

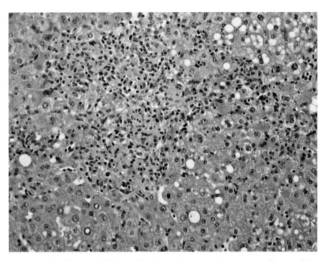

Figure 2.5.3   Drug-induced granulomatous hepatitis.

Figure 2.5.4   Lithium-induced granulomatous hepatitis with eosinophils.

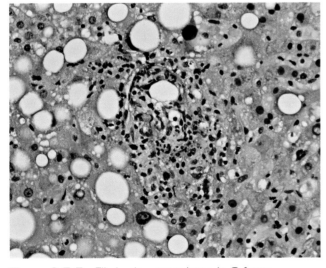

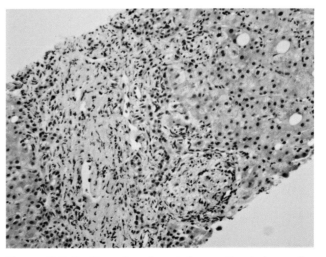

Figure 2.5.5   Fibrin ring granuloma in Q fever.

Figure 2.5.6   Granulomatous inflammation in Lyme disease.

Table 2.5.1 Different Types of Granuloma

Morphology	Common Causes
Microgranulomas	Primary biliary cirrhosis, nonspecific hepatocyte dropout including chronic hepatitis C and drug induced injury.
Epithelioid granulomas, necrotizing	Tuberculosis, MAI, fungal infection (candida, aspergillus), lymphoma.
Epithelioid granulomas, nonnecrotizing	Sarcoidosis, primary biliary cirrhosis, drug-induced injury, foreign body reaction, brucellosis, fungal infection (histoplasmosis, coccidioidomycosis, cryptococcosis), lymphoma.
Epithelioid granulomas with giant cells and eosinophils	Parasitic infection including schistosomiasis, echinococcus.
Foamy macrophage granulomas	MAI, histoplasmosis, leishmaniasis, Whipple disease.
Fibrin ring granulomas	Q-fever, CMV, EBV, toxoplasmosis, salmonellosis, drug-induced injury.
Stellate microabscess with granulomatous inflammation	Various fungal infection, bartonella, tularemia, actinomyces.
Foreign body granulomas	Talc-like substance in IV drug users, suture, thorotrast.
Lipogranulomas	Mineral oil, alcoholic and nonalcoholic steatohepatitis.

2.6 Acute Cholestasis

Cholestasis is classified as acute or chronic, and based on the localization of the interference of bile flow or formation, extrahepatic and intrahepatic cholestasis. Acute extrahepatic cholestasis is caused by obstruction to the bile ducts due to malignancy, benign bile duct stricture, bile duct compression, bile duct stones, and gallstones. Acute intrahepatic cholestasis is caused by drug-induced cholestatic liver injury, acute viral hepatitis, sepsis, paraneoplastic cholestasis, and other rare intrahepatic causes such as benign recurrent intrahepatic cholestasis and late onset of progressive familial intrahepatic cholestasis. Primary biliary cirrhosis and primary sclerosing cholangitis are considered causes of chronic cholestasis.

Drug-Induced Cholestatic Liver Injury

Drug-induced cholestatic liver injury is divided into 2 subtypes: pure (bland) cholestasis and cholestatic hepatitis. Pure cholestasis is characterized by pruritus and jaundice with generally normal or only slightly increased transaminase activities. It is often observed with a few drugs, mainly sex steroid derivatives, cytarabine, and azathioprine. Pure cholestasis is characterized by canalicular and hepatocellular cholestasis, Kupffer cell hyperplasia often containing bile pigment, and activation of sinusoidal lining cells. Inflammatory cells are virtually absent, there is no hepatocellular necrosis, and the portal tracts show minimal ductular reaction.

Cholestatic hepatitis combines cholestasis with clinical features of acute hepatitis, such as pain and hepatic tenderness, and frequently mimics the features of biliary obstruction or cholangitis. Cholestatic hepatitis shows the characteristic changes of acute hepatitis, including panlobular disarray, increased cellularity, and degenerative and regenerative changes of hepatocytes, combined with feathery degeneration, hepatocellular and canalicular cholestasis (Figures 2.6.1 and 2.6.2). In prolonged cases of cholestasis, hepatocytes form rosettes around dilated bile canaliculi. The portal tracts are slightly expanded by inflammatory cells, predominantly lymphocytes, macrophages, and scattered neutrophils. Ductular reaction and neutrophils are milder in comparison to large bile duct obstruction.

It should be noted that cholestatic hepatitis can also be caused by acute or unresolved viral or alcoholic hepatitis and rare cases of chronic viral hepatitis with cholestasis (fibrosing cholestatic hepatitis).

The prognosis of drug-induced cholestatic liver injury is generally good, although it may have a prolonged clinical course and resolve rather slowly. Ductopenia or vanishing bile duct syndrome may follow drug-induced cholestatic liver injury in a minority of patients (Figure 2.6.5).

See also "Drug-Induced Liver Injury" of this chapter for other forms of drug-induced injury.

Paraneoplastic Cholestasis

Acute cholestasis may represent a paraneoplastic syndrome in various neoplastic diseases as the result of the emission of cytokine from the neoplastic cells. Among the more common are renal cell carcinoma and lymphomas, particularly Hodgkin lymphoma. Cholestasis may precede the presentation of neoplasm. The histologic features resemble pure (bland) cholestasis without significant hepatocellular dropout (Figure 2.6.6). Kupffer cell hyperplasia containing bile pigment and activation of sinusoidal lining cells are common. The hepatocytes form rosettes around the dilated bile canaliculi. Recovery of liver function is expected after resection of tumor or eradication of lymphoma, unless severe ductopenia has occurred.

Intrahepatic Cholestasis

Mutations in canalicular transporter genes are responsible for various rare clinical forms of neonatal, pediatric, and adult forms of intrahepatic cholestatic liver diseases. Mutation in familial intrahepatic cholestasis 1 or *ATP8B1* gene (FIC1 deficiency) causes progressive familial intrahepatic cholestasis 1 (PFIC1), benign recurrent intrahepatic cholestasis 1 (BRIC1), or intrahepatic cholestasis of pregnancy 1 (ICP1); mutation in bile salt export pump (*BSEP*) gene (BSEP deficiency) causes PFIC2, BRIC2, or ICP2; and mutation in multidrug resistance protein 3 (*MDR3*) gene (MDR3 deficiency) causes PFIC3, BRIC3, or ICP3. Progressive familial intrahepatic cholestasis occurs predominantly in neonates and children, as discussed in Chapter 6; ICP is discussed in "Liver Disease in Pregnancy" of this chapter.

Benign recurrent intrahepatic cholestasis presents as multiple episodes of cholestasis in adolescents or young adult. Patients present with 3 to 4 months of jaundice, pruritus, occasional vomiting, influenza-like symptoms, and abdominal pain. Imaging study of the biliary tree is normal. Serum alkaline phosphatase (AP) levels are increased, but γ-glutamyltransferase (GGT) and transaminase activities are normal. Cholestasis resolves spontaneously and do not progress to end-stage liver disease. Episodes of cholestasis become less common later in life. Other more common causes of acute cholestasis should be excluded.

Liver biopsy demonstrates hepatocanalicular and ductular cholestasis, mild nonspecific inflammation, mild portal edema, and minimal hepatocyte dropout. GGT and CD10 immunostaining shows decrease or absent canalicular staining. Liver histology is normal during remission.

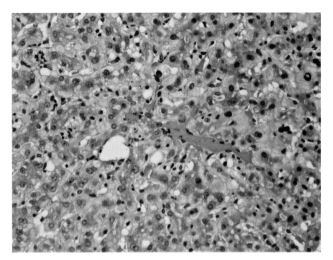

Figure 2.6.1 Drug-induced cholestatic hepatitis with hepatocanalicular bile and mild lobular necroinflammation in centrilobular area.

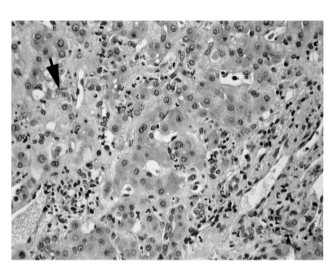

Figure 2.6.2 Cholestasis (arrow), lobular necroinflammatory activity, and mild ductular reaction in drug-induced cholestatic hepatitis.

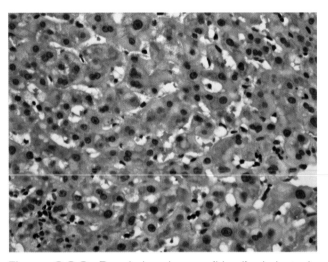

Figure 2.6.3 Drug-induced pure (bland) cholestasis caused by anabolic steroids.

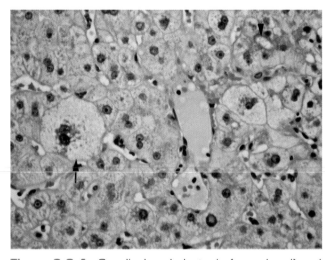

Figure 2.6.4 Canalicular cholestasis (arrowhead) and feathery degeneration (arrow) in drug-induced cholestatic hepatitis.

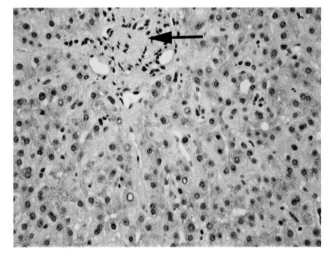

Figure 2.6.5 Ductopenia or vanishing bile duct syndrome is a rare consequence of drug-induced cholestatic injury. Portal tract without bile duct (arrow).

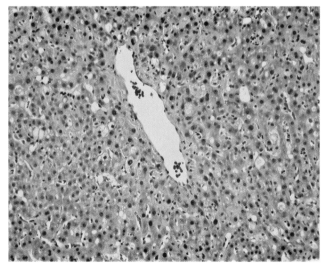

Figure 2.6.6 Hodgkin lymphoma–related acute cholestasis, histologically indistinguishable from drug-induced cholestatic injury.

Table 2.6.1   Differential Diagnosis of Acute Cholestasis

Histologic Features	Pure Cholestasis, Drug Induced	Cholestatic Hepatitis, Drug Induced	Acute Viral Hepatitis	Large Bile Duct Obstruction	Primary Sclerosing Cholangitis	Primary Biliary Cirrhosis
Hepatocanalicular cholestasis	++	++	+	+	+/−	+/−
Lobular inflammation	−	++	++	+/−	−	+/−
Panlobular hepatitis	−	++	++	−	−	−
Centrilobular hepatocyte dropout	+/−	++	++	−	−	−
Centrilobular feathery degeneration	+	+	+/−	+	−	−
Portal inflammation	−	+/−	+	+	+	++
Portal edema	−	−	+/−	++	−	−
Ductular reaction	−	+/−	+/−	++	+	+
Bile duct ectasia	−	−	−	+/−	+	+/−
Periductal fibrosis	−	−	−	−	+	−
Bile duct scar	−	−	−	−	+	−
Bile duct loss	+/−	+/−	−	−	+	+
Florid duct lesion	−	−	−	−	−	+
Periportal copper deposition	−	−	−	−	+/−	+/−

++ indicates almost always present; +, usually present; +/−, occasionally present; −, usually absent.

2.7 Alcoholic Hepatitis

Alcoholic hepatitis is characterized by fatigue, anorexia, weight loss, hepatomegaly, and in more severe cases, fever, jaundice, and vomiting. Helpful differential diagnostic points are history, large tender liver, leukocytosis, and a ratio of aspartate aminotransferase to alanine aminotransferase (ALT) greater than 1. Alcoholic hepatitis represents an acute presentation of alcoholic liver disease. The diagnosis requires history of several years of alcohol abuse, but this may be difficult to ascertain in many cases. The prognosis in alcoholic hepatitis depends largely on whether the patient continues drinking. Total abstinence from alcohol represents the most important therapeutic measure.

Pathologic Features

Alcoholic hepatitis shows marked ballooning degeneration of the hepatocytes, which often contain intracytoplasmic hyalin inclusions particularly in centrilobular areas, as the result of cytokeratin intermediate filament condensation (Figures 2.7.1 and 2.7.2). Macrovesicular or, less often, microvesicular steatosis is often present but not a requisite to the diagnosis (Figure 2.7.4). Neutrophils are the predominant infiltrate in alcoholic hepatitis, and they commonly surround ballooned hepatocytes with cytoplasmic hyalins, forming the so-called Mallory-Denk bodies. Mallory-Denk bodies are not pathognomonic to alcoholic hepatitis; they can be seen in other liver diseases including nonalcoholic steatohepatitis, drug-induced injury, Wilson disease, chronic cholestasis, and hepatocellular carcinoma. Intracytoplasmic round or oval eosinophilic inclusions may be seen, predominantly in the centrilobular areas. They represent distended mitochondria (megamitochondria).

Fibrosis occurs initially in the centrilobular area as pericellular "chicken-wire" fibrosis, which is often accompanied by fibrous thickening and obliteration of the central venule, referred to as central hyalin sclerosis. Pericellular fibrosis is usually seen prominently surrounding ballooned hepatocytes and Mallory-Denk bodies. Fibrous septa are formed from one central venule to another. Fibrosis and inflammatory infiltrates in the portal tracts and ductular reaction are initially absent but are seen in more advanced stages of alcoholic hepatitis. In severe cases, the entire lobule may be involved with hepatocellular ballooning, necrosis, and inflammation, resembling acute hepatitis with submassive necrosis and collapse. Steatosis can be absent or minimal.

Differential Diagnosis

The differential diagnoses include nonalcoholic steatohepatitis, Wilson disease, and drug-induced injury (see Table 2.7.1.). Nonalcoholic steatohepatitis is often indistinguishable from alcoholic hepatitis, and in many instances, they overlap, but in general, nonalcoholic steatohepatitis does not present acutely and shows steatosis with less neutrophilic infiltrate and Mallory-Denk bodies (Figure 2.7.5.). Drug-induced injury can mimic any form of liver disease, including alcoholic hepatitis, such as drug-induced injury due to amiodarone or hormonal chemotherapy. Without sufficient clinical information, hepatocellular carcinoma with Mallory-Denk type inclusion, rarefied cytoplasm, glycogen content, and steatosis may mimic alcoholic hepatitis, especially in core biopsy specimens (Figure 2.7.6). Other features of hepatocellular carcinoma, such as thickened cell plates, endothelial cell wrapping, bile production, polymorphism of the nuclei, and positivity for glypican 3, are helpful in distinguishing hepatocellular carcinoma from alcoholic hepatitis.

Clinically, the differential diagnosis of autoimmune hepatitis is often considered due to concurrent serum autoantibody positivity and the obscure history of alcohol intake. A biopsy of autoimmune hepatitis shows extensive hepatocellular damage, often with parenchymal collapse, accompanied by plasmacellular infiltrate with eosinophils, moderate-to-severe interface hepatitis, without Mallory-Denk bodies or significant neutrophilic infiltrate.

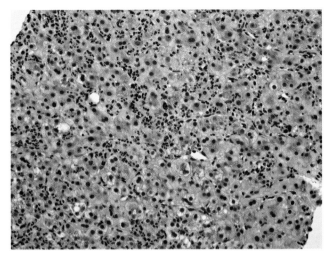

Figure 2.7.1 Alcoholic hepatitis with abundant neutrophils in the hepatic parenchyma.

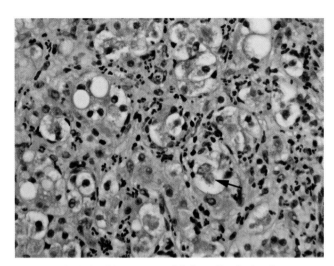

Figure 2.7.2 Numerous Mallory-Denk bodies composed of hepatocytes with cytoplasmic hyalin inclusion surrounded by neutrophils (arrow).

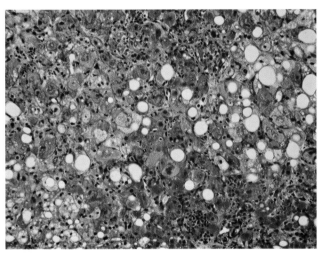

Figure 2.7.3 Trichrome stain often demonstrates preexisting pericellular fibrosis to suggest chronicity in alcoholic hepatitis.

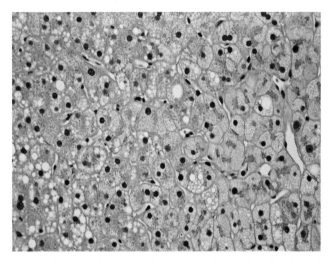

Figure 2.7.4 Medium droplet steatosis (left field) and small droplet steatosis steatosis (right field).

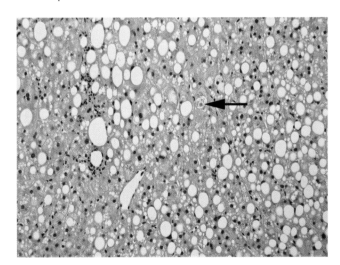

Figure 2.7.5 Mild degree of alcoholic hepatitis is indistinguishable from nonalcoholic fatty liver disease and requires clinical history to establish the diagnosis. Focal ballooning degeneration is present (arrow).

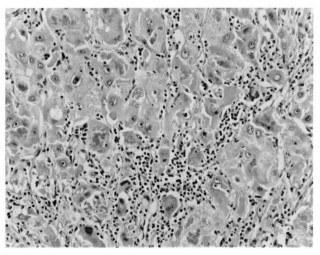

Figure 2.7.6 Hepatocellular carcinoma with Mallory-Denk inclusions and neutrophilic infiltrate, mimicking alcoholic hepatitis.

Table 2.7.1 Differential Diagnosis of Alcoholic Hepatitis

Histologic Features	Alcoholic Hepatitis	Nonalcoholic Steatohepatitis	Wilson Disease	Drug-Induced Injury
Macrovesicular steatosis	+/−	++	+/−	+/−
Microvesicular steatosis	+/−	+/−	−	+/−
Ballooning degeneration	++	+	++	+/−
Neutrophilic infiltrate	++	+	+/−	+/−
Mallory-Denk bodies	++	+/−	+	+/−
Pericellular fibrosis	++	+	+	+/−
Central hyalin sclerosis	+/−	−	−	−
Portal fibrosis	+/−	+/−	+	+/−

++ indicates almost always present; +, usually present; +/−, occasionally present; −, usually absent.

2.8 Drug-Induced Liver Injury

Drug-induced liver injury or hepatitis can mimic any form of acute hepatitis and should be considered in any patient with hepatobiliary disease. A careful history is essential and should include all drugs and supplements, prescribed and over the counter, taken over the last several months. Some may be clear-cut on the basis of known toxicity and chronology, but others may be difficult to elucidate. The latent period between drug exposure and onset of symptoms may vary from several days to a few months. There are generally no specific markers or tests for the diagnosis of drug-induced liver injury. Exposure to viral hepatitis should be ruled out because drug-induced liver injury is clinically indistinguishable from acute viral hepatitis. The list of drugs that may cause a hepatitis-like picture is very long, and virtually any drug must be considered in the differential diagnosis. Commonly used drugs, such as antibiotics, nonsteroidal anti-inflammatory drugs, antihypertensives, antidiabetic agents, anticonvulsants, lipid-lowering agents, and psychotropic drugs, may potentially be hepatotoxic.

Drug-induced liver injury is divided into intrinsic and idiosyncratic injury. Intrinsic injury is reproducible in animal models, dose related, and with clear temporal relationship, such as acetaminophen, carbon tetrachloride, phosphorus, and cocaine. Idiosyncratic injury, which represents most of the drug-induced liver injuries, is unpredictable and represents hypersensitivity reactions or genetically determined variations in drug metabolism.

Clinical Features

Drugs can reproduce practically the whole spectrum of liver diseases and should be considered in the differential diagnosis of any patient with hepatobiliary disease. In the absence of histologic data, the preferred term is *liver injury*. According to the international panel, acute drug-induced liver injuries can be classified into 3 groups using biochemical criteria based on serum ALT and AP and their ratio: acute hepatocellular injury, acute cholestatic liver injury, and mixed pattern acute liver injury. This classification has the advantage of separating types of hepatitis with different courses and prognostic features. Acute hepatocellular injury is defined by ALT over 2 times the upper limit of normal range or ALT/AP ratio of 5 or greater. Acute cholestatic liver injury is characterized by an isolated increase of AP over 2 times the upper limit of normal range or by an ALT/AP ratio of less than 2, whereas mixed pattern acute liver injury is characterized by an ALT/AP ratio between 2 and 5.

Discontinuation of the treatment is usually followed by complete recovery within 1 to 3 months. Sometimes, fulminant course occurs, often promoted by continuation of treatment despite the occurrence of jaundice. In this regard, drug-induced hepatitis is often more fulminant and fatal than acute viral hepatitis. Progression of disease following drug withdrawal has been described in rare cases.

Pathologic Features

Acute hepatocellular injury, the most common form of hepatic damage caused by drugs, generally conveys no specific clinical features and mimics acute viral hepatitis. No definite histologic changes distinguish acute drug-induced hepatitis from acute viral hepatitis; however, a few alterations may be helpful in the differential diagnosis, such as prominent eosinophils and granulomas, sinusoidal dilatation, and fatty change. Prominent eosinophilic infiltration is seen classically in chlorpromazine-induced hepatitis. In most cases, hepatocyte necrosis is spotty, but in more severe cases, sharply demarcated perivenular or confluent necrosis and progression to multiacinar and massive hepatic necrosis can occur. The degree of canalicular or hepatocellular cholestasis varies but often is more severe than in acute viral hepatitis. It may be prolonged, leads to pale swelling and feathery degeneration of the cytoplasm of the hepatocytes, and may be associated with epithelial damage of small bile ducts and mild ductular reaction. Occasionally, drug-induced hepatitis becomes chronic, leading to chronic hepatitis, for instance, after alpha methyldopa, isoniazid, and nitrofurantoin therapy.

Differential Diagnosis

In addition to acute viral hepatitis, differential diagnosis of drug-induced injury includes autoimmune hepatitis and steatohepatitis (see Table 2.8.1). Although histologically quite distinctive, both autoimmune hepatitis and steatohepatitis can be clinically difficult to distinguish from drug-induced liver injury because of the concomittant mild elevation of autoantibody titer to suggest autoimmune hepatitis or the presence of comorbidities for steatohepatitis. It should also be noted that few drugs can cause steatohepatitis or autoimmune hepatitis-like features.

Table 2.8.2 lists common drugs and their histologic patterns of liver injury.

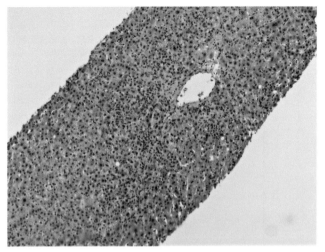

Figure 2.8.1 Panlobular inflammation in drug-induced hepatitis/injury.

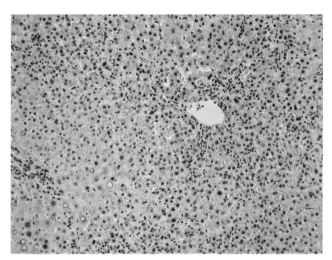

Figure 2.8.2 Predominant centrilobular necroinflammation in drug-induced injury.

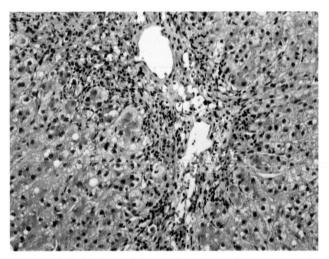

Figure 2.8.3 Centrilobular hepatocellular dropout in clonazepam-induced injury.

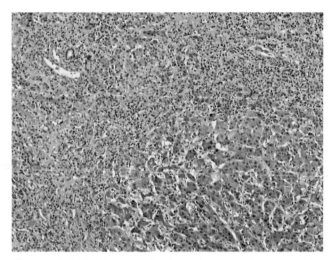

Figure 2.8.4 Submassive hepatic necrosis caused by lipid-lowering agent atorvastatin.

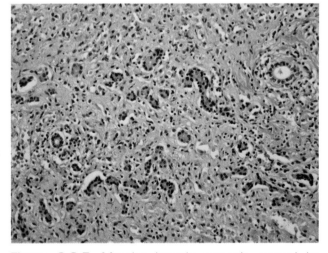

Figure 2.8.5 Massive hepatic necrosis caused by herbal supplement.

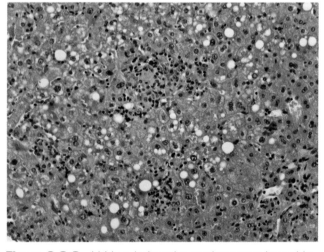

Figure 2.8.6 Lithium-induced granulomatous hepatitis.

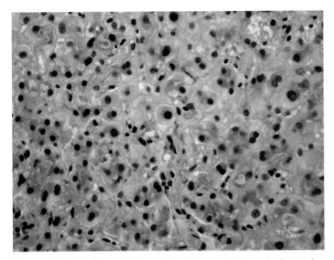

Figure 2.8.7 Drug-induced hepatocanalicular cholestasis.

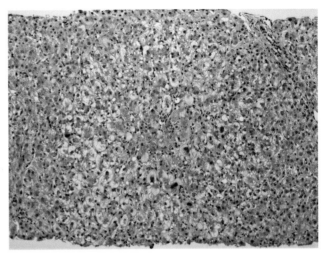

Figure 2.8.8 Rituximab-induced cholestatic hepatitis with marked feathery degeneration of the centrilobular hepatocytes.

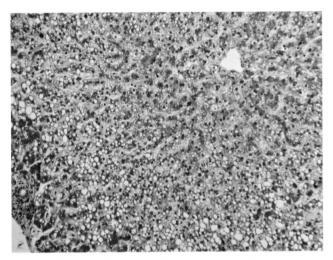

Figure 2.8.9 Valproic acid–induced small droplet steatosis (trichrome stain).

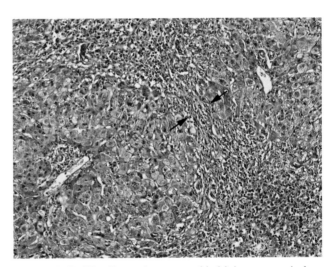

Figure 2.8.10 Central to central bridging necrosis (arrows) in *Amanita phalloides* poisoning.

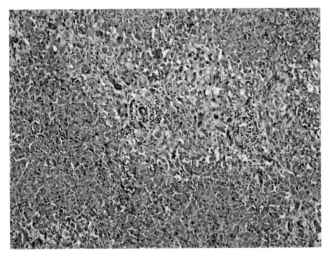

Figure 2.8.11 Eosinophilic necrosis in acetaminophen toxicity sparing periportal hepatocytes containing small droplet fat.

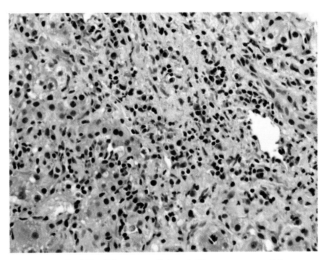

Figure 2.8.12 Plasmacellular infiltrate resembling autoimmune hepatitis in herbal supplement toxicity.

Table 2.8.1 Differential Diagnosis of Drug-Induced Hepatitis

Histologic Features	Drug-Induced Hepatitis	Acute Viral Hepatitis	Autoimmune Hepatitis	Steatohepatitis
Eosinophilic infiltrate	+	–	+	–
Lobular lymphocytic infiltrate	+	++	+	+ (minimal)/–
Portal lymphocytic infiltrate	+	+	+	+/–
Portal and lobular plasmacellular infiltrate	+	+/–	++	–
Interface hepatitis	–	+/–	+	–
Granulomas	+/–	–	–	+ (lipogranuloma)/–
Perivenular necrosis	+/–	+/–	+	–
Bridging/confluent necrosis	+/–	+/–	+/–	–
Steatosis	+/–	+/–	–	++

++ indicates almost always present; +, usually present; +/–, occasionally present; –, usually absent.

Table 2.8.2   Common Drugs and Histologic Patterns

Drug	Pattern	Comments
Antibiotics		
Beta lactams	C, H, M, G	Cholestasis may persist months/years after withdrawal, vanishing bile duct syndrome.
Tetracyclines	F, H	Dose-related. Minocycline causes hypersensitivity, ie, hepatitis, eosinophilia, dermatitis.
Macrolides	C	All erythromycin esters can produce cholestasis. Prominent portal eosinophilic infitrate.
Sulfonamides	C, H, M, G	Cotrimoxazole causes numerous forms of liver injury. Risk increased in HIV patients.
Quinolones	C, H, M, G	Mostly mild cholestatic or mixed injury. Norfloxacin causes eosinophilic necrotizing granulomatous hepatitis.
Nitrofurantoin	C, H, M, G	All types of injury. Rarely cause chronic hepatitis with features like to autoimmune hepatitis.
Chloramphenicol	C	Rare
Clindamycin	H	Rare
Antituberculosis agents		
Isoniazid	H, G	Resemble acute viral hepatitis, can be severe
Rifampicin	H	Increased risk of hepatotoxicity when combined with isoniazid
Pyrazinamide	H	Increased risk of hepatotoxicity in combination therapy
Ethambutol	M	Rare
Antifungal agents		
Azole	H, M, C	Potent inhibitors of cytochrome P450 enzymes. All have been associated with hepatotoxicity.
Terbinafine	C, H	Associated with prolonged liver injury
Amphotericin B	H	Rarely associated with hepatotoxicity
Flucytosine	H	Hepatotoxicity when used in combination with other antifungals
Antiviral agents		
Protease inhibitor	H	Ritonavir has a higher risk of hepatotoxicity.
NRTI	H, F	Zidovudine and didanosine may cause fulminant hepatic failure and microvesicular steatosis.
NNRTI	H	Nevirapine, efavirenz and delavirdine have been associated with hepatotoxicity
Antiparasitic agents		
Albendazole	H, M	Mild hepatotoxicity
Mebendazole	H, M	Mild hepatotoxicity
Thiabendazole	M	Prolonged cholestatic hepatitis, vanishing bile duct syndrome.
Pentamidine	H	High incidence of mild-to-moderate liver enzyme elevation
NSAIDs		
Aspirin	H, F	Dose-dependent, Reye's syndrome
Diclofenac	H	Women and persons with osteoarthritis may be susceptible.
Ibuprofen	H	Rarely causes vanishing bile duct syndrome
Indomemethacin	H, C	Rare massive hepatic necrosis

Table 2.8.2 *(continued)*

Drug	Pattern	Comments
Sulindac	C, H	Hypersensitivity features common, rash, nephrotoxicity, shock syndrome
Antihypertensive agents		
Methyldopa	H, C, S, G	Methyldopa-related liver injury has been well characterized.
Beta blockers	H	Low hepatotoxic potential except labetolol, which can cause severe acute hepatitis
Ca channel antagonists	H	Diltiazem also associated with cholestasis and granulomatous hepatitis
Hydralazine (I or y?)	H, C, G	
Thiazides	C	Rare
ACE inhibitor	C	Rare. Losartan may be used in treating portal hypertension.
Drugs in diabetes mellitus		
Glucosidase inhibitors	H, C	Acarbose have been associated with dose-related hepatotoxicity
Metformin	C	Rare
Human insulin	M	Rare
Sulfonylureas	C, H, G	Predominantly cholestasis
Thiazolidinediones	H	Troglitazone causes fulminant hepatic failure, rosiglitazone, and pioglitazone cause hepatocellular injury (or hepatitis?)
Lipid-lowering agents		
Statins	H, M	Elevation of liver enzymes seen in approximately 3% of recipients, dose dependent, within 3 months of therapy. Serious injury is rare.
Fibrates	H, C, MHN	Fenofibrate is associated with rare cases of autoimmune hepatitis, fibrosis, and ductopenia
Anticonvulsants		
Phenytoin	H	Focal necrosis with sinusoidal lymphocytosis
Carbamazepine	G, C	Granulomatous hepatitis, cholestasis, rarely vanishing bile duct syndrome
Valproic acid	H, S	Rarely acute liver failure with microvesicular steatosis
Psychotropic drugs		
Chlorpromazine	C	Vanishing bile duct syndrome
Haloperidol	C	Vanishing bile duct syndrome
Clozapine	H, C	Rare. May be associated with hepatic failure.
Benzodiazepine	H	May also cause chronic hepatitis
MAO inhibitors	H	Rare except with iproniazid
Tricyclic antidepressants	H, C	Amitriptyline, imipramine may cause vanishing bile duct syndrome

H indicates hepatocellular; C, cholestatic; M, mixed; G, granulomatous; F, fatty liver; MHN, massive hepatic necrosis; NRTI, nucleoside reverse transcriptase inhibitor; NNRTI, nonnucleoside reverse transcriptase inhibitor.

2.9 Bacterial, Fungal, and Parasitic Infection

Bacterial, fungal, and parasitic infections of the liver are generally secondary involvement of the liver to systemic infections. Pathologic changes include nonspecific reactive hepatitis, cholestasis, cholangitis, granuloma, necrosis, and abscess where pathogenic microorganisms occasionally colocalize in the liver and can be detected by special stains and cultures. Serologic or molecular tests are necessary in which the microorganisms are not readily visualized on liver biopsies.

Bacterial Infection

Bacterial infection causes various pathologic changes ranging from nonspecific changes, including nonspecific reactive hepatitis (see "Nonspecific Reactive Hepatitis, Mild Acute Hepatitis and Residual Hepatitis") due to circulating toxins, sepsis with ductular cholestasis (see "Sepsis"), and granulomatous inflammation (see "Granulomatous Inflammation"), to suppurative inflammation with pyogenic abscesses (see Table 2.9.1).

Suppurative hepatic inflammation is accompanied by hepatocyte necrosis, resulting in microabscesses or macroscopic pyogenic abscesses. In general, suppurative inflammation is commonly secondary infections from the biliary and gastrointestinal tract and is often polymicrobial. Associated conditions include cholangitis, inflammatory bowel disease, appendicitis, diverticulosis, and intra-abdominal malignancies. In children, pyogenic abscess may signal the presence of immunodeficiency, such as chronic granulomatous disease.

Fungal Infection

Fungal infections are generally part of disseminated systemic infection in immunocompromised patients. Hepatomegaly, elevated aminotransferases, and bilirubin are common findings. Fungi can be readily visualized on hematoxylin-eosin stain, but Grocott methenamine silver and periodic acid–Schiff stains are commonly required for identification (see Table 2.9.2). Cultures are required for further classification of the species.

Parasitic Infection

Various parasitic infections occur in the liver with different manifestations, from granulomatous inflammation, cyst, or abscess formation to biliary tree inflammation and fibrosis (see Table 2.9.3). In general, the underlying process is hypersensitivity reaction toward the parasites; therefore, common histologic features include foreign body granulomatous inflammation with eosinophilia, reactive fibrosis, and dystrophic calcification. Immunohistochemistry, serologic test, or molecular studies are often necessary for diagnosis.

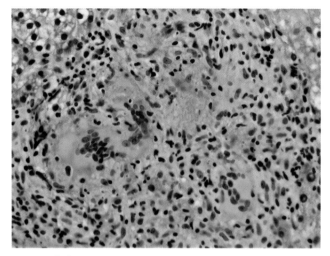

Figure 2.9.1 Tuberculous necrotizing granuloma.

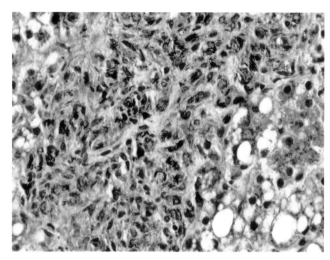

Figure 2.9.2 Numerous acid-fast bacilli (Mycobacterium avium intracellulare) identified on Ziehl-Nielsen stain.

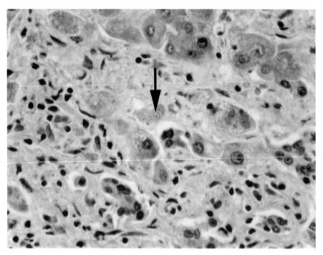

Figure 2.9.3 Lyme disease with poorly formed granulomas and macrophage containing microorganisms (arrow).

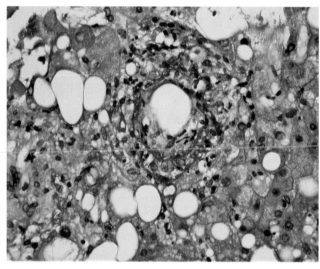

Figure 2.9.4 Fibrin ring granuloma (red ring) in Q fever (trichrome stain).

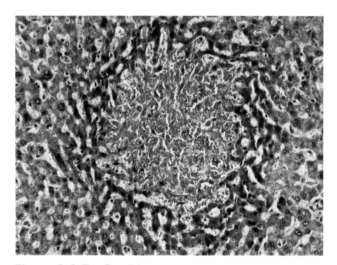

Figure 2.9.5 *Candida.*

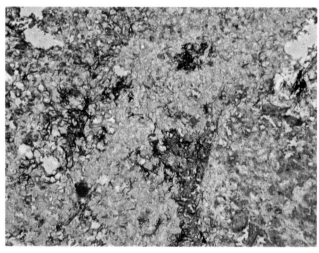

Figure 2.9.6 Syphilis spirochaete in abscess content (Steiner silver stain).

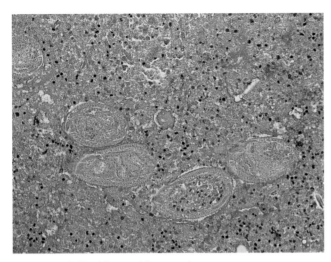

Figure 2.9.7 Visceral larva migrans.

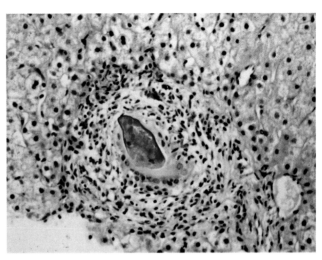

Figure 2.9.8 Schistosomiasis (periodic acid–Schiff stain after diastase digestion).

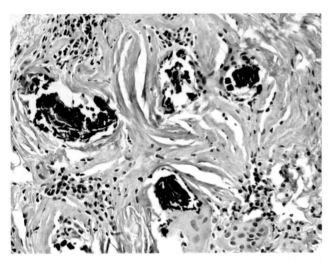

Figure 2.9.9 Calcification, fibrosis, and multinucleated giant cells in portal tract in schistosomiasis.

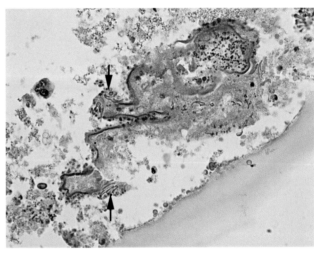

Figure 2.9.10 *Echinococcus granulosus* scolex (arrows).

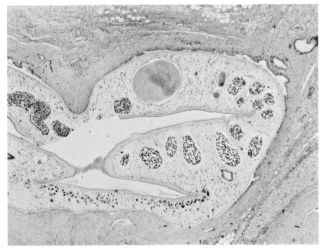

Figure 2.9.11 Liver fluke in bile duct.

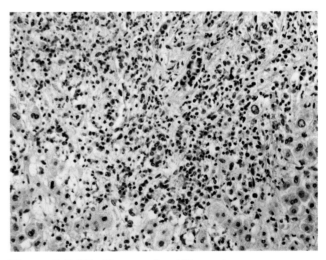

Figure 2.9.12 Hypereosinophilic syndrome.

Table 2.9.1 Pathologic Features of Various Bacterial Infections

Bacterial Infection	Pathologic Features
Pyogenic bacterial infection (*Escherichia coli, Staphylococcus aureus, Klebsiella, Proteus, Pseudomonas, Bacteroides, Fusobacterium, Salmonella, Haemophilus influenzae, Yersinia*)	Suppurative inflammation or pyogenic abscess
Typhoid fever (*Salmonella typhi*)	Nonspecific reactive hepatitis
Tularemia (*Francisella tularensis*)	Suppurative microabscesses
Bartonellosis (*Bartonella henselae, Bartonella quintana*)	Stellate microabscesses with palisading histiocytes and rim of lymphocytes; bacillary angiomatosis—peliosis
Brucellosis	Nonspecific reactive hepatitis, noncaseating granulomatous inflammation
Listeriosis (*Listeria monocytogenes*)	Microabscesses, microgranulomas
Tuberculosis (*Mycobacterium tuberculosis*)	Caseating granulomas with giant cells, accompanied by reactive hepatitis
MAI (*Mycobacterium avium-intracelllulare*)	Granulomas. Pseudosarcomatous spindle cell nodules
Leprosy (*Mycobacterium leprae*)	Foamy histiocytes in portal tract and lobules, or tuberculoid granulomas with giant cells
Rocky Mountain spotted fever (*Rickettsia rickettsii*)	Cholestasis, mixed portal inflammation, and erythrophagocytosis
Ehrlichiosis (*Ehrlichia chaffeensis*)	Reactive hepatitis with lymphohistiocytic infiltrate and cholestasis
Syphilis	Diffuse pericellular/sinusoidal fibrosis (congenital syphillis), nonspecific reactive hepatitis (acquired syphillis), nodular caseous necrosis with granuloma, and fibrosis (gumma)
Lyme disease (*Borrellia species*), Weil disease (*Leptospira*)	Nonspecific reactive hepatitis, poorly formed granulomatous inflammation
Whipple disease (*Tropheryma whippelii*)	Kupffer cell hyperplasia with PAS-positive bacilli, granuloma formation
Clostridium perfringens	Hepatitis, abscess, gas gangrene

Table 2.9.2 Pathologic Features of Various Fungal Infections

Fungal Infection	Pathologic Features
Candidiasis	Suppurative granulomatous inflammation with various degree of necrosis (microabscess). Pseudohyphae or budding yeast in the center of lesion.
Aspergillosis	Nodular infarcted parenchyma around fungi-containing blood vessels, with associated granulomaous inflammation. Septated hyphae with branches at acute angles.
Histoplasmosis	Portal lymphohistiocytic inflammation and Kupffer cell hyperplasia, mimicking tuberculosis. Small ovoid refractile intracellular yeasts with small buds in portal macrophages and Kupffer cells. Fibrous or calcified nodules in long-standing histoplasmosis (histoplasmoma).
Cryptococcosis	Suppurative granulomatous inflammation to no reaction in immunocompromised patients. Involment of the biliary tree mimics sclerosing cholangitis. Round to oval yeast with narrow-based budding in the lesion.
Blastomycosis	Microabscesses to granulomas containing yeasts with thick refractile cell wall and broad based budding.
Paracoccidioidomycosis	Microabscesses or granulomas in the vicinity of portal tracts resulting in portal fibrosis. Round to oval amphophilic yeasts with small peripheral buds resembling a ship's steering wheel.
Coccidioidomycosis	Microabscesses to granulomas with large spherules containing endospores.
Zygomycosis	Suppurative granulomatous inflammation with necrosis containing broad branching hyphae with few or no septae.

Table 2.9.3 Pathologic Features of Various Parasitic Infections

Parasitic Infection	Pathologic Features
Malaria	Dark brown congested liver with birefringent hemozoin brown pigment in Kupffer cells, portal macrophages, and erythrocytes. Erythrocytes may contain parasites.
Amoebiasis	Solitary or multiple abscesses containing red-brown paste material, associated with granulomatous inflammation and fibrous capsule. Amoebae within necrotic debris resemble large macrophages with foamy cytoplasm, round nuclei, and ingested red blood cells.
Toxoplasmosis	Cholestasis, lymphocytic infiltrate in sinusoids with occasional hepatocyte dropout containing trophozoites.
Visceral leishmaniasis	Marked Kupffer cell and portal macrophages hypertrophy containing round to oval-shaped amastigotes with nucleus and kinetoplast arranged in "double-knot" configuration.
Giardiasis	Granulomatous hepatitis and cholangitis.
Cryptosporidiasis	Cholangiopathy in patients with AIDS, do not cause significant liver inflammation.
Schistosomiasis	Lesions centered in portal vein branches caused by hypersensitivity to eggs eliciting granulomatous inflammation with multinucleated giant cells, eosinophils. Fibrosis ensues, portal tracts enlarged, and densely sclerotic (pipestem fibrosis). Schistosomal pigment resembles malarial pigment.
Clonorchiasis and opisthorchiasis	Invasion to biliary tree causes duct-like structures around large bile ducts. Eosinophilia of the smaller ducts. Biliary obstruction, recurrent cholangitis, portal fibrosis and hypertension, and cholangiocarcinoma.
Ascariasis	Focal necrosis with eosinophils and neutrophils in migratory phase to the lungs via the liver. Adult worm enters biliary tree from duodenum and causes cholangitis, duct obstruction, and abscess formation.
Toxocara canis	Visceral larva migrans with central eosinophilic abscesses containing Charcot-Leyden crystals and granulomatous inflammation.
Enterobiasis	Rare pinworm granuloma with hyalinization, peripheral inflammation, and central necrosis with eggs and worm remnants.
Strongyloidiasis	Larvae in portal veins and sinusoids. Nonspecific inflammation.

2.10 Sepsis

Sepsis leads to abnormal liver tests, including modest increases in alkaline phosphatase and aminotransferase activities, and, in severe cases, jaundice. These are caused by bacterial toxins, hepatic hypoperfusion, or infection of the liver itself. The prognosis depends on the success of treatment to overcome the sepsis; therefore, sepsis in association with persistent jaundice carries a poor prognosis and should be treated vigorously.

Pathologic Features

Cholestasis is common in sepsis (Figure 2.10.1). Initially, hepatocellular and canalicular cholestases develop in centrilobular areas accompanied by microvesicular steatosis of the hepatocytes without significant hepatocellular damage. In severe cases, cholestasis may extend to periportal hepatocytes. Neutrophils may infiltrate the sinusoids and form microabscesses. Prolonged sepsis leads to proliferation and dilatation of bile ductules and canals of Hering, filled with bile, often in the form of dense "bile concretions," so-called septic cholangitis, cholangitis lenta, or ductular cholestasis (Figures 2.10.2 and 2.10.4). Ductular cholestasis is located at the margin of portal tracts and accompanied by neutrophils. It is a common finding in sepsis and does not indicate bile duct obstruction. It may be present with or without an accompanying acute cholangitis. Centrilobular coagulative necrosis due to ischemia may be observed if the patient is in septic shock (Figure 2.10.3).

Differential Diagnosis

The differential diagnoses of sepsis include surgery-associated changes, large bile duct obstruction, drug-induced cholestatic injury, and in pediatric population, total parenteral nutrition-induced cholestatic liver disease (see Table 2.10.1). Prominent ductular cholestasis is an important feature of sepsis to an extent that is not seen in other differential diagnoses except total parenteral nutrition-induced cholestasis. In addition to ductular cholestasis, total parenteral nutrition-induced cholestasis often shows macrovesicular steatosis, and after prolonged total parenteral nutrition, progressive portal fibrosis develops. It should be noted that in decompensated cirrhosis and fulminant hepatic failure due to massive hepatic necrosis, ductular cholestasis can be found histologically without evidence of sepsis.

Surgery-associated change is characterized by collection of neutrophils in the liver parenchyma resembling microabscesses with minimal hepatocyte dropout (Figure 2.10.6) and should not be mistakenly diagnosed as sepsis. It is caused by liver exposure to free air, resulting in margination of neutrophils to the liver parenchyma.

Large bile duct obstruction results in marked portal and periductal edema, accompanied by prominent ductular reaction and neutrophils. Large bile duct obstruction is caused by malignancy or bile duct stricture or obstructing bile duct or gallstone.

Drug-induced cholestatic injury can be clinically difficult to distinguish from sepsis, because the patient is often on multidrug regimen including antibiotic at the same time, but ductular cholestasis is absent in drug-induced cholestatic injury.

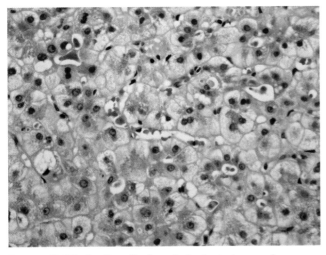

Figure 2.10.1 Canalicular cholestasis in sepsis.

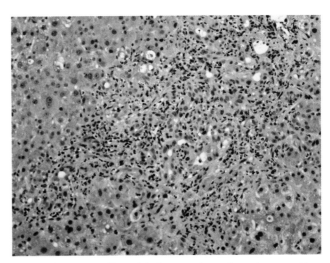

Figure 2.10.2 Portal inflammation, ductular reaction with neutrophils, and ductular cholestasis in sepsis (septic cholangitis).

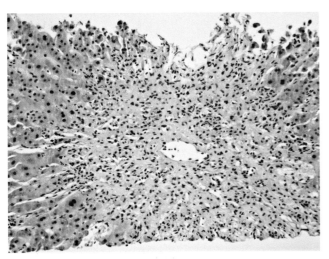

Figure 2.10.3 Shock liver with circumscribed centrilobular hepatocyte dropout.

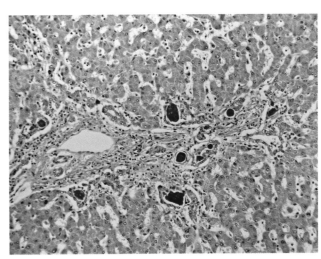

Figure 2.10.4 Ductular cholestasis in a subacute nonsuppurative cholangitis, referred as cholangitis lenta.

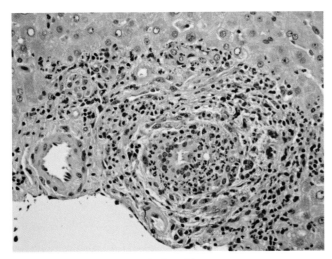

Figure 2.10.5 Acute cholangitis.

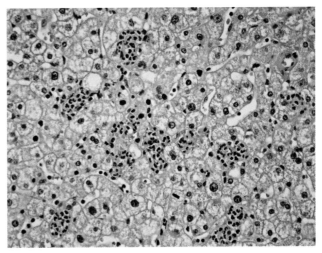

Figure 2.10.6 Clusters of neutrophils without significant hepatocellular damage in surgery-associated changes or "surgical hepatitis."

Table 2.10.1 Differential Diagnoses of Sepsis

Histologic Features	Sepsis	Surgery-Associated Changes	Large Duct Obstruction	Drug-Induced Cholestatic Injury	Total Parenteral Nutrition-Induced Cholestasis
Canalicular cholestasis	++	−	+	+	+
Hepatocellular cholestasis	+	−	+	+	+
Ductular cholestasis	++	−	−	−	+
Bile infarct	−	−	+/−	−	−
Lobular neutrophils	+	+	−	−	−
Microabscess	+/−	++	−	−	−
Microvesicular steatosis	+/−	−	−	+/−	+/−
Macrovesicular steatosis	−	−	−	+/−	+
Hepatocyte dropout	+/−	+/−	+/−	+	+/−
Centrilobular necrosis	+ (septic shock)/−	+/−	−	+/−	−
Ductular reaction	+	−	++	+/−	+
Portal inflammation	+	−	+	+/−	+
Portal neutrophils	+	−	++	+/−	+
Portal edema	+/−	−	++	−	+/−
Fibrous septa	−	−	+/−	−	+ (if prolonged)

++ indicates almost always present; +, usually present; +/−, occasionally present; −, usually absent.

2.11 Large Bile Duct Obstruction

Large bile duct obstruction or extrahepatic bile duct obstruction is caused commonly by gallstones in the common bile duct, bile duct strictures, carcinoma of the head of the pancreas, and cholangiocarcinoma. It can also be a localized change secondary to intrahepatic compression of a space-occupying lesion to a major branch of bile duct.

In large bile duct obstruction, jaundice develops slowly, and if due to gallstones, it is accompanied by constant epigastric pain or biliary colic. Pruritus is prominent. Fever develops when cholangitis complicates the bile duct obstruction. Liver enzyme test reveals a cholestatic profile, with increase in levels of conjugated bilirubin and alkaline phosphatase. Imaging techniques demonstrate dilatation of bile ducts. The diagnosis can be reliably made based on clinical and imaging findings. A liver biopsy may be helpful, particularly to assess parenchymal damage and fibrosis, but it may cause bile leak or biliary peritonitis.

Large bile duct obstruction can be relieved by surgical or endoscopic intervention with placement of drainage or stent. The prognosis depends on the underlying cause and the timing of the surgery. Early relief of the obstruction prevents hepatic fibrosis, secondary sclerosing cholangitis, and secondary biliary cirrhosis.

Pathologic Features

Large bile duct obstruction usually causes cholestasis with bile plugs in dilated bile canaliculi as well as bile pigment in the cytoplasm of the centrilobular hepatocytes and Kupffer cells (Figure 2.11.4). Hepatocytes in the area of cholestasis exhibit pale, swollen, rarefied cytoplasm, so-called feathery degeneration, accompanied by occasional eosinophilic degeneration with formation of acidophilic bodies, inflammatory cell infiltrates, and Kupffer cell enlargement. The portal tracts are enlarged, and collagen fibers are separated by edema (Figure 2.11.1). Bile ducts become tortuous and dilated, with remarkable ductular reaction at the margin or periphery of the portal tracts without extension into the adjacent parenchyma and accompanied by abundant neutrophils (Figures 2.11.2 and 2.11.3). Marginal ductular reaction is the most characteristic finding in large bile duct

obstruction. Ascending cholangitis leads to accumulation of neutrophils within the lumen of bile ducts (Figure 2.11.6).

In severe or long-standing cases, cholestasis extends from the centrilobular to the periportal areas, and bile lakes develop in the periportal areas as a result of rupture of bile ducts and ductules. Extravasation of bile leads to necrosis of hepatocytes and accumulation of pale foamy macrophages, so-called bile infarcts (Figure 2.11.5). When obstruction is not relieved, fibrous septa with ductular reaction linking adjacent portal tracts develop. Prolonged ascending cholangitis may result in secondary sclerosing cholangitis.

Differential Diagnosis

The differential diagnoses of large bile duct obstruction include sepsis, drug-induced cholestatic injury, primary biliary cirrhosis, and primary sclerosing cholangitis (see Table 2.11.1). The distinguishing features of large bile duct obstruction from the rest of the differential diagnoses are portal edema, tortuous or dilated bile ducts, abundant neutrophils accompanying ductular reaction, absence of fibrosis, and if prolonged, bile lakes, infarcts, and portal-to-portal bridging fibrosis. Sepsis causes ductular cholestasis, which is less commonly seen in large bile duct obstruction. Drug-induced cholestatic injury usually causes cholestasis, lobular inflammation, and hepatocyte dropout, and sometimes damaged bile ducts. Primary biliary cirrhosis is characterized by mixed inflammatory infiltrates including lymphocytes, plasma cells, and eosinophils; epithelioid microgranulomas; and florid duct lesions. Primary sclerosing cholangitis causes bile duct ectasia, periductal fibrosis, and bile duct scar. Prolonged large bile duct obstruction may cause secondary sclerosing cholangitis, which closely resembles primary sclerosing cholangitis, but the characteristic beading biliary tree on imaging studies is absent, and histologically, ductopenia, periductal fibrosis and bile duct scar are not as pronounced as seen in primary sclerosing cholangitis. Both primary biliary cirrhosis and primary sclerosing cholangitis do not present with remarkable canalicular and hepatocellular cholestasis, except in the late stages of the disease.

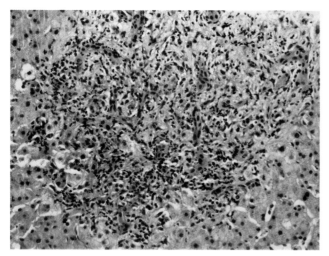

Figure 2.11.1 Portal edema and ductular reaction accompanied by neutrophils in large duct obstruction.

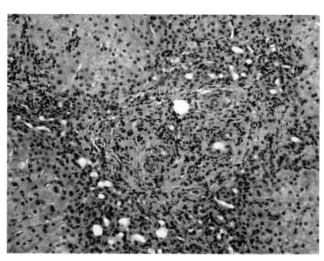

Figure 2.11.2 Marginal ductular reaction accompanied by neutrophils in large duct obstruction.

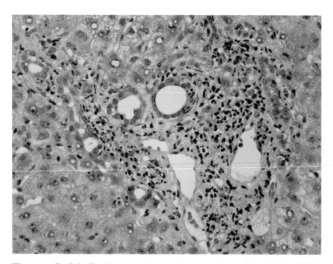

Figure 2.11.3 Large duct obstruction with dilated bile ducts accompanied by marginal ductular reaction.

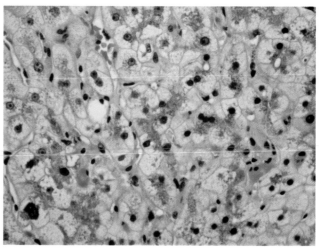

Figure 2.11.4 Hepatocanalicular cholestasis with feathery degeneration of the hepatocytes in large duct obstruction.

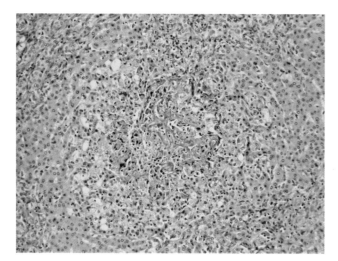

Figure 2.11.5 Bile infarct in periportal area as the result of bile ductule rupture in large duct obstruction.

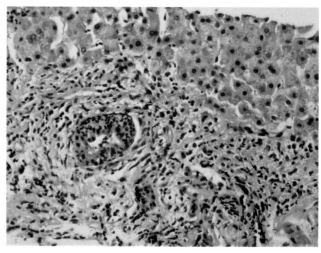

Figure 2.11.6 Acute ascending cholangitis with neutrophils in the epithelium and lumen of bile duct.

Table 2.11.1 Differential Diagnoses of Large Bile Duct Obstruction

Histologic Features	Large Bile Duct Obstruction	Sepsis	Drug-Induced Cholestatic Injury	Primary Biliary Cirrhosis	Primary Sclerosing Cholangitis
Canalicular cholestasis	+	++	+	–	–
Hepatocellular cholestasis	+	+	+	–	–
Ductular cholestasis	–	+	–	–	–
Lobular neutrophils	–	+	–	–	+/–
Lobular mononuclear inflammation	–	–	+	+	–
Microabscess	–	+/–	–	–	+/–
Microvesicular steatosis	–	+/–	+/–	–	–
Hepatocyte dropout	–	+/–	+	+/–	–
Centrilobular necrosis	–	+ (septic shock)/–	+/–	–	–
Ductular reaction	++	+	+/–	+	+
Periductal "onion skin" fibrosis	–	–	–	–	+
Epithelioid granuloma	–	–	+/–	+	–
Florid duct lesion	–	–	–	+	–
Portal lymphoplasmacytic infiltrate	–	–	+/–	++	+
Bile duct ectasia	+/–	–	–	–	+
Bile duct scar	–	–	–	–	+
Portal neutrophils	+	+	+/–	+	+
Portal edema	++	+/–	–	–	–
Fibrous septa	+ (if prolonged)/–	–	–	+/–	+/–

++ indicates almost always present; +, usually present; +/–, occasionally present; –, usually absent.

2.12 Liver Disease in Pregnancy

Pregnancy may be complicated by various liver diseases; some of them are specific to pregnancy, such as intrahepatic cholestasis of pregnancy, acute fatty liver of pregnancy, and liver injury in toxemia of pregnancy. They commonly occur in late pregnancy. Other liver diseases that affect the general population can also affect pregnancy; gallstones and Budd-Chiari syndrome are more frequent in pregnancy, and hepatocellular adenoma and hepatitis E may cause more severe complications. Acute viral hepatitis is the most common cause of acute hepatitis and jaundice in pregnancy and therefore should always be considered in the differential diagnosis.

Intrahepatic Cholestasis of Pregnancy

Intrahepatic cholestasis of pregnancy is an acquired form of cholestasis, which is observed in otherwise healthy pregnant women with a normal medical history. Intrahepatic cholestasis of pregnancy usually occurs in the second or third trimester when serum concentrations of estrogen and progesterone reach their peak. Intrahepatic cholestasis of pregnancy may be related to genetic predisposition for increased sensitivity to estrogen and progesterone metabolites, causing impaired bile salt export pump (BSEP) function. Mutations and polymorphisms in the genes coding for canalicular transporter proteins BSEP and multidrug resistance protein 3 have been associated with the development of intrahepatic cholestasis of pregnancy.

Intrahepatic cholestasis of pregnancy is the cause of jaundice in about 20% of pregnant women. Pruritus is common and may precede laboratory abnormality. In mild cases, jaundice may be absent, and pruritus is the only manifestation. In more severe cases, jaundice is accompanied by elevated conjugated bilirubin and alkaline phosphatase activity. Serum aminotransferase and γ-glutamyltransferase levels are normal or mildly elevated. Jaundice and pruritus resolve after delivery without permanent hepatic damage. The prognosis for both mother and baby is excellent. Jaundice recurs in subsequent pregnancies or after intake of oral contraceptives.

The liver only shows mild centrilobular canalicular cholestasis without hepatocellular damage, rosetting, or pseudoacinar change of the hepatocytes or portal inflammation (Figure 2.12.1).

Acute Fatty Liver of Pregnancy

Acute fatty liver of pregnancy is a rare cause of jaundice between the 31st and 38th week of pregnancy. It is a more severe condition compared to intrahepatic cholestasis of pregnancy. Acute fatty liver of pregnancy is regarded as part of systemic mitochondrial dysfunction, similar to those seen in Reye syndrome and genetic defects of mitochondrial enzymes and drug reactions.

Patients present with nausea, vomiting, and abdominal pain followed by jaundice. In severe cases, encephalopathy, ascites, renal failure, pancreatitis, and disseminated intravascular coagulation may ensue. Serum aminotransferase levels are elevated, as well as uric acid and ammonia levels. The liver appears diffusely hyperechoic on ultrasound and hypodense on computed tomography scan.

The liver parenchyma shows characteristic microvesicular steatosis with sparing of the periportal hepatocytes (Figure 2.12.2). Hepatocellular necrosis is not seen except in fatal cases. Portal and lobular lymphoplasmacellular infiltrate and mild centrilobular canalicular cholestasis may be observed.

Acute fatty liver of pregnancy carries a high mortality rate for mother and baby. Improved results are seen from early diagnosis, recognition of less severe cases, and, if indicated, early delivery. Recurrences in subsequent pregnancy are extremely rare.

Toxemia of Pregnancy

Toxemia of pregnancy occurs between the 20th and 40th weeks of pregnancy and is always associated with hypertension, proteinuria, and fluid retention. Hepatic damage is seen in patients with severe preeclampsia and eclampsia. The etiology of preeclampsia is unknown.

Patients complain of nausea, vomiting, and abdominal pain, as in acute fatty liver of pregnancy. Jaundice is rare, unless hemolysis occurs because of the underlying disseminated intravascular coagulation. Serum alkaline phosphatase and aminotransferase levels are elevated. Toxemia and acute fatty liver of pregnancy may overlap.

Liver biopsy of toxemia of pregnancy shows fibrin deposition within the periportal sinusoids and occasionally in the portal venules (Figures 2.12.3 and 2.12.4). In severe cases there may be confluent hepatocyte necrosis or wide areas of infarction. Infarction and hemorrhage may cause rupture. The portal tracts shows minimal inflammatory infiltrate.

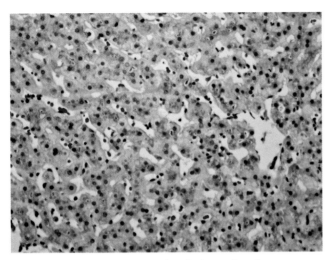

Figure 2.12.1   Intrahepatic cholestasis of pregnancy with canalicular cholestasis.

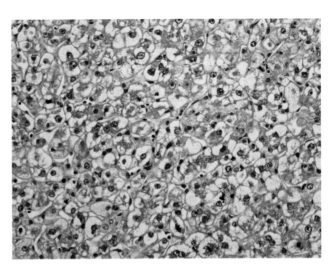

Figure 2.12.2   Diffuse microvesicular steatosis without significant hepatocellular necrosis in acute fatty liver of pregnancy.

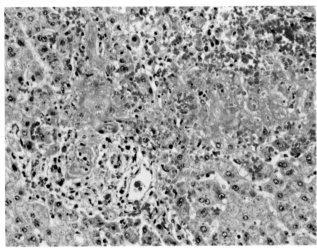

Figure 2.12.3   Toxemia of pregnancy with fibrin in periportal sinusoids and confluent hepatocyte necrosis.

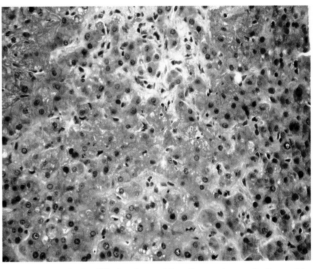

Figure 2.12.4   Fibrin deposition in periportal sinusoids in toxemia of pregnancy (trichrome stain).

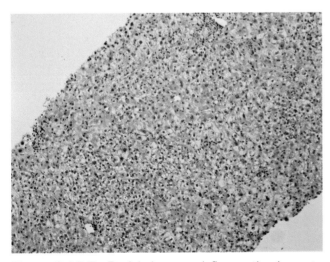

Figure 2.12.5   Panlobular necroinflammation in acute viral hepatitis.

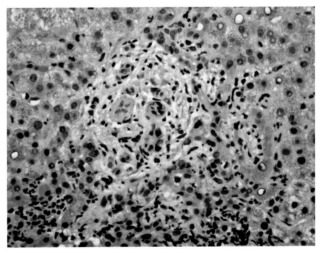

Figure 2.12.6   Portal edema and ductular reaction in large duct obstruction due to gallstones.

Table 2.12.1 Liver Diseases in Pregnancy

Histologic Features	Intrahepatic Cholestasis	Acute Fatty Liver	Toxemia	Acute Viral Hepatitis
Hepatocanalicular cholestasis	+	+/–	–	+/–
Hepatocellular damage	–	+/–	+	++
Acidophilic bodies	–	+/–	+	++
Microvesicular steatosis	–	++	–	+/–
Lobular inflammatory infiltrate	–	–	–	++
Portal inflammatory infiltrate	–	–	–	+
Fibrin thrombi in sinusoids	–	–	++	–

++ indicates almost always present; +, usually present; +/–, occasionally present; –, usually absent.

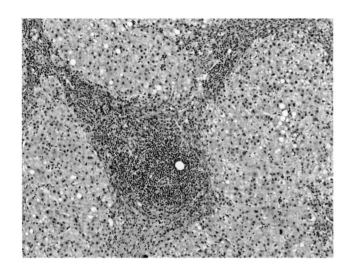

CHAPTER **3**

CHRONIC LIVER DISORDERS

3.1 Chronic Hepatitis

Chronic hepatitis is defined as a chronic inflammatory reaction in the liver. Chronic hepatitis is separated from acute hepatitis on the basis of duration, using 6 months as a cutoff. However, in clinical practice, the onset of the disease is often unknown; therefore, the practice of waiting for 6 months before proceeding with liver biopsy has been abandoned in many instances, and biopsy is performed if tests are significantly abnormal and no cause is identified. The spectrum of chronic inflammatory diseases of the liver extends from acute hepatitis to chronic hepatitis to fibrosis and finally to cirrhosis.

Chronic hepatitis may be asymptomatic or may present with a range of symptoms, particularly fatigue or malaise. Hepatomegaly with or without splenomegaly may be noted. There is variable elevation of serum aminotransferase activities. Other clinical and biochemical findings are related to the underlying cause of chronic hepatitis, such as viral hepatitis B or C infections, steatohepatitis, autoimmune liver diseases, chronic drug-induced injury, or metabolic disease such as Wilson disease. Signs and symptoms of liver failure and portal hypertension occur when chronic hepatitis has progressed to cirrhosis.

Pathologic Features

Chronic hepatitis is primarily a disease of portal tracts. Regardless of the etiology, the same basic underlying liver histology is shared to some degree. The portal tracts are expanded by various degrees of fibrosis with or without the formation of fibrous septa and by inflammatory cells, primarily lymphocytes, plasma cells, macrophages, and a few eosinophils. Extension of chronic inflammatory infiltrate from the portal tracts into the adjacent parenchyma with focal necrosis/apoptosis of the hepatocytes at the limiting plate is termed *interface hepatitis* (previously referred to as *piecemeal necrosis*) (Figure 3.1.1), usually seen in chronic viral hepatitis and autoimmune hepatitis (AIH). Interface hepatitis causes persistent damage to the liver parenchyma and gradual replacement of the hepatic parenchyma with fibrous tissue.

Hepatocyte necrosis, regeneration, and pericellular fibrosis lead to isolation of hepatocytes and formation of hepatocyte rosettes, a common feature of AIH. The severity of interface hepatitis often correlates with the degree of ductular reaction, which is accompanied by neutrophils. The lobular activity is usually less pronounced than in acute hepatitis. Scattered focal hepatocellular dropouts or spotty necrosis with lymphocytic infiltrate is usually present (Figure 3.1.2). In chronic hepatitis with severe activity, there is diffuse hepatocellular damage with ballooning degeneration, acidophilic bodies, and inflammation, but cholestasis is uncommon except in fibrosing cholestatic hepatitis. Confluent necrosis linking vascular structures (between portal tracts or portal zones and terminal venules) is called bridging necrosis, another feature of AIH. Confluent necrosis and parenchymal collapse may appear similar to those seen in acute hepatitis, but the presence of portal fibrosis and fibrous septa supports the diagnosis of chronic hepatitis. It should be emphasized, however, that there are no absolute histologic criteria to distinguish acute from chronic hepatitis; therefore, clinical and laboratory findings must be taken into account to reach the final diagnosis.

Continued interface hepatitis and the resulting fibrosis at the limiting plate lead to stellate enlargement of the portal tracts (periportal fibrosis) and eventually link adjacent portal tracts, whereas portal-central or central-to-central bridging fibrous septa in chronic hepatitis generally develops after episodes of confluent or bridging necrosis, which involves perivenular necrosis. Formation of liver cell plates that are 2 or 3 cells thick, which is best observed on silver stains for reticulin, indicates hepatocyte regeneration.

Liver Biopsy Utility

Liver biopsy in chronic hepatitis is performed for confirmation of diagnosis, suggestion of possible etiology, grading of necroinflammation, staging of fibrosis, concurrent diseases, confirmation of cirrhosis, patient management, and evaluation of treatment. There have been several grading and staging scoring systems introduced for chronic viral hepatitis and steatohepatitis. The scoring system should be used strictly for those 2 diseases and not for others. The liberal use of a scoring system in chronic hepatitis with unclear etiology leads to oversimplification and misinterpretation of the liver biopsy or obscures concomitant findings.

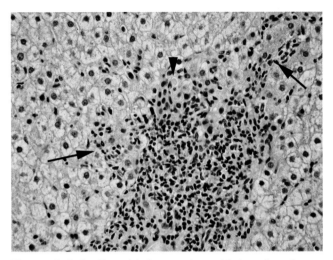

Figure 3.1.1 Portal inflammation with interface hepatitis (arrows) and acidophilic body (arrowhead) in chronic hepatitis.

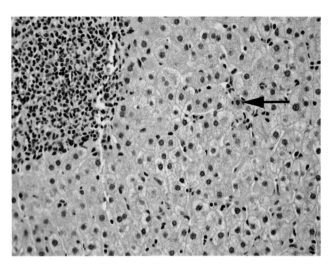

Figure 3.1.2 Mild lobular necroinflammatory activity with acidophilic body (arrow) in chronic hepatitis.

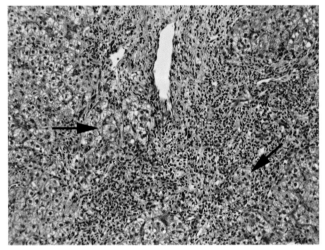

Figure 3.1.3 Expansion of portal tract due to interface hepatitis and fibrosis, resulting in entrapped hepatocytes (arrows) in fibrous stroma (trichrome stain).

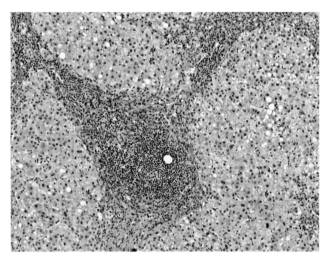

Figure 3.1.4 Cirrhosis secondary to chronic viral hepatitis C with dense lymphocytic aggregate in portal tract.

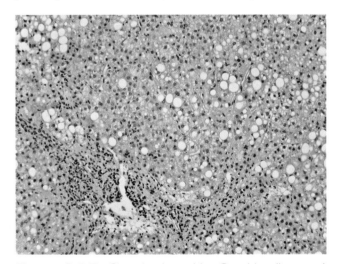

Figure 3.1.5 Chronic hepatitis C with dispersed steatosis.

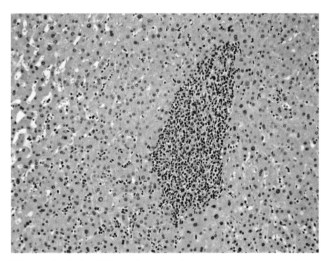

Figure 3.1.6 Diffuse large cell lymphoma involving liver, mimicking chronic hepatitis. The portal tract is expanded and the sinusoids infiltrated by monomorphic cells, and there is no interface hepatitis or hepatocellular dropout.

Table 3.1.1 Etiology of Chronic Hepatitis and Their Features

Etiology	Sex Predominance	Age Predominance	Associations	Diagnostic Tests	Histological Features	Risk of Primary Liver Cancer
Hepatitis B and D	Male	All	Asian, African, Mediteranean, homosexuals, drug abusers, immunosuppressed patients	HBsAg, HBeAg, anti-HBe, HBV-DNA; HDV-RNA, IgM anti-HDV.	Usually mild. Ground glass hepatocytes, sanded nuclei.	High
Hepatitis C	Equal	All	Blood transfusion, blood products, drug abuse	Anti-HCV, HCV-RNA.	Portal lymphoid aggregate/follicle, steatosis.	High
Autoimmune hepatitis	Female	15–30 years and post-menopausal	Autoimmune diseases	Antinuclear antibody, smooth muscle antibody, serum IgG.	Plasma cell infiltrate, severe hepatitis with bridging necrosis.	Low
Steatohepatitis	Equal	All	Obesity, diabetes, hyperlipidemia, metabolic syndrome	Physical and laboratory findings, liver histology.	Fat, rare lobular neutrophils, ballooned hepatocytes.	Low
Drug-induced chronic hepatitis	Female	Middle-aged and elderly	Isoniazid, methyldopa, nitrofurantoin, dantrolen, propylthiouracil, etc	History, liver histology.	Similar to viral or autoimmune hepatitis. Eosinophils, fat, granulomas.	Low
Wilson disease	Equal	10–30 years	Familial, hemolysis, neurological signs	Kayser-Fleischer rings, serum copper, ceruloplasmin, urinary copper, liver copper.	Ballooned hepatocytes, Mallory hyalins, glycogenated nuclei, fat, similar to steatohepatitis.	Low

3.2 Chronic Viral Hepatitis

Chronic viral hepatitis is caused by hepatitis C virus (HCV) and hepatitis B virus (HBV) with or without delta agent infection. Because of shared modes of transmission, infection with hepatitis B and/or hepatitis C is common among individuals with HIV infection. Other chronic or metabolic liver diseases, such as steatohepatitis and hemochromatosis, may also complicate the course of chronic viral hepatitis.

Chronic Hepatitis C

Chronic hepatitis C affects both women and men of all ages and typically causes mild, nonspecific symptoms. Patients can be asymptomatic or experience intermittent fatigue and malaise. The diagnosis is based on fluctuating serum aminotransferase levels and the detection of anti-HCV or HCV RNA in serum. Hepatitis C may cause mixed cryoglobulinemia type II or III and is associated with increased incidence of lymphoma. Hepatitis C may induce autoantibody formation such as antinuclear antibody (ANA) and anti–liver kidney microsomal type 1, but the titers are low; these patients with associated autoimmune conditions still resemble patients with chronic hepatitis C clinically and not those of AIH, and the diagnosis of AIH should not be rendered in this condition.

The typical overall histologic feature of chronic hepatitis C is mild. Interface hepatitis is often focal and may not involve all portal tracts or the entire circumference of the portal tracts. Lobular inflammation is mild with spotty necrosis rather than bridging or confluent necrosis. The inflammatory cells in portal tracts, in areas of interface hepatitis, and in lobules consist predominantly of mature lymphocytes. Plasma cells are rare; however, on occasion, chronic hepatitis C may exhibit fairly prominent plasma cells and represent a form of chronic hepatitis C with autoimmune features. This condition does not require immunosuppressive therapy and should not be considered as overlap syndrome.

Dense nodular aggregates of lymphocytes are often present in scattered portal tracts and are characteristic of chronic hepatitis C (Figure 3.2.1), especially in association with mild necroinflammatory activity. Lymphoid follicles with germinal centers are sometimes seen. The small bile ducts are sometimes engulfed and infiltrated by few lymphocytes, and the epithelium shows vacuolation, stratification, and eosinophilic degeneration (Figure 3.2.2). Microvesicular and macrovesicular steatosis are often present in varying degrees in chronic hepatitis C, usually mild and periportal in location but can be severe in hepatitis C genotype 3 infection (Figure 3.2.3). The triad of lymphoid aggregates or follicles, bile duct damage, and mild to moderate disperse or periportal steatosis is highly suggestive of chronic hepatitis C. There is no reliable immunohistochemical stain for hepatitis C infection.

Chronic hepatitis C has a variable course. Often, the disease is benign, but it may progress to cirrhosis after 15 to 20 years, and these patients with chronic hepatitis C are at risk of developing hepatocellular carcinoma and to a lesser extent lymphoma and intrahepatic cholangiocarcinoma. With combination treatment of interferon-α with ribavirin and promising experimental drugs such as HCV-specific protease, polymerase, or cyclophylin inhibitors, up to 40% to 60% patients with genotype 1 and 60% to 80% of patients with genotype 2 or 3 achieve a sustained virologic response, defined as undetectable HCV RNA 6 months after completion of HCV treatment.

Chronic Hepatitis B

Chronic hepatitis B varies in severity from minimal to severe activity with severe interface hepatitis and bridging or confluent necrosis. The inflammatory cells are predominantly lymphocytes, but concomitant chronic hepatitis C should be considered if lymphoid follicles and bile duct damage are seen. Hepatocytes with finely granular, eosinophilic ground glass cytoplasm are diagnostic of chronic hepatitis B (Figure 3.2.5). These cells are filled with smooth endoplasmic reticulum containing hepatitis B surface antigen (HBsAg) reactive filaments. The ground glass hepatocytes may be few and scattered or in sheets or nodules; they are seen in chronic and not acute hepatitis B infection, and their number correlated inversely with the activity of the disease. Hepatitis B core antigen (HBcAg) accumulation in hepatocyte nuclei produces "sanded" nuclei. The presence of HBsAg in ground glass hepatocytes and HBcAg in nuclei and cytoplasm of hepatocytes demonstrable by immunohistochemical staining confirms the diagnosis of chronic hepatitis B. HBsAg cytoplasmic staining can also be seen in cells without ground glass appearance. Linear membranous staining with HBsAg generally associated with a more active disease. The expression of HBcAg in the cytoplasm of hepatocytes is found in chronic hepatitis B with active viral replication and significant necroinflammatory activity.

The morphology of hepatitis B with D virus coinfection or superinfection resembles that of B infection alone, but the necroinflammatory activity is often more severe. In combined B and D virus infection, sanded nuclei may also be seen, and HDAg may be demonstrated in the nuclei and less frequently in the cytoplasm of hepatocytes by immunohistochemical stain, whereas HBcAg is negative because of suppression of HBV replication by hepatitis D virus.

An unusual rapidly progressive disease with severe parenchymal damage, extensive fibrosis, and mild inflammatory reaction, termed *fibrosing cholestatic hepatitis*, may be seen in immunocompromised patients. The parenchymal changes are characterized by marked hepatocyte swelling and cholestasis with minimal lobular inflammation. It is accompanied by marked ductular reaction at the limiting plate, combined with cholangiolitis and extensive periportal sinusoidal fibrosis. Well-developed cirrhosis, however, does not develop. The extremely high levels of HBV replication and the massive HBcAg expression in the liver, in addition to the insignificant inflammatory component, suggest a direct cytopathic effect of HBV.

Chronic Viral Hepatitis and HIV Coinfection

HIV coinfection negatively impacts the natural history of acute and chronic viral hepatitis whereby increasing the risk of chronicity and progressive fibrosis, higher viral load, and lower virologic response rates; therefore, treatment for chronic viral hepatitis is generally recommended. Progressive fibrosis may well be caused by the HIV virus stimulating hepatocyte stellate cells. Conversely, viral hepatitis itself does not alter the natural history of HIV disease but is associated with an increased risk of drug-induced liver injury related to antiretroviral therapy.

The histologic features of chronic viral hepatitis and HIV coinfection generally do not differ from those with chronic viral hepatitis only, although fibrosing cholestatic hepatitis may be encountered in these immunocompromised patients. When atypical presentation is encountered, the potential hepatotoxicity of the antiretroviral treatment should not be overlooked.

Concurrent Diseases

It is not unusual to discover concurrent diseases, such as alcoholic liver disease, steatohepatitis, drug-induced liver injury, hemochromatosis, and α-1-antitrypsin (AAT) deficiency, in the liver biopsy of patients with chronic viral hepatitis. In some patients, the concurrent disease may in fact be the predominant feature and the major contributor to fibrosis. When concurrent steatohepatitis and/or hemochromatosis is present, assessments of steatosis and/or iron accumulation should be provided; they may reduce the response to therapy in chronic viral hepatitis.

Differential Diagnosis

The differential diagnoses of chronic viral hepatitis include AIH and lymphoma. Autoimmune hepatitis shows histologic changes of severely active chronic hepatitis with numerous plasma cells, eosinophils, marked interface hepatitis, perivenular and bridging necrosis, and septal fibrosis involving all portal tracts. The overall histologic feature is more severe than chronic hepatitis C or B (except for severe cases). Lymphoma is often diagnosed as part of the workup of patients known to have lymphoma or part of fever of unknown origin workup (Figure 3.1.6).

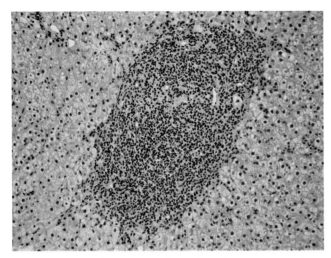

Figure 3.2.1 Dense portal lymphocytic aggregate/lymphoid follicle with germinal center in chronic hepatitis C.

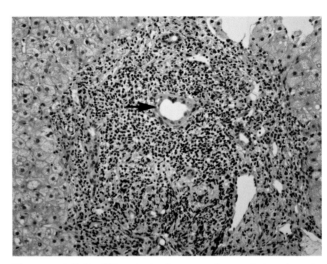

Figure 3.2.2 Bile duct damage (arrow) in chronic hepatitis C, mimicking florid duct lesion in primary biliary cirrhosis.

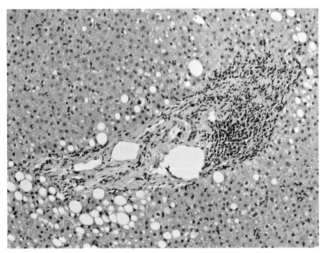

Figure 3.2.3 Mild periportal macrovesicular steatosis in chronic hepatitis C.

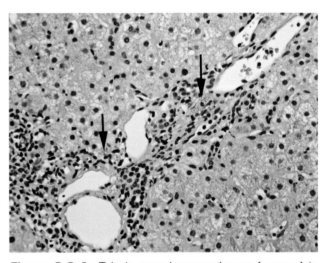

Figure 3.2.4 Talc in portal macrophages (arrows) in a patient with chronic hepatitis C and history of intravenous drug abuse.

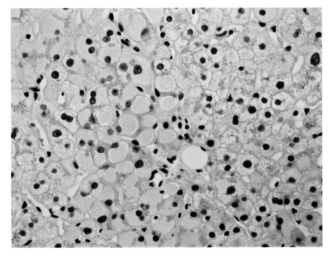

Figure 3.2.5 Ground glass hepatocytes in chronic hepatitis B.

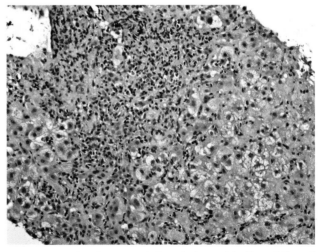

Figure 3.2.6 Combined chronic hepatitis B and C and HIV infection with severe activity.

Table 3.2.1 Differential Diagnoses of Chronic Viral Hepatitis

	Chronic HBV	Chronic HCV	Autoimmune Hepatitis	Lymphoma
Overall inflammation	Mild to severe	Mild, portal tract predominant	Severe, portal and lobular	Severe, variable portal and lobular distribution
Portal inflammation characteristics	Lymphocytic infiltrate	Dense lymphocytic infiltrate, lymphoid follicle with germinal center	Plasma cells in clusters, scattered lymphocytes, eosinophils	Expansive dense monomorphic atypical lymphoid cells compressing periportal hepatocytes
Interface hepatitis	Mild, rarely severe	Usually mild	Severe	None
Lobular inflammation characteristics	Mild, rarely severe with confluent necrosis	Usually mild, rare acidophilic bodies	Severe with centrilobular, confluent and bridging necrosis	Sinusoidal infiltrate without significant hepatocyte dropout
Other findings	Ground glass hepatocytes. Hepatocytes with sanded nuclei	Mild dispersed or periportal steatosis	Marked periportal hepatocyte regeneration and rosetting	Neoplastic lymphoid cell necrosis. Granulomatous inflammation

3.3 Grading and Staging of Chronic Viral Hepatitis

Staging is the evaluation of fibrosis, whereas grading is the evaluation of disease activity. Many different systems for scoring necroinflammatory activity and fibrosis have been developed throughout the years, mainly for chronic viral hepatitis, although lately, these systems have been used for AIH as well. The grading and staging scoring systems should be used solely for their intended purpose in chronic viral hepatitis, that is, assessment of the state of the disease at the time of biopsy, providing guidance to start treatment, predictive value for disease outcome, and as response to therapy. The grading and staging scoring systems should not be used liberally for other or unclear causes of chronic hepatitis and are not replacement for microscopic description of liver injury.

Grading and Staging Scoring Systems

The Knodell system, published in 1981, has served as a prototype for semiquantitative scoring of liver biopsy specimens. Pathologic scoring systems, such as the METAVIR, the Scheuer and Batts-Ludwig scores, and the Ishak Hepatitis Activity Index are now more commonly used in practice. These systems use 4 or 5 categories for necroinflammatory activity and 4 to 7 categories for stage of fibrosis. The Ishak score, with 7 stages, provides the most detailed fibrosis information. For patient management and prognosis, a simple staging system is best used to limit sampling error and increase reproducibility (Table 3.3.1). For clinical trials and natural history studies, more complex and detailed systems are appropriate. In addition, a pathology report should include clear verbal descriptions of the extent of fibrosis and severity of necroinflammatory activity; therefore, a scoring system can be transcribed to another preferred scoring system at a later time. Regardless of which grading and staging system is to be used, it is best to communicate to the submitting clinicians which system is used.

It is also important to realize that these systems are not to be regarded in the same fashion as biochemical laboratory tests; they were all created for the comparison of biopsies in treatment trials and not for diagnostic purposes.

In addition to stage and grade, other concurrent pathology and accurate assessments of both steatosis and iron accumulation, which may reduce response to therapy in chronic viral hepatitis, should be provided.

Liver Biopsy Size

Needle biopsies are subject to sampling error and often compounded by their small size and narrow gauge needles. Even so, small biopsies, although not ideal, are often sufficient to recognize cirrhosis, and if bridging fibrosis is recognizable, one knows that the patient has progressed to at least a higher stage of fibrosis. As a guideline, 18-gauge or wider needle biopsies are required for evaluating hepatic architecture, resulting in at least 1.5-cm needle core with 6 to 8 complete portal tracts. Surgical biopsy of the immediate 2-mm subcapsular parenchyma or adjacent to large vein or large portal tracts may mimic cirrhosis in noncirrhotic livers. Liver capsule may be seen in percutaneous liver biopsies at one end of the specimen or in the form of separate pieces of connective tissue and can be distinguished from most pathologic fibrous tissue by its density and maturity and often contain larger blood vessels and bile ducts.

Other Techniques

Noninvasive or minimally invasive alternatives are proposed as substitutes for liver biopsy and include clinical indices, cross-sectional imaging, serum biomarkers, liver stiffness measurement, and portal pressure measurement. Although these alternatives reduce the risk of liver biopsy, most alternatives to liver biopsy assess one aspect of liver disease and translate this into a numeric score; therefore, one has to realize the limitation of information that can be provided by these methods. Liver biopsy provides information about numerous variables: tissue architectural changes; necroinflammatory injury; fibrotic stage; alterations of parenchyma and bile duct epithelium; concomitant diseases; accumulation of fat, copper, and iron; and material for molecular and genetic studies.

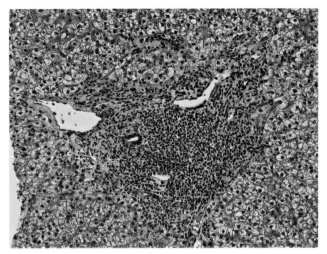

Figure 3.3.1 Portal fibrosis and periportal fibrosis (trichrome stain).

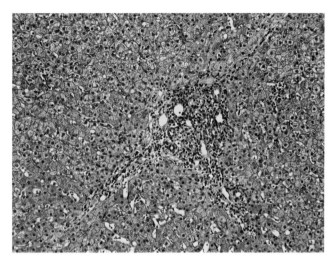

Figure 3.3.2 Portal fibrosis and fibrous septa (trichrome stain).

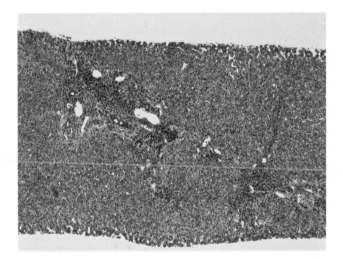

Figure 3.3.3 Bridging fibrous septa (trichrome stain).

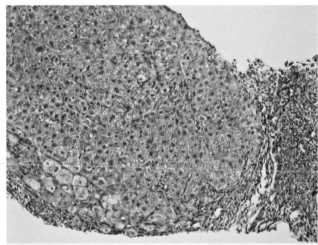

Figure 3.3.4 Liver biopsy specimen showing nodular cirrhotic liver (trichrome stain).

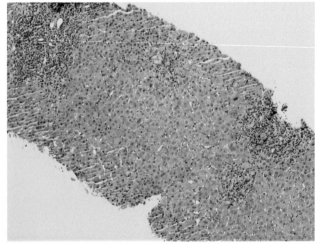

Figure 3.3.5 Mild lobular necroinflammatory activity and severe interface hepatitis involving majority of portal tracts circumferentially.

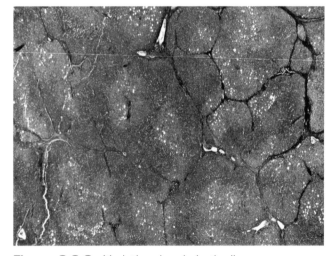

Figure 3.3.6 Variation in cirrhotic liver may cause sampling error and understaging in needle biopsy (trichrome stain).

Table 3.3.1 Semiquantitative Grading and Staging of Chronic Viral Hepatitis

Grade	Activity	Interface Hepatitis	Lobular Inflammation
0	No	No	No
1	Minimal	Focal, involving some of portal tracts	Rare acidophilic bodies, with minimal associated lymphocytic infiltrate
2	Mild	Focal, involving most of portal tracts	Mild lymphocytic infiltrate with acidophilic bodies, rare foci of parenchymal necroses
3	Moderate	Circumferential, involving majority of portal tracts	Moderate lymphocytic infiltrate with numerous acidophilic bodies and foci of parenchymal necroses
4	Severe	Circumferential, involving all portal tracts	Marked lymphocytic infiltrate with numerous acidophilic bodies, significant parenchymal necroses with focal bridging necrosis

Stage	Fibrosis	Description	
0	No	No portal fibrosis, periportal fibrosis, or fibrous septa	
1	Portal	Portal fibrous expansion	
2	Periportal	Periportal short fibrous septa with rare thin portal-portal bridging fibrous septa	
3	Septal	Bridging fibrous septa with some architectural distortion	
4	Cirrhosis	Nodules surrounded by fibrous septa	

3.4 Nonalcoholic Fatty Liver Disease

Nonalcoholic fatty liver disease (NAFLD) and its progressive form, nonalcoholic steatohepatitis (NASH), is one of the most common liver diseases in Western countries. Simple hepatic steatosis, without ballooned hepatocytes and lobular inflammation, is considered to be a benign condition without an increase in liver-related morbidity and mortality. In contrast, NASH with the added necroinflammation and fibrosis may progress to cirrhosis. The diagnosis requires a negative history of alcoholism.

Clinical Consideration

Nonalcoholic steatohepatitis represents the hepatic manifestation of the metabolic syndrome, characterized by abdominal obesity, hypertension, type II diabetes mellitus or insulin resistance, hypertriglyceridemia, and low high-density lipoprotein cholesterol. Any of the components of metabolic syndrome by itself can cause NASH. Other less common causes of NASH include gastrointestinal and pancreatic disorders, extensive bowel resection, total parenteral nutrition, Wilson disease, and drugs, particularly amiodarone, nifedipine, perhexiline maleate, glucocorticoids, and estrogens. Any debilitating disease that causes a significant catabolic state can be associated with a NASH-like disease.

The diagnoses of NASH remain ones of clinicopathologic correlation, but histologic evaluation is the only means of accurately assessing the degree of steatosis, the distinct necroinflammatory lesions, and the fibrosis of NASH and in distinguishing NASH from simple hepatic steatosis. Moreover, evaluation of liver biopsy excludes other possible causes of liver enzyme elevation in the phenotypically predisposed patient.

Pathologic Features

Nonalcoholic steatohepatitis resembles mild alcoholic hepatitis, and histologic evaluation often cannot reliably distinguish NASH from mild alcoholic steatohepatitis (ASH). Hence, it has been suggested to pathologists to discontinue the use of the "nonalcoholic," and the diagnosis should reflect the presence of microscopic lesions and pattern and extent of injury (steatohepatitis and fibrosis), and a clinical association if provided (ie, diabetes, obesity).

Steatosis varies from mild to severe and is mainly macrovesicular (Figure 3.4.1), but focal microvesicular is not uncommon (Figure 3.4.3). The minimum quantity of hepatocytes involved is not set, and small amounts of steatosis may be present in otherwise healthy individuals. It is accepted that, in adults, more than 5% to 10% steatotic hepatocytes in centrilobular distribution, accompanied by hepatocyte ballooning and inflammation, define NASH. Hepatocyte ballooning is a prerequisite feature of NASH in adults (Figure 3.4.2). Lobular inflammation is usually mild, often with neutrophils. Additional findings are glycogenated nuclei in periportal hepatocytes, lipogranulomas, scattered megamitochondria in hepatocytes, and fat cysts.

The characteristic fibrosis in NASH is the deposition of collagen in perisinusoidal spaces of zone 3 hepatocytes (Figure 3.4.4). With progression of fibrosis, fibrous septa, bridging fibrosis, and eventually cirrhosis develop (Figure 3.4.5). The presence of centrilobular perisinusoidal fibrosis in the absence of steatosis or active inflammation may indicate previous episodes of steatohepatitis. Mild and patchy portal inflammation is often seen in cases with advanced fibrosis, but excessive portal chronic inflammation raises the possibility of concurrent chronic liver disease.

Although the main process in NASH is in acinar zone 3 (centrilobular), some degree of portal and periportal fibrosis can also be seen in adults, but is more pronounced in the pediatric population (see Chapter 6).

The grading and staging system has been suggested by the Pathology Committee of the NASH Clinical Research Network, who designed and validated a feature-based scoring system that is a modification of the Brunt system (see Table 3.4.1). The system was created as a method for comparing overall change and changes in individual lesions in biopsies of patients in treatment trials and was not intended to replace the histologic diagnosis.

Differential Diagnosis

The main differential diagnosis of NASH is alcoholic liver disease and more often than not relies on the history of alcoholism. There are several features, however, that give suggestion of alcoholic liver disease, such as abundant Mallory-Denk bodies, massive infiltration of neutrophils, hepatocanalicular cholestasis, and central hyalin sclerosis.

Clinically, one of the most common differential diagnoses of NASH is AIH due to nonspecific antibodies in some patients with NASH and negative viral serology. The histology of these 2 entities is distinct. It should be noted, however, that concurrent NASH and AIH can occur.

In patients with poorly controlled type I diabetes mellitus, excessive accumulation of glycogen can occur resulting in "glycogenic hepatopathy." Hepatomegaly, abdominal pain, and elevated transaminase activities are the clinical findings, mimicking steatohepatitis. Histologically, the hepatocytes are uniformly pale and swollen due to glycogen accumulation with no or mild steatosis, minimal inflammation, and without significant fibrosis (Figure 3.4.6).

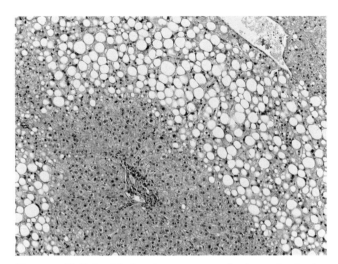

Figure 3.4.1 Moderate macrovesicular steatosis, sparing the periportal hepatocytes in nonalcoholic fatty liver disease.

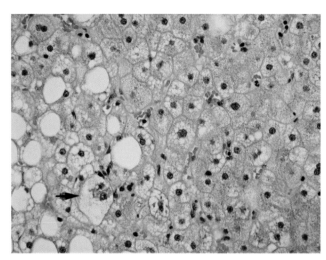

Figure 3.4.2 Hepatocyte ballooning (arrowhead) with poorly formed Mallory-Denk bodies in steatohepatitis.

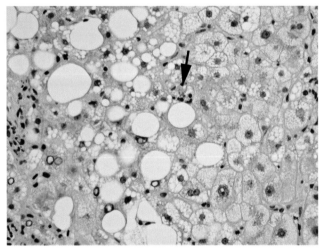

Figure 3.4.3 Mixed macrovesicular and microvesicular steatosis, hepatocytes with glycogenated nuclei, and acidophilic body (arrow) in steatohepatitis.

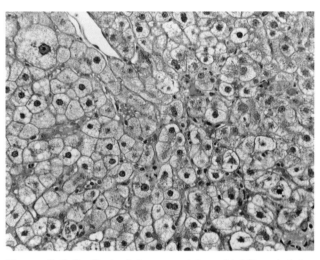

Figure 3.4.4 Pericellular or perisinusoidal fibrosis (steatofibrosis) (trichrome stain).

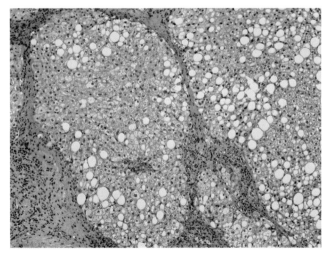

Figure 3.4.5 Cirrhosis secondary to steatohepatitis. The cirrhotic nodules show macrovesicular steatosis and are separated by relatively hypocellular fibrous bands.

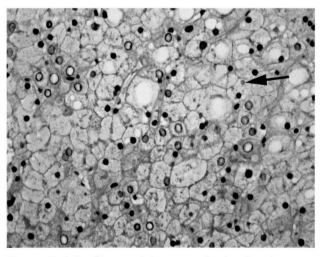

Figure 3.4.6 Glycogenic hepatopathy showing glycogen-rich hepatocytes with distinct membrane, glycogenated nuclei, and giant mitochondria (arrow) in a patient with diabetes mellitus type 1.

Table 3.4.1 Nonalcoholic Fatty Liver Disease Activity and Fibrosis Score

Activity Score (Total Score 0–8)

Steatosis (0–3)	<5% (0); 5%–33% (1); 33%–66% (2); >66% (3)
Lobular inflammation (foci/20X field) (0–3)	0 (0); <2 (1); 2–4 (2); >4 (3)
Ballooning (0–2)	None (0); few (1); many/prominent (2)

Total score ≥5 = NASH, <3 = not NASH, 3–4 = borderline

Fibrosis Score (0–4)*

1a: Mild (delicate) zone 3 perisinusoidal fibrosis

1b: Moderate (dense) zone 3 perisinusoidal fibrosis

1c: Portal fibrosis only

2: Zone 3 perisinusoidal with portal/periportal fibrosis

3: Bridging fibrosis

4: Cirrhosis

*Based on Masson's trichrome stain.

Adapted from Kleiner DE, et al. Nonalcoholic Steatohepatitis Clinical Research Network. Design and validation of a histological scoring system for nonalcoholic fatty liver disease. *Hepatology.* 2005;41(6):1313–1321.

3.5 Alcoholic Liver Disease

The development of alcoholic liver disease results from the chronic and excessive consumption of alcoholic beverages. There is a wide spectrum of histology for alcoholic liver disease that includes that of steatosis, steatohepatitis, alcoholic hepatitis (without steatosis), alcoholic foamy degeneration, cholestasis, veno-occlusive disease (VOD), central hyalin sclerosis, and micronodular cirrhosis.

Pathologic Features

Histologically, alcoholic hepatitis is characterized by swollen hepatocytes with pale or clear cytoplasm, so-called ballooning degeneration, predominantly in the centrilobular area (Figure 3.5.1). Focal necroses are also present. The ballooned hepatocytes often contain alcoholic hyalin in the cytoplasm and are surrounded by neutrophils ("satellitosis"), referred to as Mallory-Denk bodies (Figure 3.5.2). Mallory-Denk hyalin or alcoholic hyalin represents clumps or strands of intermediate filaments of the cytoskeleton, which are positive for cytokeratins 8 and 18, ubiquitin, and p62. Megamitochondria in the cytoplasm of hepatocytes are seen occasionally as globular or spindle-shaped inclusions measuring 2 to 10 μm across. The significance of megamitochondria is unknown.

In early stages, distribution of the inflammation is near the terminal hepatic venules. In more severe cases, bridging necrosis with ductular reaction and wide fibrous septa linking adjacent terminal hepatic venules are seen. Iron deposition in hepatocytes is sometimes seen in alcoholics but is usually mild and often is accompanied by hemosiderin in Kupffer cells.

Fibrosis is a common feature of alcoholic hepatitis with its most characteristic centrilobular perisinusoidal or pericellular form, so-called chicken wire type of fibrosis which may progresses to central hyalin sclerosis (Figure 3.5.3). Involvement of terminal hepatic venules results in thickening of the walls and narrowing and obliteration of their lumens (veno-occlusive disease). In more advanced cases, broad fibrous septa are formed extending from centrilobular areas to adjacent central venules or portal tracts (Figure 3.5.5), carrying arterioles into the perivenular areas. This unaccompanied arteriole should not be mistaken as a portal tract with bile duct loss. Fibrosis and inflammatory infiltration of portal tracts and ductular reaction are seen only in the more advanced stages of alcoholic hepatitis. Inflammation of portal tracts is mild, even in severe cases.

Lesions other than alcoholic hepatitis may contribute to the fibrosis or cirrhosis in alcoholics. Studies have found that alcoholic patients have a higher incidence of chronic hepatitis B or C infection. Therefore, the presence of prominent lymphoid aggregates or follicles with or without interface hepatitis, lobular inflammation, or scattered acidophilic bodies should raise the suspicion of concurrent chronic viral hepatitis.

The liver biopsy findings in alcoholic liver disease are very helpful prognostically. Extensive centrilobular parenchymal extinction and fibrosis (central hyalin sclerosis), severe hepatocellular injury including widespread Mallory-Denk bodies, cholestasis, and perivenular sclerosis represent poor prognostic indicators. Obliteration of central venules may result in portal hypertension in the absence of obvious cirrhosis. Abstinence from alcohol represents the most important therapeutic measure.

Differential Diagnosis

The differential diagnoses of alcoholic hepatitis include fatty liver disease, drug-induced phospholipidosis, Wilson disease, and chronic passive congestion. Although mild alcoholic liver disease cannot be distinguished with certainty from NAFLD, central hyalin sclerosis, obliteration of hepatic venules, and in some instances, acute cholestasis have been described in alcoholic liver disease and not in fatty liver disease. When cirrhosis occurs, regions of parenchymal extinction in alcoholic liver disease are broader than those of NAFLD. Drug-induced phospholipidosis is due to the formation of complexes between amphophilic drugs and cytosolic polar lipids that accumulate within lysosomes in many organs. A reliable clinical history in drug-induced phospholipidosis, usually related to amiodarone, tamoxifen, trimetoprim-sulfamethoxazole, and perhexiline maleate, is crucial for the differential diagnosis from alcoholic hepatitis. Drug-induced phospholipidosis shows features of acute alcoholic hepatitis with numerous Mallory-Denk bodies throughout the lobules (more than in alcoholic hepatitis), pericellular and portal fibrosis, and ductular reaction. Steatosis is inconspicuous. Wilson disease may be mild and often resembles fatty liver disease and alcoholic liver disease. Moderate to severe steatosis is common in Wilson disease; as the disease progresses, it is accompanied by enlarged hepatocytes with eosinophilic cytoplasm, diffuse ballooning of hepatocytes, Mallory-Denk hyalins, apoptotic bodies, and glycogenated nuclei. Mallory-Denk hyalins in Wilson disease are more often diffusely distributed throughout the lobule. Periportal Mallory-Denk hyalins are seen in chronic bile duct diseases such as primary biliary cirrhosis (PBC), primary sclerosing cholangitis (PSC), and biliary cirrhosis from other causes.

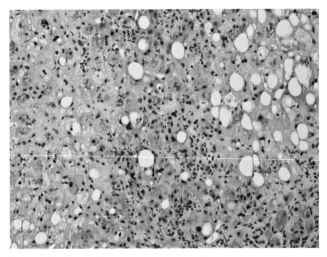

Figure 3.5.1 Steatosis, ballooned hepatocytes, Mallory-Denk bodies, and neutrophilic infiltrate in alcoholic liver disease.

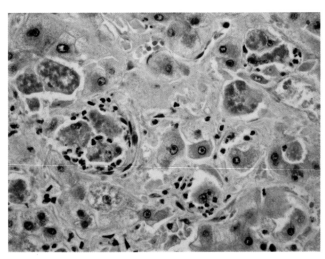

Figure 3.5.2 Mallory-Denk bodies or alcoholic hyalins with neutrophilic satellitosis.

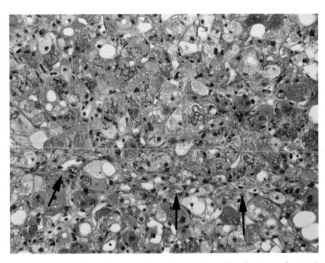

Figure 3.5.3 Central hyalin sclerosis (arrows) and pericellular "chicken wire" fibrosis in alcoholic liver disease (trichrome stain).

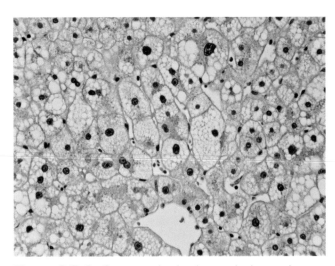

Figure 3.5.4 Severe mixed microvesicular and macrovesicular steatosis in alcoholic liver disease.

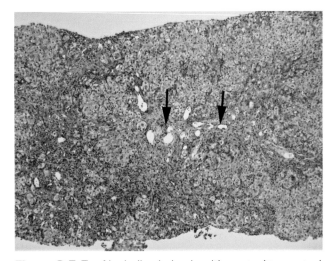

Figure 3.5.5 Alcoholic cirrhosis with central to central bridging fibrosis (arrows) (trichrome stain).

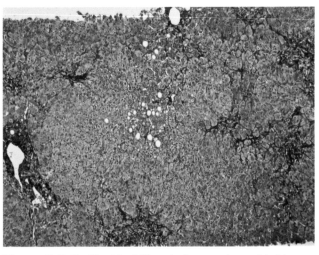

Figure 3.5.6 Residual fibrosis in a patient with history of alcoholic liver disease.

Table 3.5.1 Differential Diagnoses of Alcoholic Hepatitis

Histologic Features	Alcoholic Hepatitis	Nonalcoholic Steatohepatitis	Wilson Disease	Drug-Induced Phospholipidosis	Chronic Passive Congestion
Mallory-Denk bodies	++ (centrilobular)	+ (rare, centrilobular)/–	++ (diffuse)	++ (diffuse)	–
Neutrophilic infiltrate	++	+ (rare, in sinusoids)	+	++	–
Macrovesicular steatosis	+/–	++	+	+ (inconspicuous)/–	+ (centrilobular)/–
Microvesicular steatosis	+/–	+/–	–	+/–	+ (centrilobular)
Ballooned hepatocytes	+	+	+	+	–
Pericellular/perisinusoidal fibrosis	++	+	++	++	++
Central hyalin sclerosis	++	–	–	+/–	–
Obliteration of central venules	+	–	–	–	–
Centrilobular hemosiderin	–	–	–	–	+
Portal fibrosis	–/+ (in late stage)	+	+	+	–
Acute cholestasis	+ (when severe)/–	–	+ (when severe)/–	–	–
Sinusoidal dilatation	–	–	–	–	++
Centrilobular hepatocyte atrophy	–	–	–	–	+
Reverse lobulation	–	–	–	–	+

++ indicates almost always present; +, usually present; +/–, occasionally present; – usually absent.

3.6   Autoimmune Hepatitis

Autoimmune hepatitis is a syndrome characterized by a broad spectrum of clinical symptoms, elevated liver enzymes, (polyclonal) hypergammaglobulinemia, an immunogenetic predisposition (HLA A1, HLA-B8, HLA-DR3, or HLA-DR4), absence of viral infection, and a favorable response to immunosuppressive therapy and frequent recurrence after discontinuation of immunosuppression. Similar to other types of autoimmune diseases, AIH is due to a defect in suppressor T cells that leads to disordered immunoregulation, and production of autoantibodies and reactive immune cells, which act against hepatocyte membrane antigens. The defect may occur de novo or subsequent to a triggering episode such as hepatitis A or a variety of drug injuries.

Autoimmune hepatitis can affect patients of all ages, sexes, and races, but predominantly young women between the ages of 15 and 35 years with a second peak at menopause. The onset of the disease is usually insidious but may be acute. Liver cirrhosis is present in up to 30% of patients at diagnosis. Patients present with fatigue and jaundice, and sometimes, signs of chronic liver disease, such as spider nevi, splenomegaly, ascites, and amenorrhea. Associated autoimmune disorders such as Hashimoto thyroiditis, hemolytic anemia, rheumatoid arthritis, and others may be present.

Autoimmune hepatitis type 1 is associated with ANA with or without anti–smooth muscle antibody (SMA). Autoimmune hepatitis type 2 is associated with anti–liver kidney microsomal antibody or others. A subpopulation of patients may have an elevated antimitochondrial antibody (AMA) as well, clinically mimicking PBC. See Table 3.6.1 for the simplified diagnostic criteria for autoimmune hepatitis. The simplified criteria emphasize the importance of liver histology, autoantibody titers, IgG levels, and exclusion of viral hepatitis. Response to immunosuppressive therapy is characteristic of AIH. For those scored into probable AIH, liver biopsy is required to differentiate AIH from PBC, PSC, NASH, and drug-induced liver injury.

In children, although AIH type 1 is more common around puberty, AIH type 2 tends to present at a younger age and also during infancy. In addition, autoantibody reactivity is relatively infrequent in healthy children.

Timely diagnosis and immunosuppressive therapy contain disease activity in almost all patients, resulting in near normal or normal life expectancy. Untreated AIH has a 5-year mortality greater than 50%. For those patients that progress to cirrhosis, liver transplantation is an option, although AIH may recur within the allograft.

Histologic Features

Autoimmune hepatitis shows histologic changes of severely active chronic hepatitis. Little is known regarding the histologic changes of acute-onset AIH. Most patients with clinically acute-onset AIH actually represent a flare of previously occult chronic disease. Interface hepatitis and septal fibrosis involve all portal tracts, often with marked regeneration and rosette formation of periportal hepatocytes. Numerous plasma cells in clusters are seen within the portal and periportal inflammatory infiltrates (Figure 3.6.1). Bridging and confluent necrosis are often present, leading to broad areas of collapse surrounding large, irregular regenerative nodules (Figures 3.6.2 and 3.6.5). The presence of lobules or nodules with severe necroinflammatory activity and hepatocyte rosettes adjacent to large regenerative nodules with minimal inflammation is characteristic of AIH. Cirrhosis develops rapidly and early in untreated patients.

The typical histologic features of AIH based on the simplified diagnostic criteria for autoimmune hepatitis include interface hepatitis, lymphocytic/lymphoplasmocytic infiltrates in portal tracts and extending into the lobule, emperipolesis (active penetration by one cell into and through a larger cell), and hepatic rosette formation (Figures 3.6.3 and 3.6.4). Compatible features are histologic findings of chronic hepatitis with lymphocytic infiltration without all the features considered typical. Features are considered atypical when showing changes of another diagnosis, such as steatohepatitis.

A biopsy from a successfully treated patient may reveal the absence of significant necroinflammatory activity and interface hepatitis, including the absence of plasmacellular infiltrate (Figure 3.6.6). The hepatocytes show regenerative features with 1- to 2-cell-thick plates with expansion of the lobule and significant regression of fibrosis. When liver function test remains mildly elevated, other liver diseases such as steatohepatitis should also be considered.

Differential Diagnosis

The differential diagnoses include acute and chronic viral hepatitis, drug-induced liver injury, steatohepatitis, and Wilson disease. Chronic viral hepatitis usually has already been ruled out by viral serologic studies and therefore rarely pose a problem during the evaluation of liver biopsy. In addition, jaundice, dark urine, pruritus, poor appetite, weight loss, and high aminotransferase activities are more commonly seen in AIH than in chronic viral hepatitis. A history of prescribed and over-the-counter drug should be obtained for consideration of drug-induced injury. The presence of ceroid-containing macrophages in the perivenular area and the absence of morphological evidence of chronicity support drug-induced hepatitis rather than AIH. Some drugs may, however, cause chronic drug-induced injury that mimic AIH (see also "Chronic Drug-Induced Injury"). Patients with steatohepatitis commonly present with other clinical features including obesity, hypertension, hyperlipidemia, and diabetes mellitus. It is not uncommon, however, that these patients have an elevation of ANA as well. Wilson disease may share features of AIH; characteristically, these patients initially respond favorably but only transiently to steroids (see "Hereditary Metabolic Diseases" for a discussion on Wilson disease).

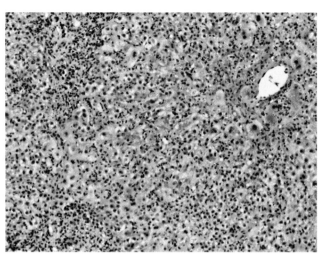

Figure 3.6.1 Severe portal and panlobular inflammation in autoimmune hepatitis.

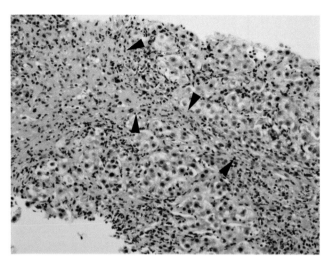

Figure 3.6.2 Autoimmune hepatitis with bridging necrosis (arrowheads).

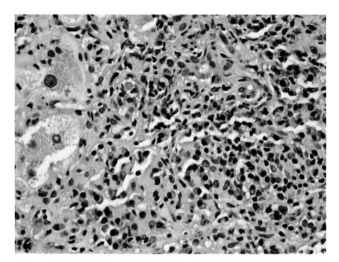

Figure 3.6.3 Autoimmune hepatitis showing sheets of plasma cells.

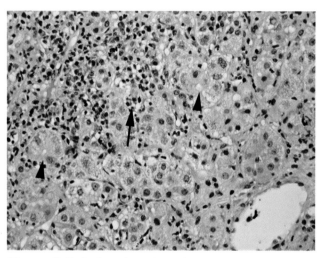

Figure 3.6.4 Interface hepatitis, hepatocyte rosette formation (arrowheads), and emperipolesis (arrow) in autoimmune hepatitis.

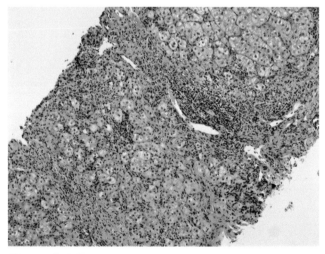

Figure 3.6.5 Autoimmune hepatitis showing areas of collapse and fibrosis with severe necroinflammatory activity surrounding irregular regenerative nodules.

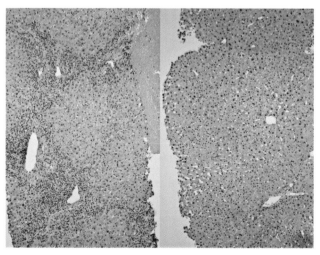

Figure 3.6.6 Biopsy specimens of a patient with autoimmune hepatitis at initial presentation (left) and during remission 3 years after (right).

Table 3.6.1 Simplified Diagnostic Criteria for Autoimmune Hepatitis

Variable	Cutoff	Points
ANA or SMA	≥1:40	1
ANA or SMA	≥1:80	
or LKM	≥1:40	2*
or SLA	Positive	
IgG	>Upper normal limit	1
	>1.10 times upper normal limit	2
Liver histology (evidence of hepatitis is a necessary condition)	Compatible with AIH	1
	Typical AIH	2
Absence of viral hepatitis	Yes	2
Total score		≥6: probable AIH
		≥7: definite AIH

*Addition of points achieved for all autoantibodies (maximum, 2 points).
ANA indicates antinuclear antibody; SMA, smooth muscle antibody; LKM, liver kidney microsomal antibodies; SLA, soluble liver antibody.
Hennes EM, et al. Simplified criteria for the diagnosis of autoimmune hepatitis. *Hepatology.* 2008;48(1):169–176.

Table 3.6.2 Differential Diagnoses of Autoimmune Hepatitis

Histologic Features	Autoimmune Hepatitis	Drug-Induced Injury	Steatohepatitis
Overall inflammation	Severe	Mild to severe	Mild
Plasma cell infiltrate	++	+/−	−
Lymphocytic infiltrate	+	+	+
Scattered lobular neutrophils	−	−	+
Portal inflammation	++	+/−	+/−
Interface hepatitis	++	+/−	−
Rosette formation	+	+/−	−
Portal fibrosis and septa	+	−	+/−
Lobular inflammation	++	+	+/−
Steatosis	−	+/−	++
Hepatocyte necrosis	++	++	+/−
Bridging and confluent necrosis	+	+/−	−
Centrilobular necroinflammation	+	+/−	+/−
Centrilobular/pericellular fibrosis	−	−	+/−
Cholestasis	+/−	+/−	−

++ indicates almost always present; +, usually present; +/−, occasionally present; −, usually absent.

3.7 Primary Biliary Cirrhosis

Primary biliary cirrhosis (PBC) is an immune-mediated chronic destructive intrahepatic bile duct disease. Almost all patients have antimitochondrial antibodies (AMAs) which react against the E2 component of the pyruvate dehydrogenase complex that accumulates in the biliary epithelium of patients with PBC.

Primary biliary cirrhosis characteristically primarily affects women between the ages of 40 and 60 years and is associated with other immunologic diseases such as keratoconjunctivitis sicca, Sjögren syndrome, Raynaud phenomenon, scleroderma, rheumatoid arthritis, lupus erythematosus, celiac sprue, and thyroiditis (CREST syndrome). Patients may be asymptomatic or present with pruritus and fatigue. Initially, jaundice is absent. The liver is usually enlarged. Characteristically, alkaline phosphatase and γ-glutamyltransferase activities, and levels of cholesterol and serum IgM are elevated. High titers of AMA in the right clinical setting are diagnostic. In later stages, the signs and symptoms are related to progressive cholestasis or cirrhosis. Progressive cholestasis causes pruritus, xanthomas, jaundice, and osteoporosis.

In summary, criteria for the diagnosis of PBC include (1) cholestatic serum enzyme pattern, (2) elevated serum IgM, (3) presence of AMA (>1:40) or PBC-specific AMA-M2 directed against the E2 subunit of the pyruvate dehydrogenase complex, and (4) histology to include florid duct lesion, granulomas, ductular reaction, and bile duct paucity.

Autoimmune cholangitis, also known as AMA-negative PBC, constitutes approximately 5% of patients with phenotypic evidence of PBC but lack high titers of AMA using standard testing. Almost all patients show positive AMA levels when using a more sensitive method of testing; therefore, autoimmune cholangitis is considered a form of PBC.

Pathologic Features

The histologic features of PBC are divided into 4 overlapping morphologic stages according to the sequence of events occurring in the portal tracts (see Table 3.7.1). The correlation between the clinical symptoms and morphologic stages is poor, or, in other words, morphologic stages do not reflect the true natural history of the disease. Regardless of stage, PBC patients if left untreated may progress to cirrhosis in a few years. In addition, the distribution may be patchy, and different morphologic stages may be observed in the same biopsy specimen.

In stage 1, "florid duct lesions" are seen involving interlobular and septal bile ducts. The damaged bile duct is surrounded by lymphocytes, macrophages, and plasma cells or granulomatous reaction, so-called nonsuppurative destructive cholangitis (Figure 3.7.1). Eosinophils are almost always present in the inflamed portal tracts. Florid duct lesion is pathognomonic for PBC (Figure 3.7.2). Granuloma can be seen in portal tracts and lobules (Figure 3.7.3).

In stage 2, bile ducts are reduced in number, and ductular reaction is noted in periportal areas. Inflammation is less intense than stage 1. Hyperplasia of hepatocytes may be present in the absence of cirrhosis, resulting in subtle nodular regenerative hyperplasia, perhaps reflecting damage of portal vein branches by granulomatous inflammation.

In stage 3, there is increasing portal fibrosis and formation of fibrous septa. Most of the small bile ducts have disappeared (Figure 3.7.4). The loss of bile ducts is recognized when hepatic artery branches in portal tracts are not accompanied by bile ducts of similar caliber. The periportal and periseptal hepatocytes show features of chronic cholestasis and cholate stasis. The cytoplasm of these cells is ballooned, pale, and rarefied (so-called feathery degeneration) and sometimes contains Mallory-Denk hyalin and increased copper deposition.

In stage 4, regenerative nodules surrounded by dense hypocellular fibrous septa are seen (Figure 3.7.5). Scattered lymphocyte aggregates in portal tracts may be observed. Hepatocellular cholestasis is always present and is usually periportal. Fibrous tissue next to the nodules is often less dense than the rest of the fibrous septa, giving rise to a pale "halo" around the nodules (Figure 3.7.6). Small bile ducts are rarely found, but large bile ducts remain and may show periductal inflammation.

A significant lymphoplasmacellular interface hepatitis, so-called sleeve necrosis (Figure 3.7.1), is often seen in PBC and by itself does not warrant the diagnosis of autoimmune feature or overlap syndrome, but it may correlate with a faster progression of fibrosis.

Differential Diagnosis

The main histologic differential diagnoses of PBC are PSC, AIH, chronic viral hepatitis, and sarcoidosis. In comparison to PSC, PBC shows lymphoplasmacellular inflammation with eosinophils, more ductular proliferation in stage 2, nodular regenerative hyperplasia, absence of periductal fibrosis, and preservation of large bile ducts but loss of interlobular and septal bile ducts in stage 4. In stage 3, the changes in PBC and PSC may be similar. Sarcoidosis may mimic the clinical and histologic presentation of PBC, but granulomas in sarcoidosis are more exuberant with reticulin fibers and fibrosis. Streaming and clustering of lymphocytes in sinusoids without significant injury of adjacent hepatocytes are seen in PBC and not in AIH. See Table 3.7.2 for the differential diagnoses of PBC.

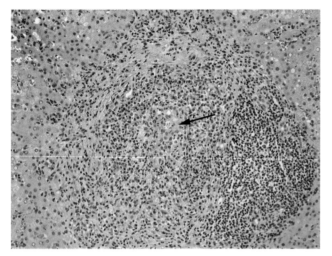

Figure 3.7.1 Dense lymphoplasmacytic infiltrate with scattered eosinophils, severely damaged bile duct (arrow), and sleeve necrosis in primary biliary cirrhosis.

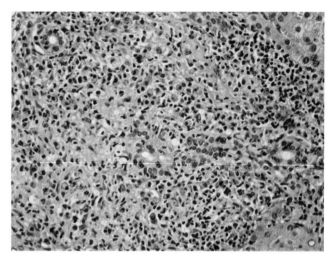

Figure 3.7.2 Florid duct lesion, the characteristic feature in primary biliary cirrhosis.

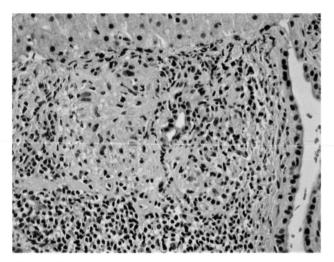

Figure 3.7.3 Epithelioid granuloma surrounding damaged bile duct in primary biliary cirrhosis.

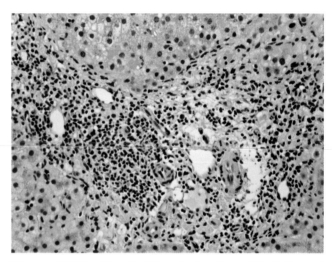

Figure 3.7.4 Bile duct is missing from this inflamed portal tract in primary biliary cirrhosis.

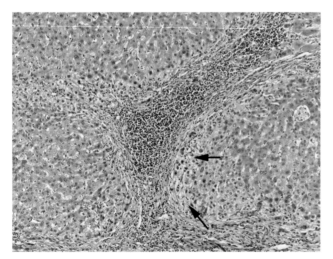

Figure 3.7.5 Cirrhosis in primary biliary cirrhosis with lymphocytic aggregates in portal tracts, bile duct loss, and periseptal feathery degeneration of hepatocytes (arrows) due to cholate stasis.

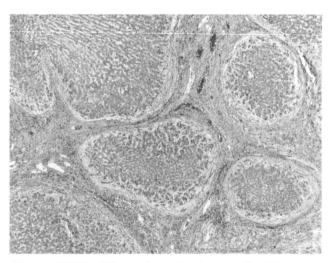

Figure 3.7.6 Biliary cirrhosis showing "halo" around the nodules and paucity of bile ducts.

Table 3.7.1 Stages of Primary Biliary Cirrhosis

Stages		Predominant Histologic Features*
1	Florid duct lesion or portal stage	Portal chronic inflammation, florid duct lesion, bile duct damage, granulomas.
2	Ductular proliferation or periportal stage	Interface hepatitis, periportal fibrosis, ductular reaction.
3	Scarring or septal stage	Bridging fibrosis, loss of bile ducts, changes of cholate stasis.
4	Cirrhosis	Biliary cirrhosis, so-called garland or jigsaw pattern with "halo."

* Features may overlap.

Table 3.7.2 Differential Diagnoses of Primary Biliary Cirrhosis

Histologic Features	PBC	PSC	Sarcoidosis	Autoimmune Hepatitis	Chronic Viral Hepatitis
Inflammatory infiltrate type	Lymphoplasmacytic with eosinophils	Lymphocytes, neutrophils	Lymphocytes, macrophages	Lymphoplasmacytic with eosinophils	Lymphocytes
Portal inflammation	++	+	+/–	++	++
Epithelioid granuloma	+	–	++	–	–
Lymphocytic cholangitis	+	+	–	–	+/–
Florid duct lesion	+	–	–	–	–
Periductal onion-skin fibrosis	–	++	–	–	–
Duct ectasia	+/–	++	–	–	–
Ductopenia	+ (stage 3,4)	+ (stage 3,4)	+/–	–	–
Small bile duct	Affected	Affected	May be affected	Unaffected	May be focally affected in chronic HCV
Large bile duct	Unaffected	Affected	May be affected	Unaffected	Unaffected
Interface hepatitis	+	– (+ in children)	–	++	+
Lobular inflammation	+	–	+/–	++	+
Cholestasis	+ (late stage)	+ (late stage)	–	+/–	–
Cholate stasis	+	+	+/–	–	–
Periportal copper deposition	+ (late stages)	+ (late stages)	+/–	–	–

PBC indicates primary biliary cirrhosis; PSC, primary sclerosing cholangitis.
++ indicates almost always present; +, usually present; +/–, occasionally present; –, usually absent.

3.8 Primary Sclerosing Cholangitis

Primary sclerosing cholangitis is a chronic biliary disorder characterized by fibrosis and inflammation involving portions of extrahepatic and intrahepatic bile ducts, resulting in obliteration of the bile ducts and eventually in biliary cirrhosis. The pathogenesis of PSC is uncertain, perhaps related to immunologic insult to subepithelial mesenchyme or microvascular damage that leads to ischemic biliary epithelium damage and secondary fibrosis, but the lack of response to immunosuppressive therapy suggests that PSC is not a straightforward autoimmune disorder.

Primary sclerosing cholangitis primarily affects adults, more common in men, between the ages of 25 and 45 years but can also occur in children. More than two thirds of patients have inflammatory bowel disease (70%-90%), particularly ulcerative colitis and less often Crohn disease. Pruritus and jaundice are present in many patients. Besides the signs and symptoms of obstruction of bile flow, patients also experience intermittent fever from bacterial cholangitis. Antimitochondrial antibodies are always absent, but antineutrophil cytoplasmic antibodies are often present (up to 70%). The diagnosis depends on the demonstration of stenosis and beading of the biliary tree on cholangiography in the absence of other causes, such as cholangiocarcinoma, lithiasis, or previous bile duct surgery. Liver biopsy is particularly helpful in the differentiation from PBC when the disease involves only the small intrahepatic bile ducts and cholangiography is noncontributory, so-called small duct PSC. It has to be realized, however, that liver biopsy may not be diagnostic if the disease involves predominantly the extrahepatic bile ducts or focally involves lobes or segments that are not sampled.

In summary, the criteria for the diagnosis of PSC include (1) cholestatic serum enzyme pattern, (2) typical cholangiographic findings of bile duct stenoses and dilatations, (3) repeated AMA negativity, and (4) compatible histology.

In children, PSC is often associated with florid autoimmune features, including elevated titers of autoantibodies, in particular ANA and anti-SMA; elevated IgG; and interface hepatitis. This condition represents an overlap syndrome with AIH and referred to as autoimmune sclerosing cholangitis (see also "Overlap Syndromes").

Primary sclerosing cholangitis is often complicated by recurrent acute cholangitis, cirrhosis, and sometimes cholangiocarcinoma. The course is variable; some patients remain asymptomatic for years, whereas others develop deep jaundice and liver failure in a few months. The prognosis is worse when large extrahepatic ducts are involved rather than intrahepatic ducts alone; therefore, small duct PSC progresses slower with lower risk of cholangiocarcinoma, but a third of patients may progress to large extrahepatic duct PSC.

Pathologic Features

Fibroinflammatory changes of the bile duct wall and periductal fibrosis, often referred to as fibrous cholangitis, result in an "onion skin" appearance (Figure 3.8.1). The inflammatory infiltrate consists predominantly of lymphocytes. Ductular reaction is present. The involved bile ducts show damage and atrophy of the epithelium and eventually are replaced by nodular dense fibrous tissue, so-called bile duct scars or fibrous obliterative cholangitis (Figure 3.8.2). Ductopenia without bile scars is seen in small portal tracts and is a common biopsy finding in patients with advanced PSC. Secondary acute cholangitis, bile duct ectasia, and cholangitic abscess may also be found.

Bile duct damage and atrophy, periductal fibrosis and bile duct scar can be found in small portal tract in small duct variant of PSC (Figure 3.8.3).

As fibrosis progresses, biliary cirrhosis may eventually occur with multifocal bile duct scar and cholate stasis (Figure 3.8.4).

Differential Diagnosis

The differential diagnoses include PBC, AIH, chronic viral hepatitis, and secondary sclerosing cholangitis. Secondary sclerosing cholangitis is not a distinct entity but rather a long-standing intrahepatic and/or extrahepatic biliary disorder with features that mimic PSC and can cause secondary biliary cirrhosis in a patient without PSC. The causes are long-standing large duct obstruction, ischemic cholangitis, bacterial or recurrent pyogenic cholangitis, IgG4-related sclerosing cholangitis, and biliary tract and pancreatic malignancy. See Tables 3.8.1 and 3.8.2 for the differential diagnoses of PSC.

Ischemic cholangiopathy (cholangitis) is focal or extensive damage of the bile ducts due to impaired blood flow and is one of the most common causes of secondary sclerosing cholangitis. It is caused by insult to the hepatic arteries in abdominal surgery or trauma, various thrombotic disorders, vasculitis, ABO-incompatible allografts, and hepatic intra-arterial chemotherapy. The initial histologic features of ischemic cholangiopathy are biliary epithelium atrophy, followed by sloughing of biliary epithelium, formation of biliary casts, and later ductopenia, fibrosis, and cirrhosis.

IgG4-related sclerosing cholangitis is a recently described member of IgG4-related diseases, which include autoimmune pancreatitis, sialadenitis, inflammatory pseudotumor, and retroperitoneal fibrosis. IgG4-related sclerosing cholangitis is responsive to corticosteroid treatment; therefore, its distinction to PSC is clinically important. It causes bile duct stricture and the inflammatory infiltrate predominantly lymphoplasmacytic with abundance of IgG4-immunopositive cells (Figure 3.8.6).

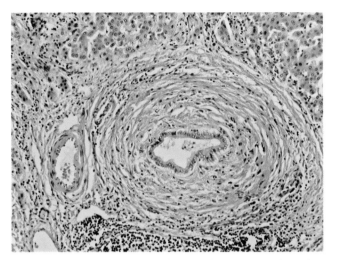

Figure 3.8.1 "Onion skin" fibrosis in primary sclerosing cholangitis.

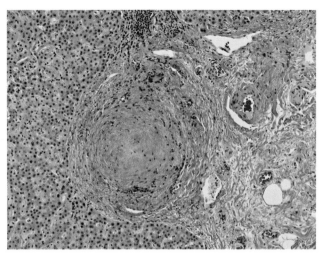

Figure 3.8.2 Bile duct scar in primary sclerosing cholangitis.

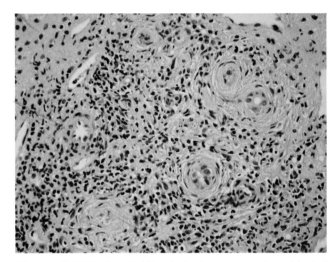

Figure 3.8.3 Small bile duct damage and periductal fibrosis in small duct variant of primary sclerosing cholangitis.

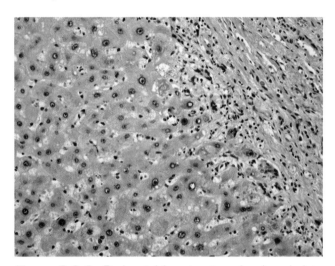

Figure 3.8.4 Periseptal hepatocytes showing cholate stasis and Mallory-Denk hyalins in biliary cirrhosis.

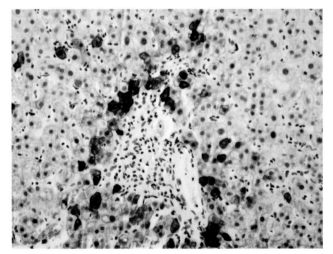

Figure 3.8.5 Cytokeratin 7 immunostain showing absence of bile duct (bile duct loss) in the portal tract and CK7 reactivity of periportal hepatocytes due to chronic cholestasis.

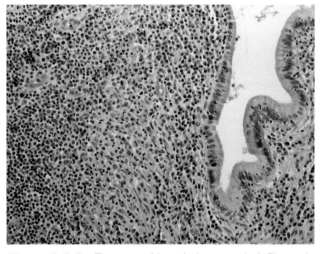

Figure 3.8.6 Dense periductal plasmacytic infiltrate in IgG4-related sclerosing cholangitis.

Table 3.8.1 Stages of Primary Sclerosing Cholangitis

Stages		Histologic Features
1	Portal stage	Portal inflammation and edema, bile duct damage, periductal fibrosis, ductular reaction
2	Periportal stage	Portal and periportal fibrosis and inflammation
3	Septal stage	Bridging fibrosis, ductopenia
4	Cirrhosis	Biliary cirrhosis, so-called garland or jigsaw pattern

Table 3.8.2 Differential Diagnoses of Primary Sclerosing Cholangitis

Histologic Features	Primary Sclerosing Cholangitis	Primary Biliary Cirrhosis	Long-Standing Large Bile Duct Obstruction	Ischemic Cholangitis	IgG4-related Sclerosing Cholangitis
Inflammatory infiltrate	Lymphocytic, neutrophils in acute cholangitis	Lymphoplasmacytic with eosinophils	Lymphocytic, neutrophils	Lymphocytic	IgG4-positive plasma cells
Intensity of inflammation	Mild	Patchy, marked	Mild	Minimal	Diffuse, marked
Lymphoid follicle	–	+/–	–	–	+/–
Interface hepatitis	+/–	+	–	–	–
Lobular inflammation	+/–	+	–	–	–
Florid duct lesion	–	+	–	–	–
Epithelioid granuloma	–	+	–	–	–
Ductular reaction	+	+	++	+	+
Periportal bile lakes and infarct	+/–	–	+/–	+/–	–
"Onion skin" periductal fibrosis	++	–	+/–	+/–	+/–
Portal edema	–	–	+ (acute)	–	+/–
Bile duct atrophy	+	–	–	++	–
Bile duct scar	+	–	–	+/–	–
Bile duct tortuosity	–	–	+	–	+/–
Cholangiectasia	++	+/–	+	–	–
Acute cholangitis & abscess	+	–	+/–	–	–
Medium bile duct loss	++	–	–	–	–
Small bile duct loss	+	++	+/–	+/–	+/–

++ indicates almost always present; +, usually present; +/–, occasionally present; –, usually absent.

3.9 Overlap Syndromes

All types of autoimmune liver diseases, AIH, PBC, and PSC, can coexist with a variety of other autoimmune diseases and/or coexist with each other. The latter is referred to as overlap syndrome. It should be realized that overlap syndrome is considerably rare and the term is best used to describe a manifestation of 2 diseases rather than 1 disease with overreaching histopathologic features. The most common overlap syndrome is AIH/PBC, followed by AIH/PSC, and then PBC/PSC as the least common.

There have been no generally accepted criteria for AIH/PBC-AIH/PSC overlap syndromes, and the diagnosis of overlap syndrome is highly controversial. The distinction between AIH and PBC or PSC as well with their overlap syndromes was not always possible on the basis of simplified diagnostic criteria for autoimmune hepatitis (see Table 3.6.1). This difficulty reflects the ongoing discussion regarding their definition and to what extent there may be overlap among these autoimmune liver diseases. In principle, for the diagnosis of overlap syndromes, compelling histologic and clinical evidence of both hepatic and biliary component should be present. The more features of AIH that are present, the more likely progressive disease will occur, and therefore, the patient will more likely benefit from—potentially life-saving—immunosuppressive therapy in addition to the conventional treatment for PBC or PSC.

Autoimmune Hepatitis/PBC Overlap Syndrome

Autoimmune hepatitis/PBC overlap syndrome represents approximately 10% of AIH or PBC cases, and the frequency varies according to the criteria used to diagnose these cases. Patients with AIH/PBC overlap syndrome present with at least 2 or 3 of the well-accepted features of each AIH and PBC, which usually translate to elevation of serum transaminase activities, cholestatic serum enzymes, hypergammaglobulinemia, AMA positivity, ANA or SMA positivity, and histologic features compatible with both AIH (moderate to severe interface and lobular hepatitis with plasmacellular infiltrate) and PBC (florid duct lesion, granuloma, ductopenia, chronic cholestasis) (Figures 3.9.1 and 3.9.2). It remains unclear whether AIH/PBC overlap syndrome represents a hepatic form of PBC or intermediate form of a continuous spectrum of the 2 autoimmune diseases or a coexistence of 2 autoimmune diseases.

Autoimmune Hepatitis/PSC Overlap Syndrome

Autoimmune hepatitis/PSC overlap syndrome occurs mainly in children, adolescents, and young adults. Patients with AIH/PSC overlap syndrome presents with characteristic clinical features of AIH, but cholangiographic findings are typical of sclerosing cholangitis; therefore, this syndrome is also referred to as autoimmune sclerosing cholangitis. Inflammatory bowel disease and positivity for antineutrophil cytoplasmic antibodies are common.

Liver biopsy shows histologic features of PSC, such as onion skin periductal fibrosis, bile duct scar, ductopenia, and features of chronic cholestasis, combined with features of AIH, such as moderate to severe interface and lobular hepatitis with prominent plasma cell component and scattered acidophilic bodies (Figures 3.9.3, 3.9.4, and 3.9.5).

Primary Biliary Cirrhosis/PSC Overlap Syndrome

Primary biliary cirrhosis/PSC overlap syndrome is rare. It combines clinical, biochemical, histologic, and cholangiographic features of both PBC and PSC (Figure 3.9.6). The exceptional rarity of this syndrome when compared to other overlap syndromes leads to the suggestion of pure coexistence of PBC and PSC rather than a true overlap syndrome.

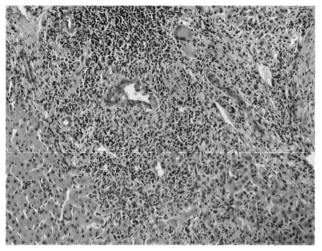

Figure 3.9.1 Autoimmune hepatitis/PBC overlap syndrome showing florid duct lesion with granulomatous reaction and prominent interface hepatitis (see also Figure 3.9.2).

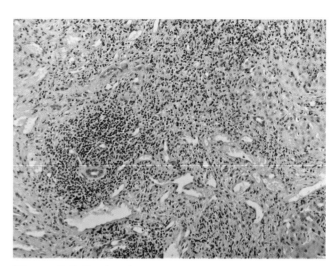

Figure 3.9.2 Autoimmune hepatitis/PBC overlap syndrome showing parenchymal collapse and plasmacellular infiltrate, similar to features of AIH alone (see also Figure 3.9.1 for bile duct damage).

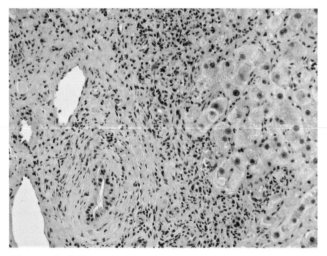

Figure 3.9.3 Autoimmune hepatitis/PSC overlap syndrome showing bile duct damage with periductal concentric fibrosis and interface hepatitis. The latter is usually not seen in PSC alone.

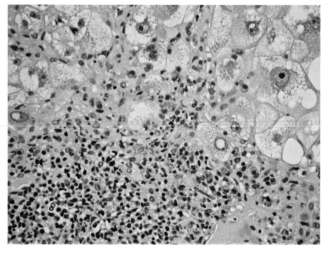

Figure 3.9.4 Autoimmune hepatitis/PSC overlap syndrome showing abundant plasma cell infiltrate, interface hepatitis, and feathery degeneration of the hepatocytes.

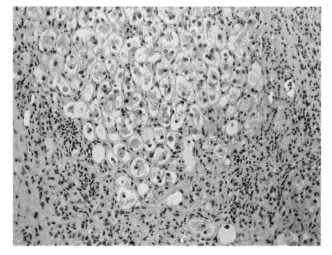

Figure 3.9.5 Autoimmune hepatitis/PSC overlap syndrome showing residual nodular parenchyma with cholate stasis (feathery degeneration).

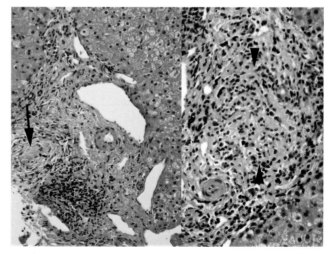

Figure 3.9.6 Primary biliary cirrhosis/PSC overlap syndrome showing bile duct scar (left, arrow) and granuloma formation (right, arrowheads).

3.10   Chronic Drug-Induced Injury

Chronic drug-induced injury may mimic other forms of chronic liver diseases, ranging from chronic viral hepatitis, AIH, steatohepatitis, alcoholic liver disease, chronic biliary disease, and liver tumor; therefore, similar to acute drug-induced injury, circumstantial evidence becomes crucial in most cases. Unfortunately, polypharmacotherapy and multiple comorbidites may hinder the implication of a single drug as the causative factor.

Drugs are responsible for less than 1% of cases of chronic hepatitis and cirrhosis. Liver disease usually develops more than a year after therapy has been started. The spectrum of clinical symptoms varies and ranges from asymptomatic elevation of aminotransferase activities to cirrhosis. The histologic and clinical features of the disease can last for very prolonged periods after discontinuation of the drug.

Autoimmune Hepatitis–Like Features

Chronic drug-induced hepatitis often mimics chronic hepatitis of other causes, both clinically and morphologically (Figure 3.10.6). The activity and fibrosis are variable. Complete serologic tests to eliminate viral and AIH and critical chronologic history of drug intake are crucial. Regardless of these, difficulties often remain in the definitive diagnosis of chronic drug-induced liver disease. The separation is especially difficult from AIH because drug-induced hepatitis often resembles AIH, and the drug may also trigger autoimmunity. Based on this feature, drug-induced chronic hepatitis can be subdivided into several categories (Table 3.10.1), including those with features resembling AIH clinically and histologically (Figure 3.10.1).

Steatosis and Steatohepatitis

Steatosis and steatohepatitis are frequent manifestations of chronic drug-induced injury. In all cases, other comorbidities such as metabolic syndrome or its component and alcoholic liver disease should be ruled out. Morphologically, in general, drug-induced steatohepatitis, such as that caused by tamoxifen, is similar to NASH, with zone 3 ballooned hepatocytes and Mallory-Denk hyalins (Figure 3.10.2). Few, such as amiodarone, may show involvement of zone 1 hepatocytes. Liver biopsies are often performed to assess methotrexate treatment effect for psoriasis or leukemia, which can cause steatosis, fibrosis, and nuclear pleomorphism (Figure 3.10.3). Other than nuclear pleomorphism, the morphologic features are indistinguishable from NASH. In these cases, other comorbidities that can cause steatohepatitis should be taken into account so that the patient can safely continue methotrexate treatment.

Phospholipidosis

Drug-induced phospholipidosis is caused by an amphophilic drug that crosses the lysosomal membrane of cells and binds with phospholipids in the acidic intralysosomal environment. The accumulation of drug-phospholipid complexes results in large lysosomes with pseudomyelin figures in hepatocytes, cholangiocytes, endothelial cells, and Kupffer cells. These characteristic lysosomal inclusions closely resemble those seen in Niemann-Pick, Tay-Sachs, and Fabry disease. Drug-induced phospholipidosis shows features of acute alcoholic hepatitis with Mallory-Denk bodies throughout the hepatic lobules, pericellular and portal fibrosis, and ductular reaction. Mallory-Denk bodies are more numerous than alcoholic hepatitis. Accumulation of phospholipids leads to enlarge, foamy, or granular cytoplasm of hepatocytes and macrophages (Figure 3.10.4), but this is difficult to discern by light microscopy.

Chronic Cholangitis and Ductopenia (Vanishing Bile Duct Syndrome)

Chronic cholangitis, with features mimicking PBC or sclerosing cholangitis, is seen in a delayed cholestatic syndrome with jaundice more than 6 months or serologic abnormalities longer than 1 year after cessation of the drug. Drug-induced cholangitis affects patients of any age or sex. Most likely, the causative drug or its metabolites trigger an immune response directed against the biliary epithelium. The portal tracts show ductular reaction with mixed inflammatory infiltrate, including neutrophils, bile duct damage, and ductopenia (vanishing bile duct syndrome). It is often accompanied by features of chronic cholestasis, such as periportal feathery degeneration or cholate stasis, Mallory-Denk hyalins, and copper deposition in periportal hepatocytes and portal fibrosis.

Vascular Injury

Drugs can cause vascular injury to different components of the hepatic vasculature, including portal vein, hepatic vein, and sinusoids. Oral contraceptives can cause periportal sinusoidal dilatation or nodular regenerative hyperplasia (Figure 3.10.5). Alkylating agents such as cyclophosphamide or busulfan can cause veno-occlusive disease. Alkaloids and radiation can lead to Budd-Chiari syndrome (BCS).

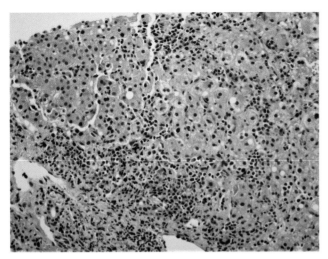

Figure 3.10.1 Autoimmune hepatitis-like phenytoin-induced hepatitis showing abundant plasma cells.

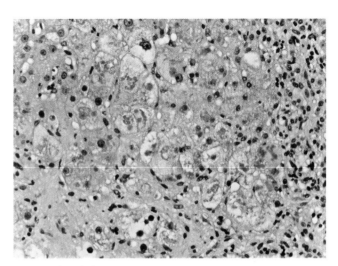

Figure 3.10.2 Amiodarone-induced steatohepatitis with ballooned hepatocytes and abundant Mallory-Denk hyalins.

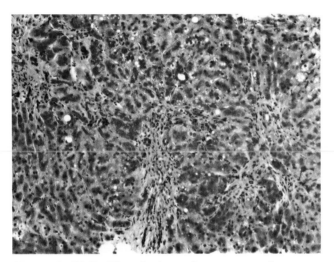

Figure 3.10.3 Fibrosis due to long-term methotrexate treatment (trichrome stain).

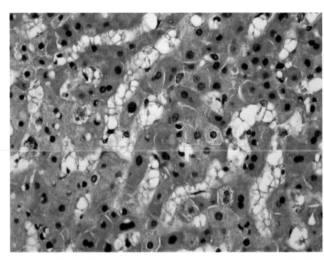

Figure 3.10.4 Drug-induced phospholipidosis with hyperplastic Kupffer cells.

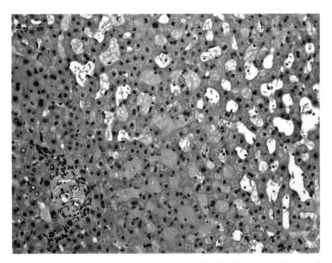

Figure 3.10.5 Periportal sinusoidal dilatation in oral hormone contraceptive injury.

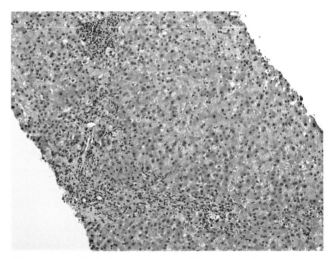

Figure 3.10.6 Chronic hepatitis due to long-term 6-mercaptopurine treatment.

Table 3.10.1 **Chronic Drug-Induced Injury**

Main Histologic Features and Drugs	Comments and Other Findings
Syndrome resembling autoimmune hepatitis	
Clometacine	ASMA, anti-DNA
Minocycline	ANA, anti-DNA
Methyldopa, nitrofurantoin, oxyphenisatin, papaverin	ANA, ASMA
Benzarone, diclofenac, propylthiouracil, fenofibrate, ecstasy	ANA
Tielinic acid, iproniazid, halothane	Anti-LKM2
Dihydralazine	Anti-CYP1A2
Halothane	Anti-carboxylesterase, anti disulfide isomerase
Iproniazid	Anti-microsomal antibody 6
Sulfonamides, etretinate	
Chronic hepatitis	
Acetaminophen, aspirin, isoniazid, lisinopril, sulphonamide, trazadone	No specific features (portal inflammation, fibrosis/cirrhosis)
Steatosis/steatohepatitis	
Valproic acid, tetracycline	Microvesicular steatosis
Corticosteroids, calcium channel blockers	Macrovesicular steatosis
Methotrexate	Macrovesicular steatosis, fibrosis
Tamoxifen, stilbestrol, didanosine, highly active antriretroviral therapy in HIV patients, irinotecan	Nonalcoholic steatohepatitis/steatofibrosis
Phospholipidosis	
Perhexiline maleate, amiodarone, tamoxifen, diethylaminoethoxyhexestrol, trimethoprim-sulfametoxazole, chloroquine, chlorpromazine	Foamy or ballooned hepatocytes, Mallory-Denk bodies, resemble alcoholic hepatitis
Chronic cholangitis	
Phenothiazines, arsenic, tricyclic antidepressants, antimicrobials, tetracycline, fenofibrate, herbal medicines (germander)	Primary biliary cirrhosis-like
Floxuridine, hepatic artery embolization	Primary sclerosing cholangitis-like
Vascular lesions	
Azathioprine, arsenic, thorothrast, vinyl chloride	Hepatoportal sclerosis
Oral contraceptives, azathioprine	Nodular regenerative hyperplasia
Oral contraceptives	Hepatic artery intimal hyperplasia
Pyrrolizidine alkaloids, azathioprine, chemotherapeutic/alkylating agents, heroin	Veno-occlusive disease
Anabolic steroids, oral contraceptives, danazol, azathioprine	Sinusoidal dilatation/peliosis

Table 3.10.2 (*continued*)

Main Histologic Features and Drugs	Comments and Other Findings
Miscellanous lesions	
Vitamin A	Stellate cell hypertrophy, fibrosis
Phenothiazine, aminopyrine	Lipofuscinosis
Excess dietary iron, alcoholism, total parenteral nutrition	Hemosiderosis
Polyglucosan or pseudo–ground glass inclusion	Phenobarbital, phenytoin, cyanamide, polypharmacotherapy
Methotrexate	Nuclear pleomorphism and hyperchromasia
Increased mitoses	Colchicine, arsenic
Oral contraceptives, anabolic steroids, estrogens	Hepatocellular adenoma
Vinyl chloride, thorotrast	Angiosarcoma
Thorotrast	Cholangiocarcinoma
Anabolic steroids	Hepatocellular carcinoma

3.11 Hereditary Metabolic Diseases

There are 3 more common inherited metabolic diseases that cause chronic liver disease in adults: hereditary hemochromatosis, Wilson disease, and α-1-antitrypsin deficiency.

Hereditary Hemochromatosis

Hereditary hemochromatosis is an autosomal recessive disease resulting in increase intestinal absorption of iron starting at birth. The most common mutation location is in chromosome 6 involving *HFE* gene, which encodes HLA class I–like molecule that regulates intestinal absorption of dietary iron. In *HFE* gene, C282Y is the most common mutation, followed by the less common H63D mutation. C282Y homozygosity causes significant iron accumulation, although the penetrance varies and is believed to be only a few percentage. H63D homozygosity and C282Y/H63D compound heterozygosity cause mild iron accumulation. The heterozygous state is at risk of iron accumulation if the condition is associated with alcohol abuse or other alterations of iron metabolism such as hemolytic anemia. Other very rare iron-related protein abnormalities involving ferroportin, hepcidin, transferrin receptor 2, and hemojuvelin are also recognized as potential causes of iron storage disease.

Overt hemochromatosis is 10 times more frequent in males than in females, with peak incidence between 40 and 60 years. Women are spared by iron loss with menstruation and pregnancy. The typical presentation is in a middle-aged man with abdominal pain, firm hepatomegaly, and normal liver function tests. Usually, there is no evidence of liver failure, ascites, or portal hypertension. Iron deposition in other organs frequently leads to signs and symptoms of cardiomyopathy, diabetes, endocrine abnormalities, infertility, arthropathy, and skin pigmentation. Serum iron, ferritin, and transferrin saturation are markedly increased.

Hereditary hemochromatosis results in a rust-brown firm liver with various degrees of fibrosis or cirrhosis. It leads to preferential loading of hepatocytes by iron. On iron stains, ferritin is dispersed in the cytoplasm and produces a diffuse bluish tint, whereas hemosiderin is present in secondary lysosomes or siderosomes and results in dense blue granules. In the initial stages of the disease in young homozygotic patients, only the periportal hepatocytes are involved, a pattern that is seen in heterozygotes throughout life, as well as in Kupffer cells, portal macrophages, bile ducts (Figure 3.11.1). There is no hepatocyte necrosis and minimal inflammation in the portal tracts and fibrous septa. Increasing portal fibrosis and periportal fibrosis, initially with preservation of the lobular architecture, result in a "holly leaf" appearance (Figures 3.11.2 and 3.11.3). Regenerative nodules and micronodular cirrhosis develop late in the disease. The combination of heavy iron overload of hepatocytes, less iron in reticuloendothelial cells, irregular fibrous septa, and partial preservation of lobular architecture is charac-

teristic of hereditary hemochromatosis (Figures 3.11.4 and 3.11.5).

Because mutation analysis confirms the diagnosis in most cases, liver biopsy is only necessary in C282Y homozygotes to assess whether there is severe fibrosis or cirrhosis to determine the protocol for subsequent follow-up. Iron can be graded semiquantitavely on a scale from 1 to 4: grade 1, minimal iron deposition in periportal hepatocytes; grades 2 and 3, intermediate iron deposition; grade 4, massive iron deposition with obliteration of lobular gradient. If necessary, iron quantification for the calculation of hepatic iron index can be performed on paraffin block after histologic examination.

Wilson Disease

Wilson disease (hepatolenticular degeneration) is an autosomal recessive disorder of copper transport that causes chronic liver disease. The gene that is involved is designated as *ATP7B* on chromosome 13, which encodes transmembrane copper-transporting ATPase. It may progress to fulminant hepatic failure or to cirrhosis. The chronic form of Wilson disease begins between the ages of 6 and 40 years and like chronic hepatitis may be asymptomatic or cause mild fatigability and malaise. The fulminant form of Wilson disease usually affects children or young adults. Kayser-Fleischer rings and neuropsychiatric symptoms, when present, are highly suggestive of the diagnosis. Serum ceruloplasmin less than 20 mg/dL, 24-hour urine copper excretion greater than 100 μg, and quantitative liver copper concentration greater than 250 μg/g dry weight are necessary for definitive diagnosis. Wilson disease should always be considered in the differential diagnosis of any chronic hepatitis, particularly in young patients.

Histologically, Wilson disease often exhibits features of chronic hepatitis or steatohepatitis (Figure 3.11.6 and 3.11.8). Inflammatory cells in portal tracts are less numerous than in chronic viral hepatitis or AIH. However, certainly in the presence of autoimmune markers, the disease can be overlooked. Lymphoid aggregates or follicles are not observed. The increased cellularity in portal tracts and fibrous septa is from ductular reaction. Macrovesicular steatosis, Mallory-Denk hyalin, abundant lipofuscin, and glycogenated nuclei are often present (Figure 3.11.7). Hepatocyte cytoplasm is dense and eosinophilic or ballooned. Severe macrovesicular steatosis or steatohepatitis with or without Mallory-Denk hyalin may be the only changes seen in the early stages of the disease and should be differentiated from ASH or NASH. Cholestasis and areas of collapse are seen in severe cases.

A special stain for copper (rhodanine) may demonstrate increased levels of copper and copper-binding proteins as granules in the cytoplasm of hepatocytes (Figure 3.11.9). In some cases, however, the stains may fail to identify copper, and quantitative hepatic tissue copper determination is necessary to confirm Wilson disease. The presence of copper granules within some cirrhotic nodules, but absent from others, or in hepatocytes away from the periportal or periseptal areas is characteristic of Wilson disease. It should be noted that the presence of copper granules in the periportal or periseptal areas is commonly seen in chronic cholestasis (cholate stasis) due to biliary disease.

α-1-Antitrypsin Deficiency

α-1-Antitrypsin deficiency is an autosomal recessive disorder marked by low serum levels of AAT protease inhibitor, leading to accumulation of AAT in periportal and periseptal hepatocytes, as eosinophilic, periodic acid–Schiff (PAS) with diastase-positive globular inclusions that measure 1 to 10 μm in diameter and surrounded by a clear halo (Figures 3.11.10 and 3.11.11). The presence of AAT in the inclusions can be confirmed by the immunohistochemical stain (Figure 3.11.12). The involved gene is located on chromosome 14q and most commonly caused by homozygosity for PiZ allele (PiZZ). The AAT globules increase in number and size with age and may be inconspicuous in children. In adults, the histologic changes are those of chronic hepatitis with varying degrees of fibrosis and cirrhosis, ductular reaction in fibrotic areas, but inflammation is rarely a prominent feature. In infants, the common presentation is cholestatic liver disease, with morphologic changes of neonatal hepatitis, that is, canalicular cholestasis, giant cell hepatocytes, and ballooning degeneration of hepatocytes, or with ductular reaction and varying degrees of fibrosis and cirrhosis. Therefore, AAT should be included in the differential diagnosis of neonatal cholestasis and extrahepatic biliary atresia in infants.

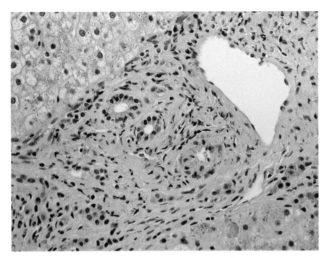

Figure 3.11.1 Marked iron deposition (brown refractive pigment) in hepatocytes, macrophages, bile duct epithelium, and portal stroma in hereditary hemochromatosis.

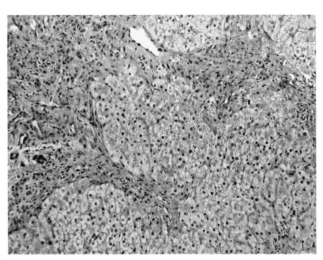

Figure 3.11.2 "Holly leaf" appearance of fibrosis in hereditary hemochromatosis.

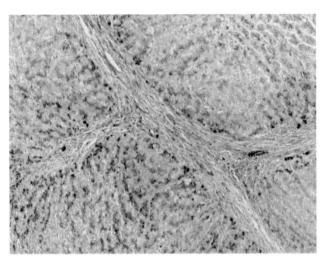

Figure 3.11.3 Perl iron stain confirms iron deposition in cirrhosis secondary to hereditary hemochromatosis.

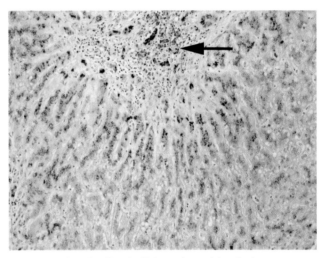

Figure 3.11.4 Grade 3 iron deposition in hepatocytes and portal macrophages (arrow).

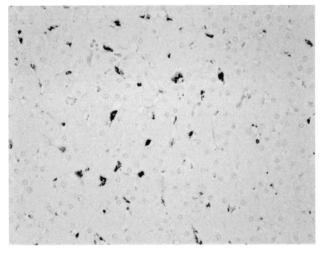

Figure 3.11.5 Iron deposition in Kupffer cells in secondary iron overload.

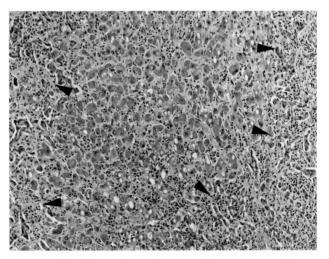

Figure 3.11.6 Wilson disease with area of collapse (arrowheads) and regenerative nodule containing hepatocytes with eosinophilic cytoplasm and Mallory-Denk hyalins and macrovesicular steatosis.

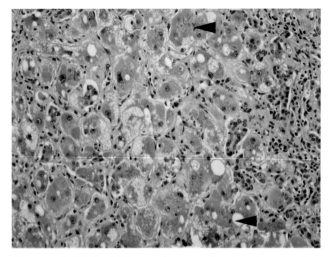

Figure 3.11.7 Wilson disease showing hepatocytes with dense eosinophilic cytoplasm, ballooning, macrovesicular steatosis, and canalicular cholestasis (arrowheads).

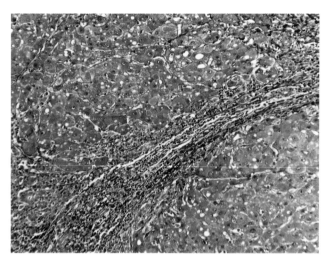

Figure 3.11.8 Cirrhosis secondary to Wilson disease (trichrome stain).

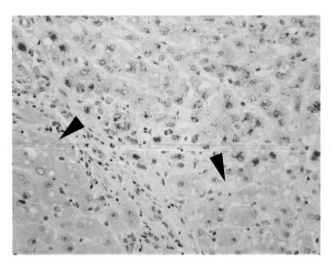

Figure 3.11.9 Abundant copper granules in hepatocytes in one nodule but absent from the next (arrowheads) is characteristic of Wilson disease (Rhodanine stain).

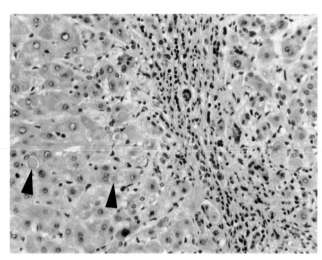

Figure 3.11.10 Eosinophilic globules in periportal hepatocytes in α-1-antitrypsin deficiency.

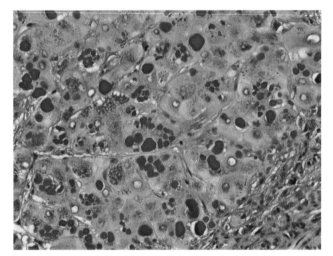

Figure 3.11.11 α-1-Antitrypsin granules and globules in hepatocyte cytoplasm in α-1-antitrypsin deficiency (D-PAS reaction).

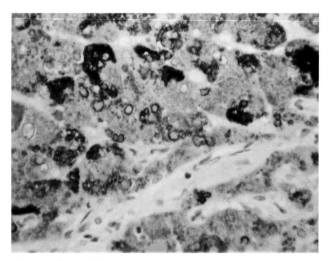

Figure 3.11.12 Immunohistochemical stain confirms the presence α-1-antitrypsin intracytoplasmic globules. Typically, only the outer ring of the globules is stained.

3.12 Diagnosis of Cirrhosis

Cirrhosis is defined as a diffuse process with fibrosis and nodule formation, resulting in significant disturbance of lobular architecture and hepatic circulation. It is the end stage of many liver diseases of various etiologies. The pathogenesis of cirrhosis involves progressive collagen deposition, arteriolization of parenchymal sinusoids, obliteration of portal and hepatic veins, parenchymal extinction, shunt formation, vascular thrombosis, and hepatocyte regeneration.

Cirrhosis is initially thought to be irreversible, but reversibility in early cirrhosis is increasingly considered a feasible option. Resorption of the fibrous tissue results in the "reversal or regression" phenomenon of fibrosis.

A cirrhotic patient usually presents with signs and symptoms of chronic liver disease, portal hypertension, splenomegaly, hypersplenism, ascites, esophageal varices, hepatic encephalopathy, hepatic insufficiency leading to cholestasis, and defects of synthetic and excretory liver functions.

Pathologic Features

Grossly, cirrhosis is a diffuse process characterized by parenchymal nodules, usually with evidence of regeneration, surrounded by connective tissue. The cirrhotic liver is firm and nodular and may be normal in size, enlarged, or shrunken.

Morphologically, cirrhosis has been classically classified as micronodular (fairly homogenous nodules up to 3 mm), macronodular (variable nodules larger than 3 mm surrounded by fibrous septa of varying thickness), or mixed pattern (both micronodules and macronodules); the latter represents the most common form. It has to be realized, however, that this classification is not a precise indication of the etiology of cirrhosis, for example, alcoholic micronodular cirrhosis becomes macronodular during inactive disease and hepatitis C cirrhosis often progresses from initial macronodular toward micronodular cirrhosis. There are 2 uncommon variants of cirrhosis: incomplete septal cirrhosis and postnecrotic cirrhosis. Incomplete septal cirrhosis (often referred to as "regressed fibrosis") is a regressed form

of cirrhosis often associated with portal hypertension but with normal hepatocellular function. It is frequently missed when biopsy specimens are thin and shorter than 2 cm. Postnecrotic cirrhosis is the fibrotic stage of severe acute hepatitis causing large contiguous regions of parenchymal extinction and lesser regions of regenerative hepatocytes.

Liver biopsy represents the best method for the confirmation of cirrhosis (see Table 3.12.1). Connective tissue or reticulin stains are essential for the evaluation of liver biopsies, particularly small transjugular liver biopsy or aspiration biopsy (Figure 3.12.1). Aspiration biopsy often extracts the parenchymal fragments and leaves behind the fibrous septa (Figure 3.12.2). Regenerative nodules are composed of hepatocytes that form 2-cell-thick plates as a result of regeneration. Normal liver parenchyma consists of single cell plates. The nodules are surrounded by fibrous septa that contain various numbers of inflammatory cells, ductular reaction, and dilated vascular or lymphatic channels. The hepatocytes may show various alterations including large cell change, oncocytic change, steatosis, cholestasis, cholate stasis/feathery degeneration, or Mallory-Denk bodies. Small cell change is a preneoplastic condition. In incomplete septal cirrhosis, thin fibrous septa extend from the portal tracts into the parenchyma but often do not connect with other portal tracts or hepatic venules. Portal tracts are variably attenuated, and vascular channels appear relatively increased, although the portal vein often is obliterated or narrowed. "Differential regeneration" and irregular orientation of hepatocyte plates to portal tracts and hepatic venules are suggestive of nodules. Postnecrotic cirrhosis results in misshapen liver with large regenerative regions of liver parenchyma separated by very broad regions of parenchymal scar.

Differential Diagnosis

There are chronic liver diseases that can cause clinical sign and symptoms of cirrhosis (see Table 3.12.2). They should be considered when evaluating liver biopsies in patients with clinical cirrhosis.

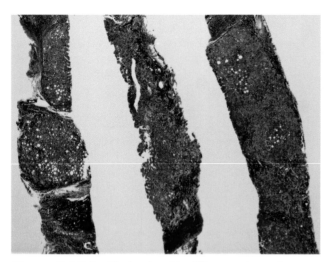

Figure 3.12.1 Cirrhosis with different sizes of regenerative nodules.

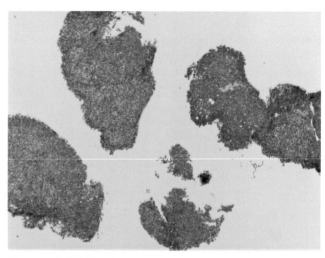

Figure 3.12.2 Fragmentation of biopsy specimen in cirrhosis (trichrome stain).

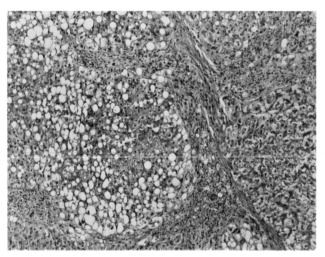

Figure 3.12.3 Cirrhosis secondary to steatohepatitis with steatotic regenerative nodules and hypocellular fibrous septa.

Figure 3.12.4 Alcoholic micronodular cirrhosis.

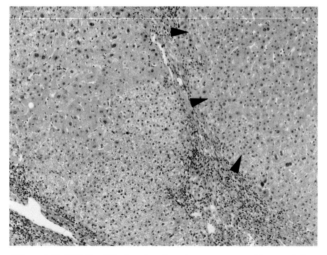

Figure 3.12.5 Cirrhosis showing regenerative nodules with variation of regenerative activity of hepatocytes and concentric hepatocyte plates (arrowheads).

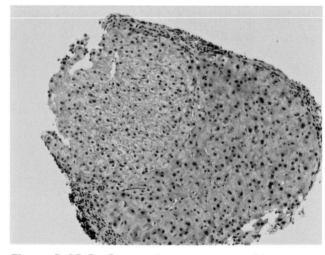

Figure 3.12.6 Concentric arrangement of hepatocyte plates and "differential regeneration" of hepatocytes suggestive of cirrhosis.

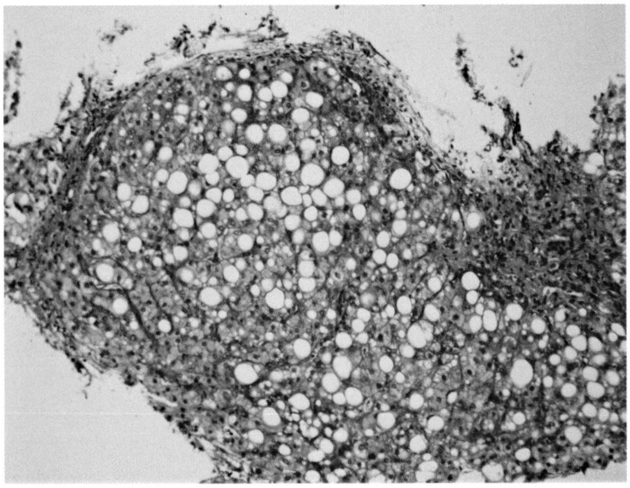

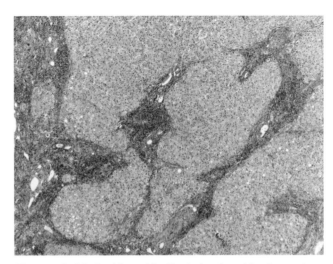

Figure 3.12.7   Connective tissue rim over more than half of circumference of nodule in cirrhosis (trichrome stain).

Figure 3.12.8   Hepatitis C cirrhosis with dense lymphocytic infiltrate in portal tracts.

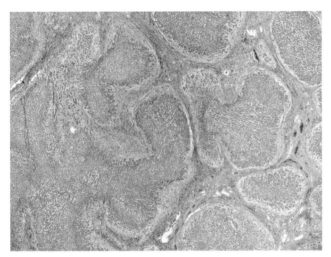

Figure 3.12.9   Mosaic or "jigsaw puzzle" pattern in biliary cirrhosis.

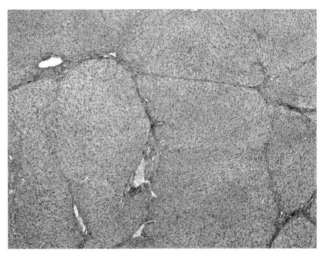

Figure 3.12.10   Regressed fibrosis in patient successfully treated for chronic hepatitis B, showing delicate fibrous septa and absence of inflammation.

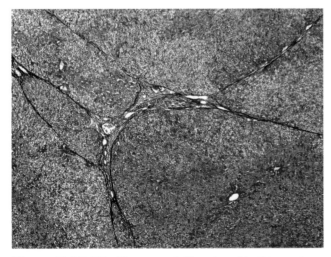

Figure 3.12.11   Regressed fibrosis with thin mature fibrous septa, irregular arrangement of portal tract and hepatic veins, and absence of interface hepatitis and lobular necroinflammatory activity.

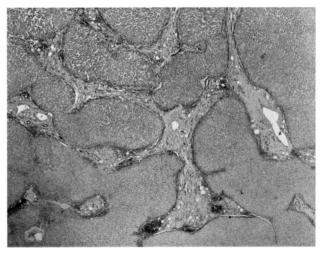

Figure 3.12.12   Postnecrotic cirrhosis after acetaminophen toxicity. The parenchymal nodules are separated by broad fibrous bands.

Table 3.12.1 Diagnosis of Cirrhosis

Definite Features of Cirrhosis	Suggestive Features of Cirrhosis	Suggestive Features of Incomplete Cirrhosis/Regressed Fibrosis
Parenchymal nodules surrounded entirely by fibrous tissue.	Fragmentation of a needle biopsy specimen into round parenchymal pieces	Fragmentation of a needle biopsy specimen into expansive sheets of liver parenchyma without portal tracts and without obvious central hepatic venules
Fibrous septa linking portal tracts and central venules. Septa between portal tracts or between central venules in advanced fibrosis.	Connective tissue rim over more than half of the circumference of a parenchymal fragment	Delicate remnants of mature fibrous septa
	Fibrous septa extending from portal tracts into parenchyma without reaching the central venules	Irregular arrangement of portal tracts and hepatic veins
	Concentric arrangement of hepatocyte plates, particularly at the periphery of parenchymal fragments	Irregularity of parenchymal atrophy and hyperplasia (nodular regeneration)
	Variations in the degree of regenerative activity of hepatocytes resulting in differences in nuclear and cell size, plate thickness ("differential regeneration") and compression of adjacent liver tissue	Regenerative activity of hepatocytes resulting in differences in plate thickness
	Variations between nodules in the content of fat, glycogen iron, lipofuscin, copper, bile or inflammatory cells	Absence of interface hepatitis or lobular necroinflammatory activity
	Disproportion between portal tracts and central venules with reduction in number, absence or hypoplasia of portal tracts and increased number of hepatic veins	Absence of fat or ballooning degeneration of hepatocytes

Table 3.12.2 Conditions Mimicking Cirrhosis

Diagnosis	Histologic Features
Alcoholic central hyalin sclerosis	Severe extinction of centrilobular hepatocytes replaced by fibrosis, chicken-wire fibrosis, Mallory-Denk bodies, neutrophils. No regenerative nodules, portal tracts initially normal.
Long standing severe congestive heart failure	Centrilobular dilatation of sinusoids and central venules, followed by perisinusoidal fibrosis, hepatocyte atrophy containing small droplet fat or lipofuscin pigment. No regenerative nodules.
Secondary biliary cirrhosis from prolonged bile duct obstruction	Portal and perilobular fibrosis, dilated bile ducts with periductal fibrosis, cholate-stasis in periportal hepatocytes. No regenerative nodules.
Hepatic schistosomiasis	Fibrous obliteration and thickening portal vein branches, extensive dense portal fibrosis (so-so called pipestem fibrosis), thin-walled vascular channels in portal tracts and septa. Granuloma with schistosoma eggs, hemozoin pigment in Kupffer cells and portal tracts.
Hypervitaminosis A	Extensive fibrosis along sinusoids. Hepatic stellate cell hyperplasia containing fat globules and scalloping of the nuclei.
Myeloproliferative disorders	Extramedullary hematopoiesis accompanied by fibrosis of the sinusoids.
Congenital hepatic fibrosis	Dense fibrous septa separating islands of normal liver parenchyma. Elongated or cystic well-formed bile duct structures in the periphery of portal tracts or scattered throughout fibrous septa.
Veno-occlusive disease	Congestion of centrilobular and midzonal region with occlusion of central venules by loose fibrous tissue.
Nodular regenerative hyperplasia	Hyperplastic parenchymal nodule without fibrous septa, compression of surrounding parenchyma with congestion.
Hepatoportal sclerosis	Portal fibrosis, thickening, absence or marked narrowing of portal veins, localized engorgement of periportal sinusoids, parenchymal atrophy accompanied by sinusoidal dilatation.
Portal vein thrombosis	Portal vein fibrosis or obliteration, centrilobular hepatocyte atrophy with sinusoidal dilatation, reverse lobulation.
Gaucher disease	Accumulation of pale macrophages in portal tracts and sinusoids with striated cytoplasmic appearance.
Sarcoidosis	Multiple often coalescing nonnecrotizing epithelioid granulomas with associated fibrosis.

3.13　Fibropolycystic Disease of the Liver

Fibropolycystic disease of the liver is a group of congenital diseases caused by embryonal ductal plate malformation that includes congenital hepatic fibrosis, polycystic liver disease, Caroli disease, and biliary microhamartoma (von Meyenburg complex). The defect "cholangiociliopathy" allows the possibility that different diseases are expressed alone or in various combinations in the same liver. In addition, different family members of a proband may exhibit different abnormalities of the biliary tree.

Fibropolycystic diseases clinically result in 3 effects depending on which abnormality predominates: space-occupying lesions (polycystic liver disease), portal hypertension (congenital hepatic fibrosis), and cholangitis (Caroli disease). Biliary microhamartomas do not give rise to liver abnormalities or symptoms but may be seen in association with other forms of fibropolycystic disease. Cholangiography and other imaging methods of liver and bile ducts and liver biopsy are important for the diagnosis. Polycystic disease of the kidneys is associated to a variable extent. Cholangiocarcinoma may complicate this disease.

Congenital Hepatic Fibrosis

Congenital hepatic fibrosis occurs both in sporadic form and familial form with autosomal recessive inheritance. It is often associated with autosomal recessive polycystic kidney disease, which may manifest in early life, whereas the liver disease is diagnosed between ages 3 and 10 years or even later.

In congenital hepatic fibrosis, islands of normal liver parenchyma are separated by broad or narrow septa of dense mature fibrous tissue containing elongated or cystic well-formed bile duct structures, sometimes filled with inspissated bile (Figures 3.13.1 and 3.13.2). Portal tracts are incorporated in the fibrous bands and may contain normal or ectatic interlobular bile ducts in the center. Portal vein branches are hypoplastic or completely absent. The parenchymal islands vary in shape like mosaic and maintain a normal vascular relationship with central venules. The hepatocytes are arranged in regular plates rather than regenerative 2-cell-thick plates forming true nodules as in cirrhosis. There is no inflammation in the parenchyma or in the fibrous septa. Inflammation, cholestasis, and/or cholangitis should raise the possibility of associated Caroli disease or choledochal cyst.

Congenital hepatic fibrosis must be distinguished from cirrhosis. Because liver function is preserved in congenital hepatic fibrosis, the prognosis is considerably better following portacaval shunt to relieve portal hypertension.

Caroli Disease

Caroli disease may affect different parts of the intrahepatic biliary tree and is seen alone or in combination with other forms of fibropolycystic liver disease, particularly congenital hepatic fibrosis (Caroli syndrome). It is characterized by segmental saccular dilatations of the intrahepatic bile ducts, surrounded by extensive fibrosis (Figure 3.13.3). The dilated ducts connect with the main duct system. Therefore, bile duct cysts in Caroli disease often contain inspissated bile or bile stones and show chronic inflammatory infiltrate and neutrophilic infiltrate from recurrent ascending cholangitis or abscess formation (Figure 3.13.4). Acute inflammation is often superimposed with ulceration of the bile duct epithelium and pus in the lumen mixed with bile and mucus. When the epithelium of the cystic bile ducts is preserved, it is often columnar and hypertrophic.

Antibiotic treatment may be required for cholangitis. Recurrent drainage of the bile ducts may be required to remove calculi. Localized involvement may be treated by resection. Liver transplantation may be an option in diffuse disease.

Polycystic Liver Disease

Polycystic liver disease causes nodular enlargement of the liver, but hepatic function is normal. It may involve the liver diffusely or restricted to one lobe, usually the left lobe. The cysts measure up to 10 cm in diameter filled with clear or rarely hemorrhagic fluid. The cysts in polycystic liver disease are not connected with the main biliary system. The cysts are lined by low cuboidal or flattened biliary epithelial cells (Figure 3.13.5). They do not contain bile, and there is no associated cholangitis. Frequently, microhamartomas are also present.

Polycystic liver disease is compatible with long life. The prognosis depends on the associated polycystic renal disease. Aspiration of the cysts or surgical resection may be considered for large cysts.

Biliary Microhamartomas

Biliary microhamartomas are common in patients with congenital hepatic fibrosis and polycystic liver disease. Biliary microhamartomas (von Meyenburg complexes) are located in or close to portal tracts and rarely exceed 3 mm in diameter. They represent solitary or multiple small nodules of dense collagen containing many interconnecting mature bile duct structures lined by cuboidal biliary epithelium, which often contain inspissated bile (Figure 3.13.6). Biliary microhamartomas do not require treatment.

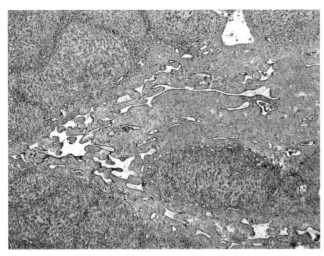

Figure 3.13.1 Broad and thin mature fibrous septa containing elongated and dilated interconnecting bile duct structure, separating islands of normal liver parenchyma, in congenital hepatic fibrosis.

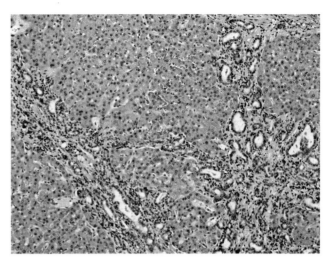

Figure 3.13.2 Congenital hepatic fibrosis with interconnecting dilated bile duct structure in mature fibrous septa.

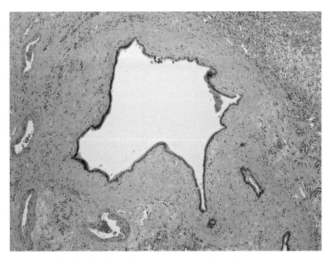

Figure 3.13.3 Cystic bile duct in Caroli disease.

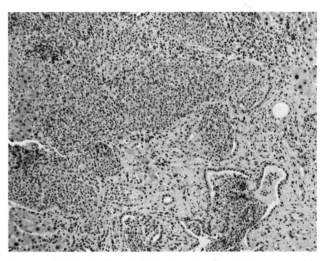

Figure 3.13.4 Cystic bile duct in Caroli disease with acute cholangitis.

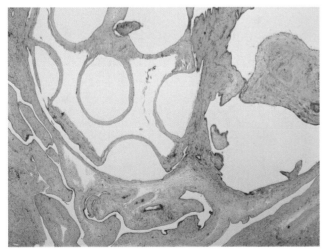

Figure 3.13.5 Multiple cysts lined by flat to cuboidal biliary epithelium in polycystic liver disease.

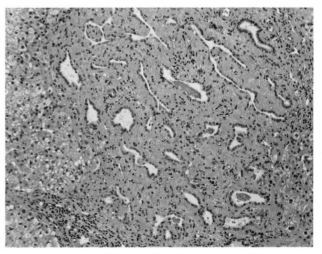

Figure 3.13.6 Biliary microhamartoma (Meyenburg complex) composed of small bile duct structures lined by cuboidal biliary epithelium containing inspissated bile.

Table 3.13.1 Fibropolycystic Disease of the Liver

Characteristics	Congenital Hepatic Fibrosis	Caroli Disease	Polycystic Liver Disease	Biliary Microhamartoma
Genetic mutation	Fibrocystin gene	Not identified	Polycystin-1 and polycystin-2 genes (*PKD1*, *PKD2*)	Not identified
Age, sex	3-10 years old, rarely later age	Any age, M>F	Adult, F>M	
Clinical features	Portal hypertension, splenomegaly, large firm liver	Recurrent fever, jaundice, abdominal pain, hepatomegaly	Abdominal pain, hepatomegaly	Asymptomatic
Inheritance	Sporadic, autosomal recessive	Autosomal recessive or dominant	Autosomal dominant	Sporadic, autosomal recessive or dominant
Association	Autosomal recessive polycystic kidney disease, Caroli disease	Congenital hepatic fibrosis	Autosomal dominant polycystic kidney disease	Congenital hepatic fibrosis, polycystic liver disease
Liver enzyme activities	Normal	Cholestatic	Normal	Normal
Communication with biliary tree	No	Yes	No	No
Cyst features	Persistent cystic duct plate remnants in periphery of portal tracts	Dilated segmental bile ducts, often wrapping hepatic artery	Multiple large cysts, massively replacing liver parenchyma	Dilated or tortuous small ductular structures embedded in hyalinized stroma, near or in portal tracts
Cyst content	Inspissated bile	Bile, inflammatory cells, pus	Clear fluid	Inspissated bile

3.14 Outflow Problem

Although there are different etiologies, pathogeneses, and location, anatomical or functional venous outflow obstruction results in similar clinical symptoms. In severe acute stage, patients present with sudden onset of high-protein ascites, painful hepatomegaly, and mild jaundice. In chronic form, patients present with an enlarged tender liver, ascites, and other signs and symptoms of portal hypertension as seen in cirrhosis. Causes of venous outflow obstruction include Budd-Chiari syndrome (BCS) and veno-occlusive disease (VOD). Chronic passive congestion of the liver may become so severe that it resembles BCS or VOD. Alcoholic central hyalin sclerosis produces extensive centrilobular fibrosis that may mimic outflow problem.

There are similarities in gross and histologic features in BCS, VOD, and severe chronic passive congestion: nutmeg liver, centrilobular sinusoidal dilatation, extravasation of red blood cells to the space of Disse, atrophy of centrilobular hepatocytes, centrilobular hemosiderin deposition in Kupffer cells, preservation and regenerative hyperplasia of periportal hepatocytes, and unremarkable portal tracts.

Budd-Chiari syndrome

Budd-Chiari syndrome is characterized by occlusion of large hepatic veins or intrahepatic or suprahepatic portion of the inferior vena cava. Budd-Chiari syndrome occurs in patients with hypercoagulable states, particularly myeloproliferative disorders, acquired and inherited thrombophilias, and oral contraceptives (primary BCS); malignant neoplasms such as renal cell carcinoma or hepatocellular carcinomas growing into the inferior vena cava; trauma; or membranous obstruction of the inferior vena cava (secondary BCS).

In both BCS and VOD, the liver is dark red and enlarged with rounded edges. The cut surface shows dark red areas with centrilobular congestion and congestive bridges surrounding pale brown parenchyma, which represents reverse lobulation and results in a nutmeg appearance. Regenerative hyperplasia leads to yellow to pale brown nodular areas. Thickened hepatic veins may be demonstrable. Caudate lobe enlargement is a characteristic finding in BCS.

Budd-Chiari syndrome causes severe dilatation and congestion of centrilobular and midzonal sinusoids with extravasation of red blood cells into the space of Disse and hepatic plates (Figure 3.14.1). This results in compression and loss of hepatocytes with formation of blood lakes. The periportal hepatocytes are relatively preserved, and the portal tracts are intact. Chronic BCS leads to extensive centrilobular fibrosis with fibrous bridges to adjacent centrilobular areas (Figure 3.14.2). Hemosiderin deposition is noted in Kupffer cells in the centrilobular areas. The central venules are patent and dilated.

Veno-occlusive disease

Veno-occlusive disease is characterized by occlusion of the central hepatic venules and sublobular hepatic veins as the result of endothelial damage from, among others, pyrrolizidine alkaloids in herbal teas, radiation to the liver, or chemotherapy, particularly in association with bone marrow transplantation.

The gross findings in VOD are similar to those of BCS, except for the presence of occlusion that may be seen in hepatic venules or veins of VOD cases.

Veno-occlusive disease causes dilatation and congestion of centrilobular and midzonal sinusoids with extravasation or red blood cells into the space of Disse, similar to those seen in BCS, but in VOD, the central hepatic venules and sublobular veins show subintimal edema, fibrin deposition, and partial to complete occlusion of the lumen by loose fibrous tissue (Figures 3.14.3 and 3.14.4). Venous occlusion may be focal and difficult to find in biopsy specimens. In chronic stage, fibrous tissue is deposited in centrilobular sinusoids with formation of fibrous bridges to adjacent centrilobular areas and is referred to as "sinusoidal obstruction syndrome."

Chronic Passive Congestion

Chronic passive congestion is seen in patients with congestive heart failure due to coronary artery disease, cardiomyopathy, valvular diseases, and constrictive pericarditis. It may lead to cardiac cirrhosis.

Patients with chronic passive congestion present with mild jaundice, right upper abdominal pain, enlarged tender liver, and ascites similar to the other 2 disorders, but features of portal hypertension are usually absent, except for splenomegaly. Cardiac problems are usually the major manifestations.

Chronic passive congestion is characterized by dilatation and congestion of central venules and centrilobular sinusoids with compression of the hepatocytes (Figure 3.14.5). The latter contain increased amount of lipofuscin, fat globules, and sometimes bile pigments in the cytoplasm or bile plugs in canaliculi. In severe, long-standing cases, centrilobular hepatocytes are replaced by fibrous tissue. The central venules, however, remain patent, although the wall may be thickened and the surrounding sinusoids are engorged. All of this results in reversed lobulation with normal portal tracts surrounded by unaffected parenchyma (Figure 3.14.6). Eventually, fibrous bridges form between adjacent centrilobular areas, but regenerative nodules and true cirrhosis are extremely rare.

In some patients, intracytoplasmic PAS-positive globules can be seen in a centrilobular congested area, morphologically similar to those of α-1-antitrypsin globules but in centrilobular and not in periportal location (see "Intracytoplasmic Inclusions").

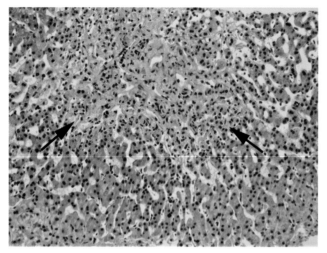

Figure 3.14.1 Centrilobular necrosis in Budd-Chiari syndrome (arrows) with midzonal sinusoidal dilatation.

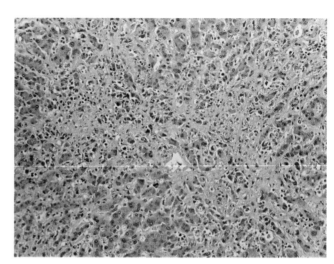

Figure 3.14.2 Chronic Budd-Chiari syndrome with centrilobular fibrosis, congestion, hepatocyte atrophy, and hemosiderin in Kupffer cells.

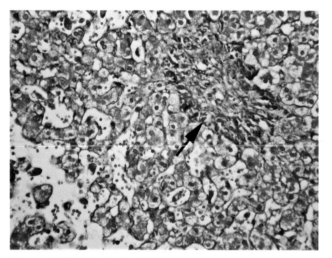

Figure 3.14.3 Occluded central venule (arrow) in veno-occlusive disease (trichrome stain).

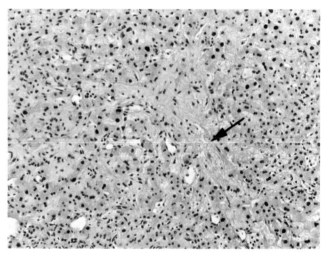

Figure 3.14.4 Occluded central venule (arrow) and sinusoidal fibrosis in radiation-induced veno-occlusive disease.

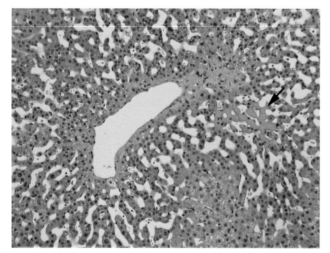

Figure 3.14.5 Chronic passive congestion with dilated and thickened central venule, centrilobular sinusoidal dilatation, small droplet fat in centrilobular hepatocytes, and extravasation of red blood cells to the space of Disse (arrow).

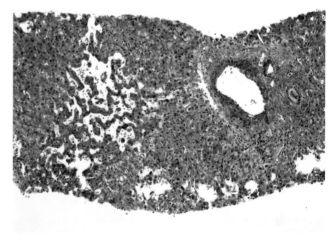

Figure 3.14.6 "Cardiac sclerosis" with centrilobular sinusoidal dilatation, fibrosis, and reverse lobulation of parenchyma.

Table 3.14.1   Differential Diagnosis of Outflow Problem

Histologic Features	Chronic Passive Congestion	Budd-Chiari Syndrome	Veno-Occlusive Disease	Alcoholic Central Hyalin Sclerosis
Centrilobular congestion	+	++	+	–
Extravasation of red blood cells	+ (when severe)/–	++	+	–
Central venule dilatation	+	+	–	–
Central venule thickening	++	++	+	++
Central venule occlusion	–	+/–	+	++
Sinusoidal dilatation	++	+	+	–
Centrilobular steatosis	+	–	–	++
Reverse lobulation	+	+	+	–
Centrilobular hemosiderosis	+	++	++	–
Mallory-Denk bodies	–	–	–	++

++ indicates almost always present; +, usually present; +/–, occasionally present; –, usually absent.

3.15   Intracytoplasmic Inclusions

There are 3 common morphologic categories of intracytoplasmic inclusions associated with various chronic liver diseases, metabolic liver diseases, and drug-induced liver injury: (1) globular eosinophilic inclusions, (2) coarse eosinophilic inclusions, and (3) ground glass–like inclusions. In addition, many of these inclusions are often exaggerated in hepatocellular carcinoma, necessitating the differential diagnosis of hepatocellular carcinoma when inclusions are present in abundance and a neoplasm is suspected.

Globular Eosinophilic Inclusions

Inclusions in this category are characterized by single or multiple, round to oval eosinophilic intracytoplasmic globules, including α-1-antitrypsin (AAT) inclusions, passive congestion inclusions, and giant mitochondria.

α-1-antitrypsin inclusions are predominantly periportal or periseptal in location (Figure 3.15.1). The globules are larger, multiple, and more easily identified on hematoxylin-eosin in older individuals or cirrhotic liver due to AAT deficiency. Immunohistochemical stain for AAT is confirmatory and more sensitive than PAS-D stain (Figures 3.15.2 and 3.11.12).

Passive congestion inclusions demonstrate similar characteristics and positivity for PAS and PAS-D stains as AAT, but passive congestion inclusions are predominantly located in the congested centrilobular region and often concurrent with fat vacuoles as the result of hypoxia (Figures 3.15.4 and 3.15.5). Passive congestion inclusions tend to be more regular in size when compared with AAT inclusions.

Giant mitochondria or megamitochondria are round to spindle-shaped inclusions, often present in alcoholic liver disease and to a lesser extent in NASH. In alcoholic liver disease, they are predominantly distributed in a centrilobular area and associated with hepatocyte ballooning. In NASH, they can be seen in the periportal area. They are similar in color to AAT inclusions on H&E–stained slides but usually no more than 1 to 2 giant mitochondria per hepatocytes (Figure 3.15.3).

Irregularly Shaped Eosinophilic Inclusions

Mallory-Denk hyalins are the only irregularly shaped eosinophilic inclusions identified in hepatocytes (Figure 3.15.6). They represent clumps or strands of intermediate filaments of the cytoskeleton, which are positive for cytokeratins 8 and 18, ubiquitin, and p62. Mallory-Denk hyalins are the hallmark of ASH and NASH. They are also seen in a variety of other chronic liver disorders with chronic cholestasis and/or cholate stasis, particularly late stages of PBC and PSC; in Wilson disease; in drug-induced liver diseases; and in hepatocellular carcinoma.

Ground Glass–Like Inclusions

Inclusions in this category include HBsAg inclusions, fibrinogen inclusions, Lafora bodies, and Lafora-like bodies or polyglucosan inclusions. They are characterized by finely granular, pale eosinophilic ground glass–like appearance, often surrounded by a "halo" and when large becomes crescentic and displaces hepatocyte nucleus to the periphery. Other eosinophilic changes that can be confused with ground glass hepatocytes are hepatic oncocytes and induction cells.

Hepatitis B surface antigen accumulates in the smooth endoplasmic reticulum producing the classic pale, finely granular "ground glass hepatocytes," encountered in patients with chronic hepatitis B, and their presence can be detected by immunohistochemical stain for HBsAg and orcein or Victoria blue stain (Figure 3.15.7).

Fibrinogen inclusion varies from round deeply eosinophilic inclusion to finely granular pale eosinophilic inclusion, seen in fibrinogen storage diseases (Figure 3.15.10). In hepatocellular carcinoma and fibrolamellar carcinoma, fibrinogen inclusions are referred as "pale bodies."

Lafora bodies in hepatocytes are seen in patients with progressive familial myoclonic epilepsy (Figure 3.15.8). They are identified by their content of mucopolysaccharides. Lafora-like bodies or polyglucosan inclusions fundamentally are non–membrane-bound intracytoplasmic glycogen that can be encountered in various liver diseases, such as glycogenosis type IV, cyanamide aversion therapy for alcohol abuse, and polyglucosan body disease (Figure 3.15.9). The term *pseudo–ground glass* for these inclusions was previously used in patients with polypharmacotherapy.

Induction bodies are pale ground-glass–like cytoplasmic inclusion seen in drug-induced injury, particularly barbiturates, chlorpromazine, or azathioprine that cause induction of cytochrome P450, resulting in increase of smooth endoplasmic reticulum. They are located in the periportal or centrilobular area (Figure 3.15.12).

Hepatic oncocytes (also known as oncocytic hepatocytes) are hepatocytes with distinctively dense, finely granular, and strongly eosinophilic cytoplasm due to densely packed mitochondria, resembling oncocytes in other exocrine or endocrine glands (Figure 3.15.11). Hepatic oncocytes are found only in cirrhosis of various etiologies. They are located primarily adjacent to the periportal or periseptal area and are often surrounded by fibrous tissue.

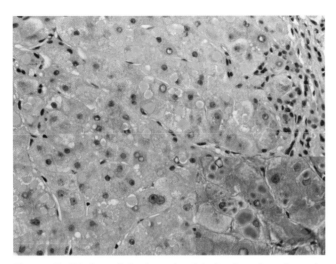

Figure 3.15.1   α-1-Antitrypsin globules in α-1-antitrypsin deficiency are faintly eosinophilic, better visualized on trichrome stain (inset) or PAS-D stain.

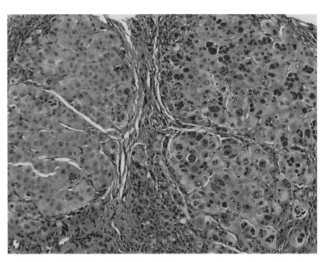

Figure 3.15.2   PAS-D stain shows irregular distribution of α-1-Antitrypsin globules in cirrhotic nodules.

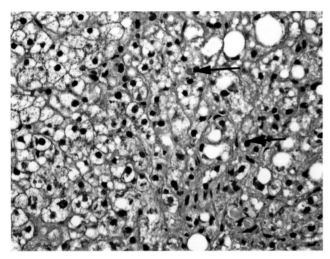

Figure 3.15.3   Giant mitochondria (arrows) are better visualized in ballooned hepatocytes in steatohepatitis.

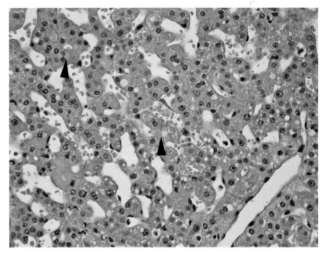

Figure 3.15.4   Chronic passive congestion showing centrilobular eosinophilic globules (arrowheads) in hepatocytes in the area of congestion.

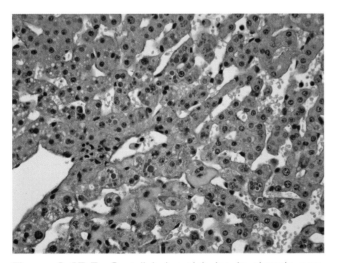

Figure 3.15.5   Centrilobular globules in chronic passive congestion are positive for PAS-D, similar to α-1-antitrypsin globules.

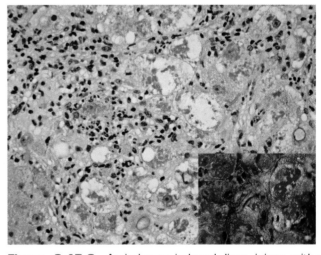

Figure 3.15.6   Amiodarone-induced liver injury with numerous irregularly shaped Mallory-Denk hyalins. Mallory-Denk hyalin is red in trichrome stain (inset).

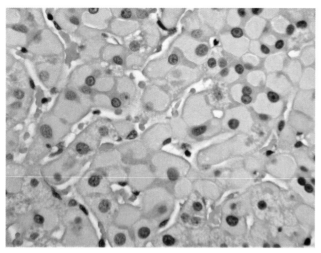

Figure 3.15.7 Chronic hepatitis B showing numerous ground glass hepatocytes.

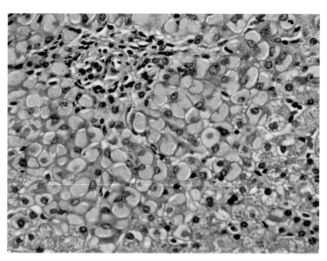

Figure 3.15.8 Lafora bodies in myoclonus epilepsy consisting of predominantly non–membrane-bound mucopolysaccharide deposition.

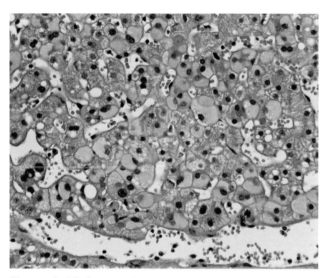

Figure 3.15.9 Polyglucosan bodies or pseudo–ground glass hepatocytes in polypharmacotherapy.

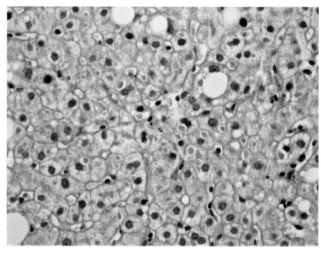

Figure 3.15.10 Fibrinogen pale eosinophilic inclusion in fibrinogen storage disease (PAS-D stain).

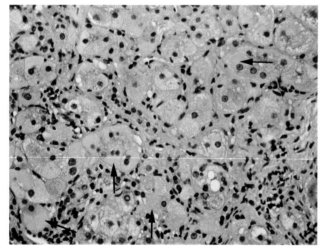

Figure 3.15.11 Numerous hepatic oncocytes or oncocytic hepatocytes (arrows) in cirrhosis as the result of densely packed mitochondria may be confused with ground glass hepatocytes in chronic hepatitis B.

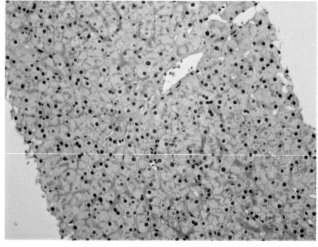

Figure 3.15.12 Increased in smooth endoplasmic reticulum producing pale ground glass-like hepatocytes "induction cells" in drug-induced injury.

Table 3.15.1 Intracytoplasmic Inclusions

	Location	Trichrome	PAS-D	PTAH	Orcein or HBsAg	Colloidal Iron	Ultrastructure	Associated Conditions
Globular eosinopilic inclusion								
α-1-Antirypsin inclusion	Periportal	red	+	–	–	–	Finely granular material in dilated endoplasmic reticulum or in membrane-bound vacuoles	α-1-Antitrypsin deficiency, cirrhosis caused by other conditions
Giant (or mega-) mitochondria	Centrilobular (alcoholic), periportal (nonalcoholic)	red	–	+	–	–	Dilated mitochondria with crystalloid bodies	Alcoholic and nonalcoholic steatohepatitis
Passive congestion inclusion	Centrilobular	red/blue	+	–	–	–	Microfibrillar material with occasional rod-shaped material in lysosomes	Chronic passive congestion
Coarse eosinophilic inclusion								
Mallory-Denk hyalin	Centrilobular (steatohepatitis), periportal (chronic cholestasis)	red/purple	–	–	–	–	Cytokeratin intermediate filament	Alcoholic and nonalcoholic steatohepatitis, Wilson's disease, drug induced injury, hepatocellular carcinoma
Ground glass-like inclusion								
Hepatitis B surface antigen inclusion	Azonal	light red	–	–	+	–	Hepatitis B surface antigen in smooth endoplasmic reticulum	Chronic hepatitis B infection
Fibrinogen	Azonal	gray/light blue	–	+/–	–	–	Dilated rough endoplasmic reticulum with tubular fingerprint-like structures	Fibrinogen storage disease, hepatocellular carcinoma (pale bodies)
Lafora(-like) bodies or polyglucosan inclusion	Azonal	light red	–	–	–	+	Intracytoplasmic glycogen granules, non membrane bound	Polypharmacotherapy, polyglucosan body disease, glycogenosis type IV, myoclonus epilepsy (Lafora's disease), cyanamide aversion therapy for alcohol abuse
Hepatic oncocytes	Periseptal or periportal in cirrhosis	red	–	+	–	–	Densely packed mitochondria	Cirrhosis of various etiologies
Induction hepatocytes	Periportal or centrilobular	light red/gray	–	–	–	–	Increased smooth endoplasmic reticulum	Drug-induced injury

PAS indicates periodic acid–Schiff; PAS-D, periodic acid–Schiff with diastase digestion; PTAH, phosphotungstic acid hematoxylin; HBsAg, hepatitis B surface antigen; +, positive; –, negative; +/–, weakly positive.

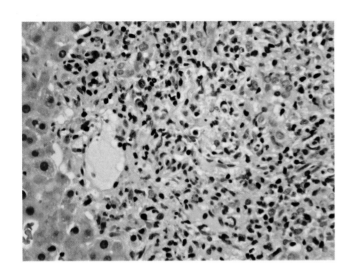

CHAPTER 4

TRANSPLANT LIVER DISORDERS

4.1   Donor Liver Evaluation

The donor liver is frequently subjected to frozen section analysis, prompted by clinical history of the donor, circumstances surrounding donor death, or macroscopic appearance of the organ such as a grossly fatty liver, which raises uncertainty on the suitability of the donor organ for transplantation.

Liver Biopsy Size and Preparation

A 2.0-cm-long needle core from the anterior inferior edge of the liver is adequate in most cases, when the anticipated changes are diffuse. It is crucial that the biopsy is freshly obtained to reduce preservation artifacts, which result in underestimation or overestimation of the degree of steatosis or necrosis. In addition, biopsies kept in saline are significantly impacted by this medium, resulting in clumping of the cytoplasm and edema of the extracellular spaces. Routine hematoxylin & eosin–stained frozen section is adequate to determine the type and severity of steatosis and pathology in donor liver.

Cadaveric Donor Liver Evaluation

Although the criteria of a donor liver evolve over time, transplantation is currently contraindicated when infectious disease, sepsis, malignant tumor, or severe macrovesicular steatosis involving 60% or more of the parenchyma is detected. Other criteria considered include age of donor more than 60 years, extended cold ischemia (>12 hours), donation after cardiac death, extended intensive care unit stay, and history of malignancy.

Because recurrent hepatitis C virus (HCV) infection is universal after liver transplantation and its progression is not affected by the HCV status of the donor, HCV-positive donor organs with mild inflammation and nonbridging fibrosis have been increasingly used for recipients with end-stage HCV liver disease (Figure 4.1.6).

Severe macrovesicular steatosis (Figure 4.1.1) commonly results in primary graft nonfunction, caused by lysis of the steatotic hepatocytes. In less than severe macrovesicular steatosis, the recipient surgeon decides the risk-to-benefit ratio of using the less-than-optimal organ for transplantation in a particular recipient.

Microvesicular steatosis (or often referred to as small droplet steatosis) is not a contraindication for donor liver because it is often found after a short period of warm ischemia and other insults and does not reliably predict posttransplant function (Figure 4.1.2).

Living Donor Liver Evaluation

Living donor liver transplantation has been increasingly taking the place of cadaveric liver transplantation to supplement the significant shortage of cadaveric donors. To minimize the risk of donation, donor evaluation is considerably more thorough, and therefore, unexpected pathologic findings are less common. The most common donor biopsy abnormality is fatty liver disease, and in general, less than 30% macrovesicular steatosis is preferred. Mild iron overload in periportal hepatocytes (1+ on a scale of 0-4) does not detract donation.

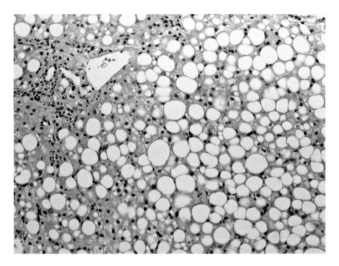

Figure 4.1.1   Severe steatosis disqualifies donation.

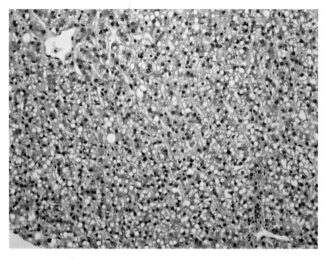

Figure 4.1.2   Diffuse microvesicular steatosis (small droplet steatosis) due to warm ischemia.

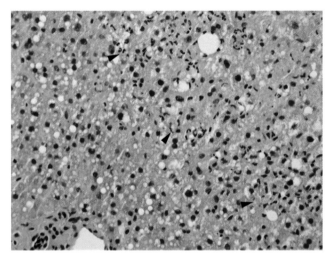

Figure 4.1.3   Centrilobular coagulative necrosis (arrowheads) with neutrophils due to hypotensive shock, in the background of microvesicular steatosis (small droplet steatosis).

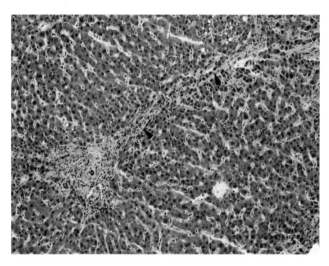

Figure 4.1.4   Donor liver with portal fibrosis and fibrous septum (arrowheads).

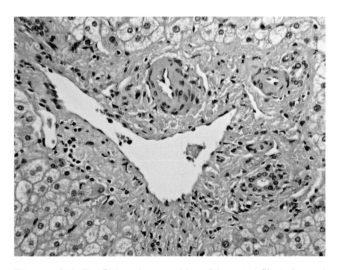

Figure 4.1.5   Older donor with mild portal fibrosis and thickened hepatic artery.

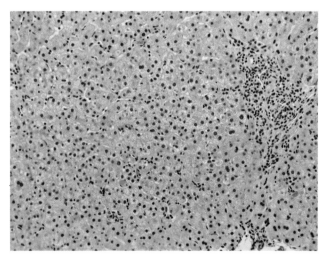

Figure 4.1.6   Chronic hepatitis C with low grade and stage in donor liver.

Table 4.1.1 Common Findings in Donor Liver Evaluation

Conditions or Findings	Pathologic Features	Significance
Fatty liver disease	Macrovesicular steatosis, ballooning degeneration, rare neutrophils	>60% disqualifies organ
Prolonged warm ischemia	Microvesicular steatosis	Does not reliably predict posttransplant function
Prolonged cold ischemia (>12 h)	No definite pathologic changes	Higher frequency of biliary problem and graft failure
Prolonged intensive care unit stay	Nonspecific reactive hepatitis, ductular reaction	No significance, does not predict posttransplant function
Hypotensive shock	Centrilobular coagulative necrosis to diffuse necrosis	Diffuse necrosis causes graft failure
Older donor	Centrilobular lipofuscinosis, thickened hepatic arteries, portal fibrosis, parenchymal atrophy	Generally older donor livers do not function as well as younger donor livers. Rapid fibrosis in HCV-positive recipient
Chronic B or C viral hepatitis	Low inflammation grade and fibrosis stage are common	HBV- or HCV-positive donors with low grade and stage are triaged to HBV- or HCV-positive recipients. Severe activity and high stage disqualify donor
Malignant liver tumor	Hepatocellular carcinoma, cholangiocarcinoma	Disqualify donor
Benign liver tumor	Hepatocellular adenoma	Disqualify donor
	Focal nodular hyperplasia, biliary hamartoma, bile duct adenoma, cavernous hemangioma	No significance. Liver can be used after tumor is excised
Granuloma	Localized or diffuse granulomata. Foreign body type granuloma or infectious granuloma	Workup for infectious granuloma should be considered posttransplant

4.2 Preservation Injury

The term *preservation injury* is used to describe the organ damage that results from the effects of cold and warm ischemia followed by reperfusion. Preservation is one of the causes of liver allograft failure within the first few weeks after transplantation. Livers harvested from a donor with preexisting diseases, who are older, hemodynamically unstable, or after cardiac death are relatively more susceptible to preservation injury. Excessive manipulation during organ harvest, prolonged cold ischemic time (>12 hours) and warm ischemic time (>120 minutes), or complicated vascular reconstruction often compounds the problem. Other causes of early allograft failure include vascular thrombosis and biliary tract complications (see Table 4.2.1).

Severe early graft dysfunction is characterized by various degrees of encephalopathy, coma, renal failure associated with lactic acidosis, persistent coagulopathy, poor bile production, and marked elevations of aminotransferase activities. Otherwise, the clinical signs and symptoms and the timing of less severe preservation injury are similar to those of acute rejection. Liver biopsy is required for definitive diagnosis. Comparison with previous biopsy and correlation with the clinical course are useful to determine the precise cause of allograft dysfunction.

Severe preservation injury leading to early allograft failure is clinically referred to as primary graft dysfunction, which is divided into initial poor function (IPF) and primary nonfunction. The IPF is characterized by aspartate aminotransferase greater that 2000 IU/mL and prothrombin longer than 20 seconds in the first week after transplantation. Primary nonfunction is defined as death or need for retransplantation within 2 weeks after transplantation in patients with IPF and is associated with clinical features of severe acute liver failure.

Hyperacute rejection is a rare cause of early graft dysfunction and may present as severe preservation injury both clinically and pathologically.

Pathologic Features

Preservation injury results from ischemic damage of the liver and is best seen after reperfusion of the donor liver. The predominant inflammatory cells are neutrophils and then followed by mononuclear cells, predominantly macrophages (Figures 4.2.1 to 4.2.3). The degree of severity ranges from microvesicular steatosis, accumulation of neutrophils in the sinusoids and around central venules, as seen in "surgical" hepatitis, to more extensive centrilobular hepatocyte dropout. Functional cholestasis is always seen in more severe injury. The portal tracts show mild to moderate ductular reaction (Figure 4.2.4). Centrilobular/zonal or confluent coagulative necrosis of the hepatocytes may be followed by collapse of the reticulin framework and triggers hepatocyte regeneration. The changes may persist for several months after transplantation.

Reperfusion of donor liver with macrovesicular steatosis leads to impaired sinusoidal blood flow and results in lysis of fat-containing hepatocytes and release of lipid droplets into the sinusoids, resulting in large fat globules accompanied by local fibrin deposition, neutrophils, and congestion. Fat globules will eventually resolve within several weeks.

Differential Diagnosis

The differential diagnosis of preservation injury includes hyperacute rejection, acute rejection, biliary tract complication, and ischemia secondary to vascular complication. The diagnosis of hyperacute rejection can be confirmed by demonstrating the presence of granular IgG, IgM, C3, and fibrinogen within sinusoids by immunofluorescence stainings on fresh frozen sections. In contrast to acute rejection, preservation injury involves mainly the parenchyma, and the predominant inflammatory cells are neutrophils and, later on, macrophages. Mixed inflammation and edema of the portal tracts, endotheliitis, and bile duct damage usually seen in acute rejection are not seen in preservation injury (Figures 4.2.5 and 4.2.6). In severe acute rejection, parenchymal injury and inflammation are seen. Hepatocyte ballooning, necrosis, and dropout are observed in centrilobular areas with endotheliitis of central venules. The inflammatory infiltrate similar to that in portal tracts is of mixed cellularity.

Biliary tract complications cause changes in portal tracts that consist of portal edema, ductular reaction, and sometimes acute cholangitis. Ductular reaction is more prominent than in preservation injury. Mixed inflammatory cell infiltrate and endotheliitis characteristic of acute rejection are not seen.

Ischemia secondary to vascular complication typically has a coagulative pattern in random or zonal distribution, without cholestasis. It should be noted that ischemia may also cause ischemic cholangitis.

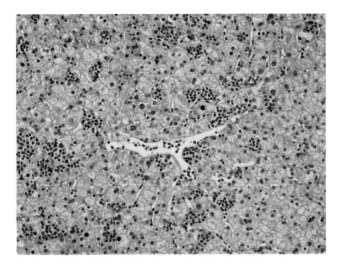

Figure 4.2.1 Preservation/reperfusion injury with clusters of neutrophils around central venule.

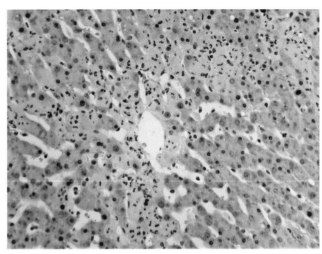

Figure 4.2.2 Preservation/reperfusion injury with centrilobular coagulative necrosis of the hepatocytes.

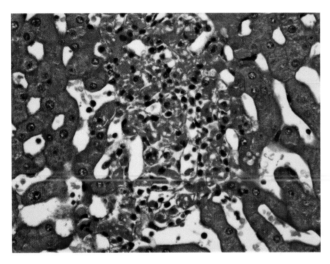

Figure 4.2.3 Focus of preservation injury with necrotic hepatocytes (trichrome stain).

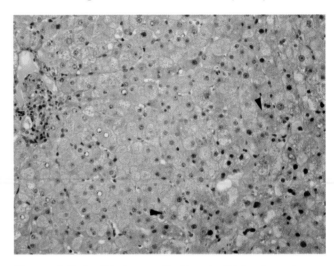

Figure 4.2.4 Bile in canaliculi and mild feathery degeneration of centrilobular hepatocytes (arrowheads) are seen in functional cholestasis.

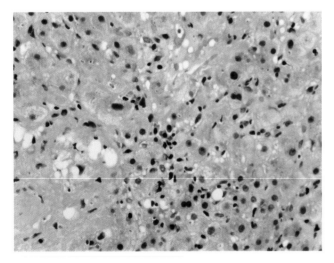

Figure 4.2.5 Mixed lobular inflammatory infiltrate and cholestasis in acute rejection.

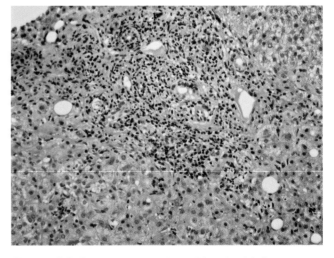

Figure 4.2.6 Acute rejection with mixed inflammatory infiltrate and bile duct damage in the portal tract.

Table 4.2.1 Liver Allograft Pathology According to Peak Time After Transplantation

Time	Diagnosis	Risk	Comments
0-1 mo	Preexisting donor liver lesions	Donor with steatosis or nonfibrotic chronic viral hepatitis	Recognized in pretransplant donor biopsies
	Preservation injury	Older donor, long cold or warm ischemic time, reconstruction of vascular anastomoses	Recognized in postperfusion biopsies. Poor bile production. Frequently coexist with other early post transplant complications, such as rejection
	Hyperacute rejection	ABO-incompatible donor	Uncommon, several hours after reperfusion
	Acute rejection	Increased in younger or female recipients	Common
	Ischemia	Complicated arterial anastomosis, pediatric recipients with small-caliber vessels, donor atherosclerosis	Usually caused by hepatic artery thrombosis, less commonly due to portal vein thrombosis
1-12 mo	Acute rejection	Inadequately immunosuppressed recipients	
	Chronic rejection	Severe or persistent acute rejection, inadequately immunosuppressed recipients	Bimodal distribution with early peak during first posttransplant year
	Biliary complications	Arterial insufficiency or thrombosis, complicated biliary anastomosis, recipients with PSC, anastomotic stricture	Present with features of acute or chronic biliary obstruction
	Opportunistic infections	Overimmunosuppressed recipients. Seropositive donors to seronegative recipients	CMV hepatitis is the most common, other organisms are rarely seen
	Venous outflow obstruction	Difficult hepatic vein reconstruction, cardiac failure	First several weeks after transplantation
	Recurrent disease	HBV, HCV or AIH recipients	Recurrent hepatitis C is frequent
>12 mo	Recurrent disease	HBV, HCV, AIH, PSC, PBC, NASH, alcoholic steatohepatitis	Hepatitis C (80%). PBC, PSC, AIH (less common, 20-50%). Alcohol, hepatitis B (uncommon, <20%)
	Immune-mediated hepatitis	Unknown. More frequent in children	May represent a form of rejection
	De novo NASH	Drugs or immunosuppressive therapy	Often incidental finding
	Vascular complications	Anastomosis complication of hepatic artery. Poor flow of portal vein	Portal vein thrombosis/insufficiency may cause zonal steatosis, atrophy, nodular regenerative hyperplasia, or portal hypertension
	Biliary complications	Arterial insufficiency or ischemia. Anastomotic stricture. CMV infection	Nonanastomotic strictures occuring late posttransplant are usually associated with preservation-related risk factors
	Acute or chronic rejection	Noncompliant or inadequately immunosuppressed patients. Patients with infections, PTLD, malignant tumors, etc	Acute rejection—rare. Chronic rejection represent second peak of bimodal distribution
	Idiopathic post transplant hepatitis and nonspecific changes	Unknown. Some may represent late onset acute rejection or AIH	Some cases may represent a form of rejection
	Malignancy: hepatocellular carcinoma, cholangiocarcinoma	Recurrence related to size, grade, stage of these tumors	De novo hepatocellular carcinomas have been reported

4.3 Vascular and Biliary Tract Complications

Vascular Complications

Hepatic Artery and Portal Vein Thrombosis

Vascular complication is the most common cause of allograft failure and frequently by hepatic artery thrombosis. Hepatic artery thrombosis usually occurs within several days posttransplantation or within 1 to 3 years posttransplantation. Unlike native livers, an allograft is devoid of collateral arterial circulation and therefore is susceptible to ischemia. Extrahepatic and intrahepatic bile ducts are the first to be affected by ischemia. Bile duct ischemia results in ulceration, strictures, obstruction, cholangitic abscesses, poor wound healing, bile leak, and biliary sludge syndrome, collectively referred to as ischemic cholangitis or ischemic cholangiopathy.

Most hepatic artery thrombosis does not produce significant problems and symptoms. The symptoms, when present, are related to hepatic infarcts, abscesses, and impaired bile flow, such as abdominal pain, fever, bacteremia, bile peritonitis, and jaundice.

The diagnosis of hepatic artery thrombosis requires hepatic arteriogram. Needle biopsy may not be diagnostic because thrombosis most commonly affects the hilum and large branches. When the effect of the thrombosis is severe, liver biopsy may show coagulative necrosis, ballooning degeneration of centrilobular hepatocytes, ductular reaction with or without ductular cholestasis, and acute cholangitis (Figures 4.3.1 and 4.3.2). Chronic ischemia leads to centrilobular hepatocyte atrophy and sinusoidal dilatation.

Portal vein is less commonly thrombosed. The incidence of complications is increased in reduced-size and living donor transplant (see below for "small-for-size" graft syndrome). Complete portal vein thrombosis may result in massive hepatic necrosis/failure or portal hypertension with massive ascites and edema. Partial portal vein thrombosis can cause liver atrophy, zonal or panlobular steatosis, nodular regenerative hyperplasia, or seeding by intestinal bacteria resulting in milliary/small abscesses and intermittent fever.

Hepatic Vein and Vena Cava Complications

Hepatic vein and vena cava stenosis or thrombosis resemble Budd-Chiari syndrome, in which the symptoms include hepatic enlargement, tenderness, ascites, and edema. The risk is slightly increased in reduced-size and living donor allografts due to complexity of reconstruction of the venous outflow tract or creation of alternative anastomosis.

Acute changes include congestion and hemorrhage involving the hepatic venules and centrilobular sinusoids, similar to those of Budd-Chiari syndrome (Figures 4.3.3 and 4.3.4). If outflow obstruction is prolonged, perivenular fibrosis and nodular regenerative hyperplasia develop.

Biliary Tract Complication

Biliary tract complication manifests either early after transplantation as bile leak or later as biliary stricture and obstruction. It is twice as common after living donor transplant as compared with cadaveric transplant. Bile leaks are usually associated with hepatic artery thrombosis and are rarely due to technical reasons. Patients may present with peritonitis. The diagnosis is made using hepatobiliary iminodiacetic acid scan and cholangiography. Patency of the hepatic artery should be evaluated.

Biliary obstruction may result from bile sludge and cast formation, or stricture at the anastomosis site. Cholangitis is often the presenting problem.

Biliary tract complication causes changes in portal tracts that consist of portal edema, ductular reaction accompanied by neutrophils, and sometimes acute cholangitis. Centrilobular cholestasis is commonly present. Chronic biliary tract complication results in chronic portal inflammation, ductular reaction without neutrophils, bile duct atrophy, and patchy small bile duct loss, mimicking chronic rejection.

"Small-for-Size" Graft Syndrome

Small-for-size graft syndrome or portal hyperperfusion occurs when transplanted donor segment is less than 30% of the expected liver volume of the recipient or less than 0.8% of recipient body weight, or in severely cirrhotic recipients with hyperdynamic portal circulation and high portal venous blood flow. Increased portal venous flow diminishes hepatic artery flow, predisposing to arterial thrombosis and ischemic cholangitis. In addition, splanchnic congestion increases portal venous endotoxin levels that can contribute to liver dysfunction and cholestasis.

Patients present with cholestasis, coagulopathy, and ascites, usually within the 1 to 2 weeks posttransplantation, mainly as the result of splanchnic congestion. Hepatic arteriogram may demonstrate arterial narrowing, thrombosis, and poor liver filling.

Early changes include denudation and rupture of portal and periportal microvasculature, resulting in hemorrhage into portal and periportal connective tissue. If the allograft survives, reparative changes follow. Endothelial cell proliferation, subendothelial edema, and myofibroblastic proliferation result in luminal obliteration or recanalization of thrombi. In needle biopsies, these changes may not be present. In early stages, the liver parenchyma may show nonspecific changes such as centrilobular canalicular cholestasis, steatosis, hepatocyte atrophy, congestion, mild ductular reaction, and ductular cholestasis. In late biopsies, obliterative venopathy and nodular regenerative hyperplasia are noted due to small portal vein branch occlusion.

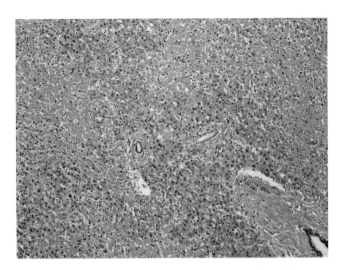

Figure 4.3.1 Extensive coagulative necrosis with preservation of periportal hepatocytes due to hepatic artery thrombosis.

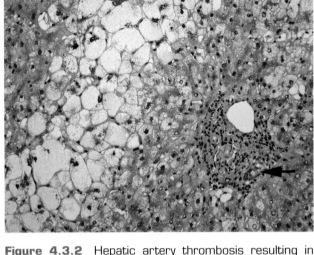

Figure 4.3.2 Hepatic artery thrombosis resulting in bile duct injury (arrow) and centrilobular cholestasis with feathery degeneration.

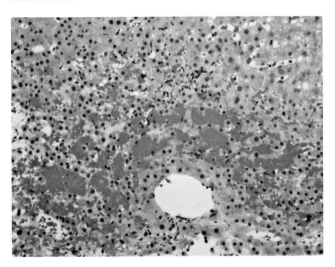

Figure 4.3.3 Centrilobular congestion and hemorrhage due to venous outflow problem.

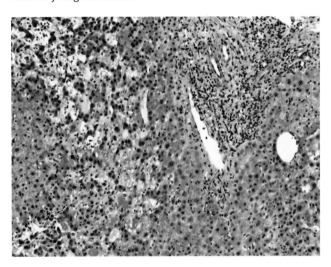

Figure 4.3.4 Centrilobular hepatocyte atrophy, hemorrhage, and iron deposition in venous outflow problem.

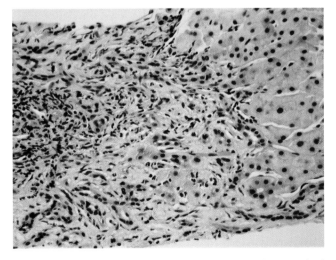

Figure 4.3.5 Biliary tract complication with marginal ductular reaction in living donor liver transplantation.

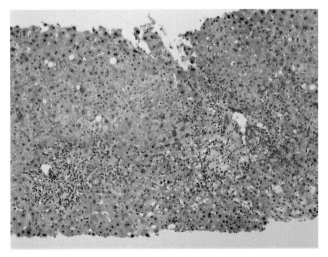

Figure 4.3.6 Severe acute rejection with mixed inflammatory infiltrate in the portal tracts and centrilobular area with hepatocyte dropout.

Table 4.3.1 Differential Diagnosis of Early Allograft Failure

Histologic Features	Preservation Injury	Ischemia	Biliary Tract Complication	Acute Rejection
Portal edema	–	–	++	+
Ductular reaction	+ (severe)/–	+/–	++	+/–
Immunoblasts	–	–	–	++
Mixed portal inflammation	–	–	–	+
Mixed lobular/perivenular inflammation	–	–	–	+
Periportal hepatocyte regeneration	+	+	–	–
Centrilobular steatosis and ballooning degeneration	+	+	–	–
Centrilobular hepatocyte injury	+	++	–	+/–
Centrilobular feathery degeneration/canalicular cholestasis	+/–	–	+	+/–
Endotheliitis	–	–	–	++

++ indicates almost always present; +, usually present; +/–, occasionally present; –, usually absent.

4.4 Acute Rejection

Liver rejection is categorized into antibody-mediated (hyperacute/humoral), acute, and chronic. Antibody-mediated rejection is rare due to ABO-incompatible graft and occurs within the first several weeks after transplantation. Acute rejection occurs at any time after transplantation but is most common within the first month after transplantation. Chronic rejection develops directly from severe or persistent and unresolved acute rejection, or subclinical acute rejection.

Acute rejection is the most common cause of early posttransplant liver dysfunction. It occurs within the first month of transplantation and can be observed as early as 2 to 3 days after transplantation, but it is uncommon after 2 months unless the patient is inadequately immunosuppressed. Late-onset acute rejection (more than 1 year after transplantation) is usually associated with inadequate immunosuppression and often leads to allograft failure.

Clinical findings are often absent in early or mild acute rejection. In severe rejection, patients may experience fever, malaise, abdominal pain, hepatosplenomegaly, and increasing ascites. Bile output is diminished. Elevation of serum bilirubin level and of alkaline phosphatase and γ-glutamyltransferase activities is greater than the rise of aminotransferase activities. Peripheral blood leukocytosis and eosinophilia are also frequently present.

Patients with indeterminate or mild acute rejection without significant liver function abnormalities are usually not treated, but patients with moderate or severe rejection or with significant liver function abnormalities should be treated with increased immunosuppression because of the risk of graft failure and chronic rejection.

Pathologic Features

Acute rejection has 3 characteristic histologic features:

1. Enlarged and edematous portal tracts with mixed inflammatory cell infiltrate (Figure 4.4.1). The inflammatory infiltrate consists predominantly of mononuclear cells, that is, immunoblasts (activated lymphocytes), lymphocytes, plasma cells, and macrophages, with scattered neutrophils and eosinophils and is usually confined to portal triads in milder rejection.

2. Endotheliitis of the portal veins with infiltration of inflammatory cells, particularly lymphocytes, beneath and adhering to the endothelial cells (Figure 4.4.3). The lumen of portal veins may be filled with inflammatory cells that obscure the vessels. Endotheliitis often involves the central venules as well, with necroinflammatory changes in the surrounding liver parenchyma, so-called central perivenulitis (Figure 4.4.5).

3. Degeneration and inflammation of interlobular bile ducts (rejection cholangitis) (Figures 4.4.2 and 4.4.3). Bile ducts are invaded by lymphocytes, and the biliary epithelial cells show vacuolization, ballooning, or eosinophilia of the cytoplasm and nuclear pyknosis, as well as regenerative changes including mitotic activity.

In addition to the above features, the liver parenchyma may show sinusoidal cell activation and an increased number of mononuclear inflammatory cells. Cholestasis of various degrees is always present. In severe acute rejection, parenchymal injury and inflammation are seen. Hepatocyte ballooning, necrosis, and dropout are observed in centrilobular areas with endotheliitis of central venules (Figure 4.4.6). The mixed inflammatory infiltrate is similar to that in portal tracts.

Differential Diagnosis

The differential diagnosis of acute rejection depends on the time period of its occurrence after transplantation. In the first months, acute rejection must be distinguished from preservation injury and vascular or biliary complications. Later on, acute rejection may be difficult to distinguish from acute hepatitis of various etiologies or recurrent viral hepatitis B or C and autoimmune hepatitis (AIH) or immune-mediated hepatitis.

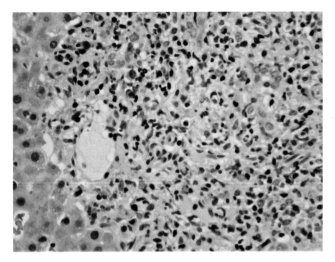

Figure 4.4.1 Mixed inflammatory cell infiltrate including eosinophils in acute rejection.

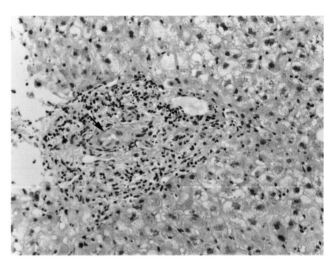

Figure 4.4.2 Bile duct injury (arrow) in acute rejection.

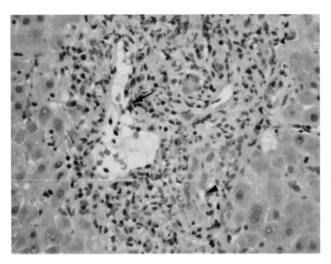

Figure 4.4.3 Endotheliitis of portal vein (arrow) and bile duct damage (arrowhead) in acute rejection.

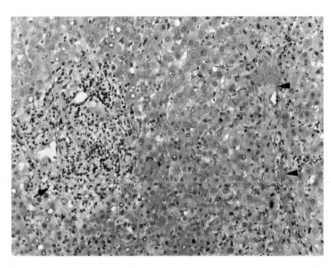

Figure 4.4.4 Portal tract (arrow) and perivenular (arrowheads) inflammation with similar inflammatory infiltrate in severe acute rejection.

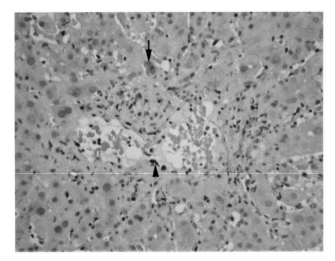

Figure 4.4.5 Endotheliitis of central venule (arrowhead) accompanied by hepatocyte dropout (arrow) in acute rejection.

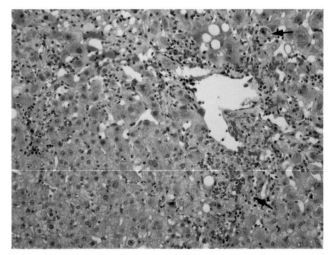

Figure 4.4.6 Endotheliitis of the central venule and foci of hepatocyte dropout and necrosis (arrows) in severe acute rejection.

Table 4.4.1 Banff Grading System of Acute Allograft Rejection

Rejection	Grade	Criteria
Indeterminate		Portal inflammatory infiltrate that fails to meet criteria of acute rejection
Mild	I	Inflammatory infiltrate in a minority of portal triads, generally mild, and confined to portal spaces
Moderate	II	Inflammatory infiltrate expanding most or all portal triads
Severe	III	As above for moderate, with spillover of inflammation into periportal areas, moderate to severe perivenular inflammation extending into hepatic parenchyma and associated with perivenular hepatocyte necrosis

Table 4.4.2 Acute Rejection Activity Index (RAI)*

Category	Criteria	Score
Portal inflammation	Mostly lymphocytic inflammation involving, but not expanding, minority of portal triads	1
	Expansion of most or all portal triads, by a mixed infiltrate containing lymphocytes with occasional blasts, neutrophils, and eosinophils	2
	Marked expansion of most or all portal triads by a mixed infiltrate containing numerous blasts and eosinophils with spillover into periportal parenchyma	3
Bile duct inflammation/damage	Minority of ducts are cuffed and infiltrated by inflammatory cells and show only mild reactive changes, such as increased nucleus-to-cytoplasm ratio of epithelial cells	1
	Most, or all, ducts are infiltrated by inflammatory cells. More than an occasional duct shows degenerative changes, such as nuclear pleomorphism, loss of polarity, and cytoplasmic vacuolization.	2
	Score 2, plus most or all ducts showing degenerative changes or luminal disruption	3
Venous endothelial inflammation	Subendothelial lymphocytic infiltration involving <50% of portal and/or hepatic venules	1
	Subendothelial lymphocytic infiltration involving >50% of portal and/or hepatic venules	2
	Score 2, plus moderate or severe perivenular inflammation extending into perivenular parenchyma and associated with perivenular hepatocyte necrosis	3

*Banff schema for grading liver allograft rejection: an international consensus document. *Hepatology.* 1997;25:658-63.
Total RAI score is the sum of all component scores for portal inflammation, bile duct inflammation/damage, and venous endothelial inflammation.
Total RAI score: 1-2, indeterminate for acute rejection; 3-4, mild rejection; 5-6, moderate rejection; >6, severe rejection.

4.5 Chronic Rejection

Chronic rejection occurs weeks to years posttransplantation, frequently after 3 to 4 months. It may develop after an unresolved episode of severe acute rejection, multiple episodes of acute rejection, or mild, clinically unapparent persistent acute rejection. Chronic rejection potentially causes irreversible damage to bile ducts, arteries, and veins and eventually results in allograft failure, typically within the first year.

Chronic rejection causes progressive loss of bile ducts, resulting in a slowly progressive cholestatic picture until the patients become deeply jaundiced. Alkaline phosphatase and γ-glutamyltransferase activities and bilirubin levels are markedly elevated. A hepatic angiogram showing pruning of branches of hepatic arteries with poor peripheral filling supports the diagnosis, and liver biopsy is confirmatory.

Chronic rejection can be categorized into early and late chronic rejection. Early chronic rejection implies that there is a significant potential for recovery. Limited potential for recovery and retransplantation should be considered in late chronic rejection.

Pathologic Features

The main features of chronic rejection are ductopenia and obliterative arteriopathy. The portal tracts in chronic rejection show mild inflammation and consist predominantly of lymphocytes, especially around the remaining and damaged bile ducts. Eosinophils are usually not found. Instead of edema that is usually seen in acute rejection, mild to moderate portal fibrosis is present in chronic rejection. Loss of small bile ducts is observed. Duct loss is determined by calculating the percentage/ratio between the number of bile ducts and the number of hepatic artery branches in at least 20 portal tracts. Caution should be applied in assessing bile duct numbers, particularly in small biopsies with fewer than 10 portal tracts, because bile duct loss can be patchy in distribution. A finding of fewer than 80% of portal tracts with bile ducts is suggestive of ductopenia; bile duct loss in less than 50% of portal tracts is seen in early chronic rejection, whereas bile duct loss in greater than 50% of portal tracts confirms the diagnosis of ductopenia and is seen in late chronic rejection. Although bile duct loss in early chronic rejection is not significant, many of them may show "senescence" change, characterized by atrophy of the bile duct,

eosinophilic cytoplasm, uneven nuclear spacing, nuclear enlargement, and hyperchromasia (Figure 4.5.1). Duct loss results in cholestasis, which is seen in centrilobular areas and often is greater than in acute rejection (Figure 4.5.2). Ductular reaction is unusual in chronic rejection.

Obliterative arteriopathy involves medium and large branches of hepatic arteries. These arteries show subintimal accumulation of lipid-laden macrophages or foam cells, which may cause narrowing or obliteration of these vessels (Figure 4.5.4). Because obliterative arteriopathy does not involve the small branches, usually it is not seen in needle biopsy specimens. Its consequences however may be reflected in the biopsy specimen, such as centrilobular hepatocyte degeneration and necrosis and/or centrilobular fibrosis (Figure 4.5.4). Clusters of foamy macrophages may also be present in the lobules (Figure 4.5.5).

In addition to ductopenia and obliterative arteriopathy, in early rejection, the centrilobular areas show mononuclear inflammation consisting of lymphocytes and plasma cells, hepatocyte dropout, and accumulation of ceroid-laden macrophages. Spotty acidophilic necrosis of hepatocytes, so-called transitional hepatitis, may occur during the evolution from early to late chronic rejection. Late chronic rejection is characterized by perivenular fibrosis and occasional obliteration of hepatic venules and central-to-central bridging fibrosis. Other features of late chronic rejection include centrilobular hepatocyte ballooning and dropout, hepatocanalicular cholestasis, nodular regenerative hyperplasia-like changes, and intrasinusoidal foam cell clusters.

Differential Diagnosis

The differential diagnosis of chronic rejection includes acute rejection, biliary tract complication, cholestatic drug-induced injury, and outflow obstruction. The differentiation between acute and chronic rejection is important because chronic rejection does not respond to an increase in immunosuppressive medication, and overimmunosuppression should be avoided.

In addition to bile duct damage, acute rejection shows endotheliitis and portal edema with mixed inflammatory infiltrate, including immunoblasts, lymphocytes, plasma cells, neutrophils, and eosinophils (Figure 4.5.6). There is no bile duct loss in acute rejection.

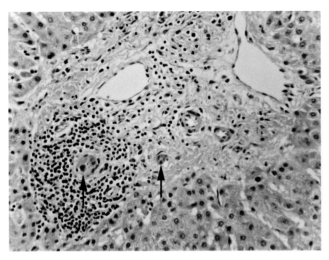

Figure 4.5.1 Chronic rejection with mild portal inflammation and senescence change of the bile duct (arrows).

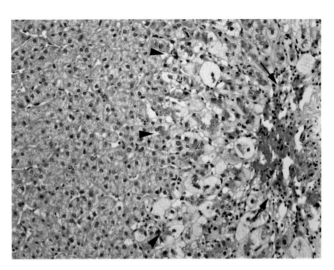

Figure 4.5.2 Chronic rejection with centrilobular hepatocyte dropout (arrows) and centrilobular cholestasis with feathery degeneration (arrowheads).

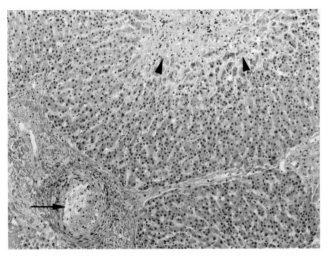

Figure 4.5.3 Chronic rejection with obliterative arteriopathy (arrow) and centrilobular hepatocyte dropout (arrowheads).

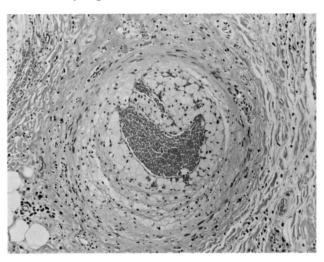

Figure 4.5.4 Obliterative arteriopathy with subintimal accumulation of lipid-laden macrophages or foam cells.

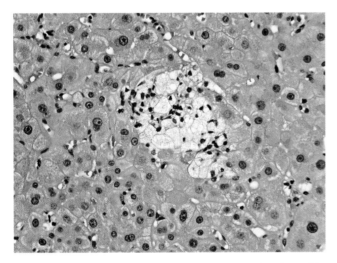

Figure 4.5.5 Accumulation of foam cells in sinusoids in chronic rejection.

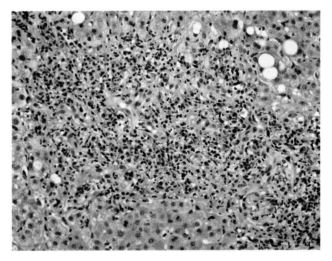

Figure 4.5.6 Acute rejection with mixed portal inflammatory infiltrates. The bile duct and portal vein are obscured by bile duct damage and endotheliitis.

Table 4.5.1 Early and Late Chronic Allograft Rejection*

Features	Early Chronic Rejection	Late Chronic Rejection
Small bile ducts (<60 μm)	Bile duct loss in <50% of portal tracts. Degenerative change involving the majority of bile ducts: eosinophilic transformation of the cytoplasm, nuclear hyperchomasia, uneven nuclear spacing, ducts partially lined by epithelial cells	Bile duct loss in >50% of portal tracts. Degenerative changes in remaining bile ducts
Terminal hepatic venules and zone 3 hepatocytes	Intimal/luminal inflammation. Lytic zone 3 necrosis and inflammation. Mild perivenular fibrosis	Focal obliteration. Variable degree of inflammation. Severe perivenular fibrosis (central-to-central bridging fibrosis)
Portal tract hepatic arterioles	Occasional loss, involving <25% of portal tracts	Loss involving ≥25 % of portal tracts
Other	"Transitional" hepatitis with spotty necrosis of hepatocytes	Sinusoidal foam cell accumulation; marked cholestasis
Large perihilar hepatic artery branches	Intimal inflammation, focal foam cell deposition without luminal compromise	Luminal narrowing by subintimal foam cells fibrointimal proliferation
Large perihilar bile ducts	Inflammation-associated degeneration and focal foam cell deposition	Mural fibrosis

*Demetris A, et al. Update of the International Banff Schema for Liver Allograft Rejection: working recommendations for the histopathologic staging and reporting of chronic rejection. An international panel. *Hepatology.* 2000;31:792-799.

4.6 Acute Hepatitis

Acute hepatitis after liver transplantation is caused by viral hepatitis, drug-induced injury, or immune-mediated hepatitis. It can occur a few weeks or months after transplantation.

Clinical Findings

Acute hepatitis after liver transplantation has a variety of presentations ranging from asymptomatic rise of serum aminotransferase activities to gastrointestinal and influenza-like symptoms with or without jaundice.

Pathologic Features

Acute viral hepatitis affects predominantly the hepatic lobule resulting in diffuse necroinflammatory changes. Because posttransplant patients are closely monitored, particularly early after transplantation, biopsy specimens with milder changes than in classic acute viral hepatitis in the general population are often encountered. Increased parenchymal cellularity, due to activation of sinusoidal lining cells, particularly Kupffer cells, and infiltration of sinusoids by lymphocytes and macrophages are seen. Scattered individual hepatocytes undergo eosinophilic or ballooning degeneration throughout the lobules. Endophlebitis of the central venule may be observed. Cholestasis, intracellular or canalicular, is mild. Portal tracts are infiltrated by lymphocytes.

The morphologic changes of drug-induced injury are generally similar to those described in native liver, except for immunosuppresive drugs that may cause specific disorders in the allograft. For example, short-term use of azathioprine may cause centrilobular necrosis and fibrosis, cholestatic hepatitis, or veno-occlusive disease (VOD), whereas long-term use may cause nodular regenerative hyperplasia. Cyclosporine can cause self-limited cholestasis. Tacrolimus may cause centrilobular necrosis, but toxicity nowadays is rare because of low dosing and monitoring of blood levels.

Immune-mediated hepatitis may histologically resembles drug-induced injury; therefore, clinical correlation is required to establish the diagnosis.

Differential Diagnoses

The differential diagnoses of acute hepatitis include acute rejection and chronic hepatitis. Acute rejection shows 3 characteristic changes in the portal tracts that are not seen in acute hepatitis, that is, (1) portal edema with mixed inflammatory infiltrate and immunoblasts, (2) endotheliitis of portal veins, and (3) bile duct damage. The inflammatory infiltrate in acute hepatitis consists of lymphocytes without immunoblasts, distributed throughout the lobule. In comparison, foci of parenchymal necroses and inflammation in the acute rejection are predominantly centrilobular. Endotheliitis of portal veins and rejection cholangiopathy are absent in acute hepatitis.

Recurrent chronic viral hepatitis is characterized by portal chronic inflammation, various degrees of portal fibrosis, interface hepatitis, and mild lobular necroinflammatory activity. The features are similar to non–transplant-related chronic viral hepatitis.

Table 4.6.1 Differential Diagnosis of Acute Hepatitis in Liver Allograft Biopsies

Histologic Changes	Acute Viral Hepatitis	Fibrosing Cholestatic Hepatitis	Drug-Induced Injury	Acute Rejection
Portal/periportal changes				
Portal inflammation	+	+	+	++
Inflammatory cells	Predominantly lymphocytes	Lymphocytes and neutrophils	Lymphocytes and plasma cells, eosinophils	Mixed infiltrate, with immunoblasts, eosinophils and neutrophils
Portal edema	–	–	+/–	++
Bile duct damage/ inflammation	–	–	–	++
Ductular reaction	+/–	++	+/–	+/–
Endotheliitis	+/–	–	+/–	++
Fibrosis	–	++	–	–
Lobular changes				
Severity of inflammation	++	+	++	+/–
Distribution of inflammation	Random, spotty to confluent necrosis	Random	Random, spotty necrosis to confluent necrosis	Centrilobular/perivenular necrosis
Acidophilic bodies	++	+/–	+	+/–
Central venulitis	+	–	+/–	++
Cholestasis	+/–	++	+/–	+/–

++ indicates almost always present; +, usually present; +/–, occasionally present; –, usually absent.

4.7 Recurrent Diseases

Recurrent diseases, with longer posttransplant survival, have become an increasingly important cause of late graft dysfunction and have become the leading cause of graft failure in patients surviving more than 12 months posttransplant.

Histopathologic features of recurrent disease are generally similar to those occurring in the native liver but may be affected by transplant-related pathology, and the features may overlap, such as in HCV with acute rejection, primary biliary cirrhosis (PBC) with acute or chronic rejection, and primary sclerosing cholangitis (PSC) with ischemic cholangitis. The effects of immunosuppressive therapy should also be considered; for example, autoimmune liver diseases are likely to be prevented from recurring or progress more slowly, whereas viral infections are more aggressive and may be associated with atypical histological features not usually observed in immunocompetent individuals.

Recurrent Hepatitis B

Nearly all patients with hepatitis B virus (HBV) who showed active viral replication before transplantation will reinfect their allograft. Hyperimmunoglobulin and/or antiviral therapy is used to decrease the risk of recurrent infection and progressive liver disease. The acute phase of recurrent hepatitis B usually manifests 6 to 8 weeks after transplantation. The most common clinical feature is mild elevation of liver function tests. Nausea, vomiting, jaundice, and hepatic failure signal severe recurrent disease.

The acute phase of recurrent hepatitis B shows features of acute hepatitis with a small percentage of patients develop bridging or even submassive necrosis, particularly when the level of immunosuppression is abruptly lowered. Chronic hepatitis is characterized by portal lymphocytic infiltrate and persistent lobular necroinflammatory activity. The hepatocytes may show ground-glass cytoplasm and/or sanded nuclei corresponding to HBV surface and core antigen expression. Fibrosing cholestatic hepatitis can occur in recurrent hepatitis B, usually associated with marked expression of HBV core and/or surface antigen (Figure 4.7.3). The features include cholestasis, prominent hepatocyte ballooning, portal tract expansion/edema with prominent ductular reaction at marginal zones, and fibrosis (Figures 4.7.2 and 4.7.3). Fibrosing cholestatic hepatitis is associated with high rate of graft failure. Other causes of cholestasis, including biliary obstruction, chronic rejection, and drug-induced toxicity, should be excluded.

Recurrent Hepatitis C

Recurrence of chronic hepatitis C is universal in HCV-positive posttransplant patients. Although recurrent hepatitis C evolves slowly, up to 30% to 50% of patients are cirrhotic 5 to 10 years posttransplantation. The presence of fibrosis at the first year posttransplantation has been shown to be predictive for subsequent fibrosis progression and graft failure. Although the histological changes are mostly similar to those in native liver, recurrent hepatitis C tends to show more severe necroinflammatory activity, which can include areas of confluent and bridging necrosis and rapid progression of fibrosis to cirrhosis (Figures 4.7.4 to 4.7.6). A grading and staging scoring system that has been used for native liver biopsies should also be applied to posttransplant biopsies. Cholestatic variant of recurrent hepatitis C can be seen in HCV-positive patients with high serum and intrahepatic levels of HCV-RNA, usually due to overimmunosuppression. Cholestatic variant of recurrent hepatitis C is characterized by prominent lymphocytic infiltration, hepatocyte ballooning and dropout and extensive ductular reaction, but less fibrosis than fibrosing cholestatic hepatitis B (Figures 4.7.7 and 4.7.8).

The distinction between recurrent hepatitis C and acute rejection is often difficult, and the changes may reflect a combination of both conditions. In most cases, recurrent hepatitis C predominates, and rejection-related changes are minimal or mild, requiring no antirejection therapy. Increased immunosuppression should only be considered in moderate rejection or when there are features suggestive of progression to chronic rejection.

Recurrent PBC

Primary biliary cirrhosis recurs in up to 50% of patients, but it tends to have a mild subclinical disease with normal or near-normal liver enzyme activities. Antimitochondrial antibody level remains elevated in most patients after transplantation. Therefore, the diagnosis of recurrent PBC often requires biopsies. As with the native liver, the inflammatory change with florid duct lesion in recurrent PBC is often patchy involving some of the portal tracts. In some cases, features of nonspecific or autoimmune-like chronic hepatitis may precede or occur in conjunction with the diagnostic florid duct lesions (Figure 4.7.11). Other findings include periportal edema, portal fibrosis, ductular reaction, cholatestasis, accumulation copper or copper-associated protein in periportal hepatocytes, and patchy small bile duct loss. Cirrhosis or graft failure rarely occurs.

Recurrent Primary Sclerosing Cholangitis

Primary sclerosing cholangitis recurs in up to 30% of patients. Recurrent PSC is more frequently clinically symptomatic than recurrent PBC and may progress to graft failure. Recurrent PSC usually manifests more than 6 months posttransplantation. As in the native liver, the diagnostic periductal "onion-skin" fibrosis for PSC is rarely seen in liver allograft biopsies (Figure 4.7.12). Therefore, the diagnosis is often based on compatible findings of chronic cholestasis, ductopenia, ductular reaction, and biliary fibrosis occurring in the absence of other identifiable causes. The distinction between recurrent PSC and ischemic biliary complications or chronic rejection can be difficult and requires exclusion of other causes of biliary complications and supported by characteristic cholangiographic findings of PSC.

Recurrent AIH

Autoimmune hepatitis recurs in approximately 20% to 30% of patients. The diagnosis is based on a combination of biochemical, serological, and histological changes and in some cases, on response to immunosuppressive therapy. The diagnostic utility of autoantibody testing alone in establishing the diagnosis of recurrent AIH is uncertain, as autoantibodies have been found in posttransplant patients for other conditions.

The histologic features of recurrent AIH are similar to those in the native liver, including plasma cell–rich infiltrate, presence of eosinophils, variable interface hepatitis and lobular inflammation, and occasional areas of confluent or bridging necrosis. Lobular inflammation may precede the typical portal inflammation and interface hepatitis.

Recurrent Alcoholic Liver Disease

Recidivism is not uncommon (up to 30%) in patients transplanted for alcoholic liver disease, but serious graft complications are rare. A high γ-glutamyltransferase/alkaline phosphatase ratio identifies potential recidivism. Centrilobular steatosis, mixed but predominantly macrovesicular, is the most common finding in liver biopsy, which may progress to steatohepatitis, alcoholic hepatitis, and steatofibrosis (Figure 4.7.9).

Recurrent Nonalcoholic Fatty Liver Disease

Nonalcoholic fatty liver disease (NAFLD) may recur in up to 40% of patients, particularly those who were transplanted for "cryptogenic" cirrhosis or having risk factors for NAFLD (Figure 4.7.9). Immunosuppressive drugs and other transplant-related factors may exacerbate NAFLD.

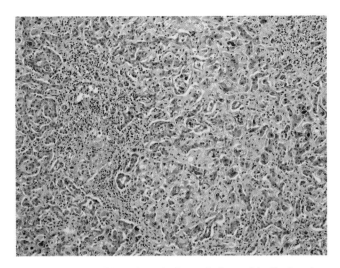

Figure 4.7.1 Fibrosing cholestatic hepatitis B showing marked cholestasis, ductular reaction, and fibrosis.

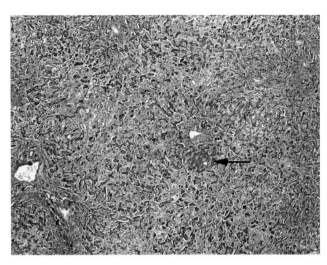

Figure 4.7.2 Extensive ductular reaction with fibrosis replacing liver parenchyma with cluster of residual hepatocytes (arrow) in fibrosing cholestatic hepatitis B.

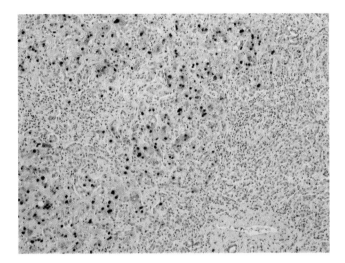

Figure 4.7.3 HBcAg immunostain shows diffuse nuclear and cytoplasmic positive staining in fibrosing cholestatic hepatitis B.

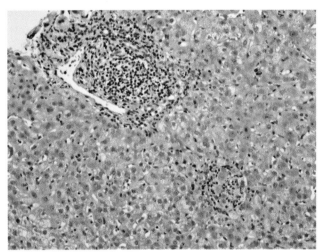

Figure 4.7.4 Recurrent hepatitis C with dense portal lymphocytic aggregate and mild lobular necroinflammatory activity.

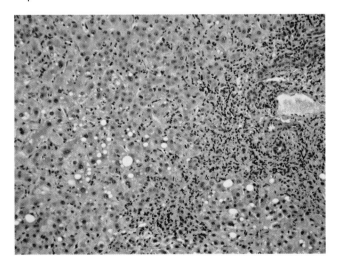

Figure 4.7.5 Recurrent hepatitis C with severe interface hepatitis, lobular necroinflammatory activity, and cholestasis.

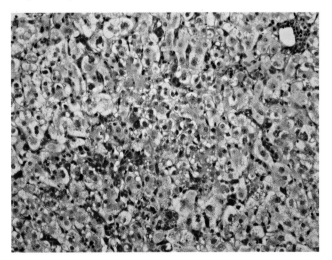

Figure 4.7.6 PAS-D stain shows numerous lobular PAS-D–positive macrophages in recurrent hepatitis C with severe lobular necroinflammatory activity.

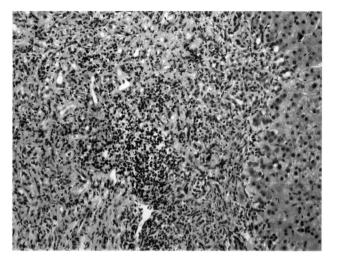

Figure 4.7.7 Cholestatic variant of chronic hepatitis C with extensive ductular reaction.

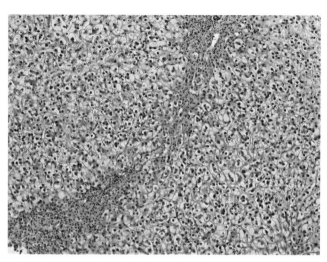

Figure 4.7.8 Marked ductular reaction and hepatocyte ballooning in cholestatic variant of chronic hepatitis C.

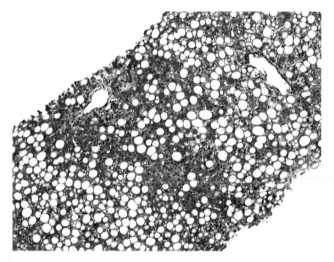

Figure 4.7.9 Recurrent fatty liver disease with severe macrovesicular steatosis (trichrome stain).

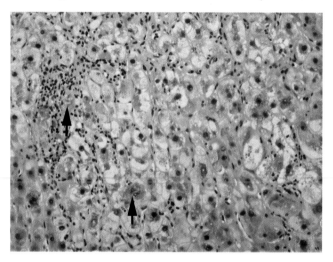

Figure 4.7.10 Recurrent alcoholic liver disease with marked ballooning degeneration of the hepatocytes and Mallory-Denk bodies (arrows).

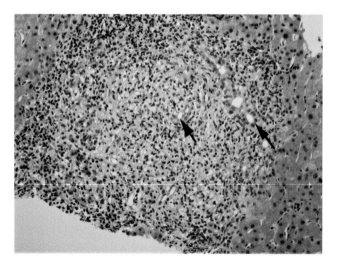

Figure 4.7.11 Recurrent primary biliary cirrhosis showing expansion of portal tract by lymphoplasmacellular infiltrate with eosinophils around damaged bile ducts (arrows) (florid duct lesion).

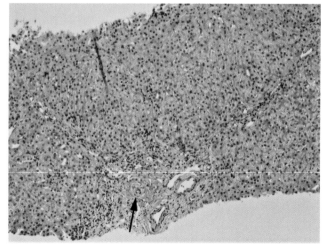

Figure 4.7.12 Recurrent primary sclerosing cholangitis with periductal fibrosis (arrow).

4.8 Immune-Mediated Hepatitis and Other Findings in Late Posttransplant Biopsies

Immune-Mediated Hepatitis

Immune-mediated hepatitis, also known as de novo autoimmune hepatitis (AIH), is chronic hepatitis with biochemical, serological, and histological features of AIH in patients transplanted for diseases other than AIH. Serological profile, high titers of antinuclear antibodies and/or anti–smooth muscle antibodies, similar to AIH type 1 is most common. A higher frequency of immune-mediated hepatitis has been reported in children (up to 10%) compared to adults (1%-2%), possibly related to interference of immunosuppressive drugs with normal T-cell maturation.

Several studies have noted the overlap features between immune-mediated hepatitis and liver allograft rejection, including the presence of antibodies in an otherwise typical cases of acute or chronic rejection, and the development of donor-specific antibodies to glutathione-S-transferase T1 (GSTT1) occurring in the setting of donor mismatch for GSTT1 is highly predictive of the development of immune-mediated hepatitis; all of which suggest that immune-mediated hepatitis is a form of rejection.

Histological features are generally similar to those seen in AIH in native liver and recurrent AIH in liver allograft, but lobular inflammatory changes tend to be more prominent and occur more frequently as a presenting feature, before typical portal inflammatory changes are seen (Figures 4.8.1 to 4.8.4).

Idiopathic Posttransplant Chronic Hepatitis

Idiopathic (unexplained) posttransplant chronic hepatitis occurs in up to 50% of biopsies from long-term liver allograft survivors with no obvious cause and without clinical or serologic evidence of viral hepatitis, autoimmunity, or drug-induced hepatitis. Normal or minor abnormalities of liver tests are frequently encountered, commonly in the form of mild elevation of aminotransferase activities.

Histological findings include a predominantly mononuclear portal inflammatory infiltrate with variable interface hepatitis. Bile duct damage, ductopenia, or endotheliitis are absent or minimal. Lobular inflammation is commonly present, tends to be more prominent in the centrilobular/perivenular areas, and may be associated with foci of parenchymal necroses. Progression to fibrosis or cirrhosis has been reported.

Some cases may have overlap features with acute or chronic rejection, whereas others are associated with autoantibodies but lack other diagnostic features of immune-mediated hepatitis, which suggest that idiopathic posttransplant chronic hepatitis may represent a form of late rejection and may respond well to increased immunosuppressive therapy.

Architectural or Vascular Changes

Architectural and vascular changes of varying degrees have been documented in up to 80% of late liver allograft biopsies, including mild portal lymphocytic infiltrate without bile duct damage or ductopenia, thickening of hepatocyte plates with pseudorosette formation, nodular regenerative hyperplasia, sinusoidal dilatation, and sinusoidal fibrosis. These changes are encountered after the exclusion of primary and recurrent disorders and cannot be attributed to any particular cause.

Many cases are mild and clinically asymptomatic, but up to 50% develop signs of portal hypertension, in some cases leading to graft failure, necessitating retransplantation.

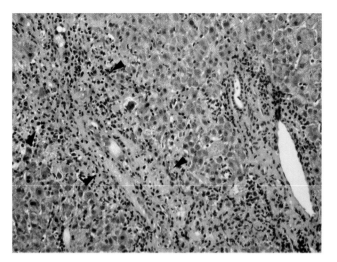

Figure 4.8.1 Immune-mediated hepatitis with plasma cell infiltrate and centrilobular necrosis (arrowheads).

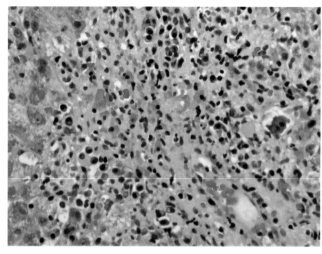

Figure 4.8.2 Centrilobular prominent plasma cell infiltrate and hepatocyte dropout in immune-mediated hepatitis.

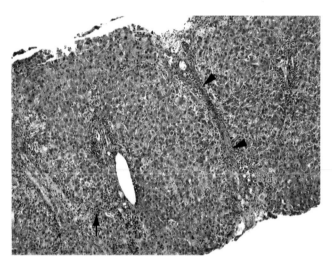

Figure 4.8.3 Immune-mediated hepatitis with portal-to-central bridging necrosis (arrow) and central-to-central bridging necrosis and fibrosis (arrowheads).

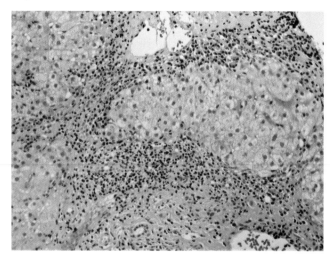

Figure 4.8.4 Immune-mediated hepatitis with severe interface hepatitis and cirrhosis. The inflamed septa are rich in plasma cells.

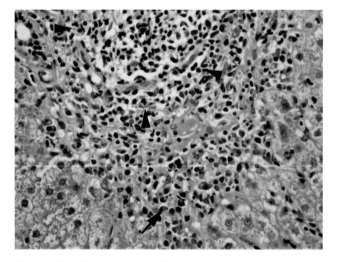

Figure 4.8.5 Recurrent chronic hepatitis C with plasma cell infiltrate (arrow). Dense portal lymphocytic aggregate typical for chronic hepatitis C is noted (arrowheads).

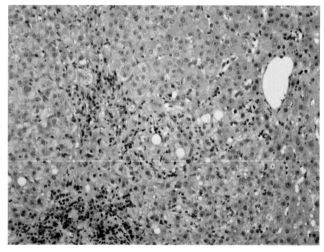

Figure 4.8.6 Late acute rejection with plasma cells and eosinophils.

4.9   Opportunistic Infections

Cytomegaloviral Hepatitis

Cytomegaloviral (CMV) hepatitis is the most common opportunistic infection in liver allograft specimen. It is either a primary infection of donor liver from transfused blood or secondary from reactivation. The infection presents 1 to 4 months posttransplantation, usually after increased immunosuppression. It may become chronic and lead to bile duct loss/vanishing bile duct syndrome. Diagnosis is by isolation of virus from urine or saliva or by rising levels of complement-fixing antibodies and CMV IgM antibodies. Liver biopsy is useful in the diagnosis of CMV hepatitis. Cytomegaloviral hepatitis usually responds well to treatment with antiviral drug gancyclovir and reduction of immunosuppressive drugs whenever possible.

Cytomegaloviral hepatitis results in characteristic histologic lesions, that is, small clusters (more than 10 cells) of neutrophils (so-called microabscesses) (Figure 4.9.1) or a collection of macrophages and lymphocytes surrounding a necrotic hepatocyte ("microgranuloma"). Eosinophilic or amphophilic nuclear and basophilic cytoplasmic inclusions within enlarged endothelial, bile duct epithelial, or parenchymal cells are diagnostic (Figure 4.9.3). Portal tracts may contain mononuclear inflammatory cells surrounding bile ducts with inclusions. In contrast to the findings in acute rejection, endotheliitis and rejection cholangiopathy are not seen. Immunohistochemical staining to localize CMV antigens is useful in confirming the diagnosis (Figure 4.9.2). Cytomegaloviral antigens may be detected in infected cells even in the absence of microabscesses or viral inclusions. In return, parenchymal microabscesses have also been seen in cases with no evidence of CMV infection; suggested causes include other infections (bacterial, viral, or fungal), graft ischemia, and biliary obstruction/cholangitis.

Herpes Simplex Viral Hepatitis

Herpes simplex viral (HSV) hepatitis may have a clinical presentation similar to that of CMV hepatitis, but jaundice is rare and fulminant liver failure is more frequent. It can occur as early as 3 days after transplantation. It is usually part of a generalized herpetic disease that involves infant, person with AIDS, immunosuppressive treatment, or organ transplantation and rarely affects immunocompetent individuals. Mucocutaneous lesions are not always present. Herpes simplex viral hepatitis has a variable course depending on the other organs involved and the severity of the involvement. Acyclovir is effective in treatment of HSV infection.

Herpes simplex viral hepatitis results in well-circumscribed areas of lytic or coagulative necrosis of hepatocytes ("punched out" lesions) with varying inflammatory response. These areas of necroses are nonzonal, with hepatocyte ghosts intermixed with neutrophils and necrotic debris. In severe cases, the necrotic areas coalesce resulting in massive hepatic necrosis with isolated islands of noninfected hepatocytes (Figure 4.9.4). Viral inclusions in HSV hepatitis are in hepatocytes at the margins of necrotic areas. They are eosinophilic intranuclear inclusions surrounded by a clear halo characteristic of Cowdry type A inclusions. Nuclear inclusions, however, are often absent in severe hepatitis. Initially, inclusions may be basophilic without halo (Cowdry type B). Immunohistochemical staining for herpes simplex viruses types I and II is a sensitive and fast method to confirm the diagnosis. Other methods include electron microscopy and viral culture.

Epstein-Barr Viral Hepatitis

Epstein-Barr viral (EBV) hepatitis presents as a flu-like syndrome with fever, sore throat, and lymphadenopathy, which resembles classic mononucleosis syndrome. Hepatosplenomegaly often is found. The increase of serum aminotransferase activities is usually mild. Jaundice when present is mild and transient. Leukocytosis with atypical lymphocytes in peripheral blood and IgM anti-EBV antibodies are present. The differentiation between EBV hepatitis, posttransplant lymphoproliferative disease, and acute rejection may be difficult both clinically and pathologically. Epstein-Barr viral hepatitis may resolve or progress to lymphoproliferative disease. Reduction of immunosuppressive drugs is the treatment of choice and is usually effective. Monitoring of peripheral blood for EBV nucleic acid is used to preempt manifestations.

In EBV hepatitis, mononuclear inflammatory cells are abundant. They consist predominantly of atypical lymphocytes, which infiltrate portal tracts and sinusoids (Figure 4.9.6). These cells are not in contact with hepatocytes but are often in single-file arrangement in the sinusoids. Sinusoidal lining cells are enlarged and prominent. Hepatocellular damage is mild or absent, and most hepatocytes appear normal. Epstein-Barr viral antigen may be demonstrable by immunohistochemical staining in the cytoplasm of rare atypical lymphocytes. In situ hybridization for EBV-encoded small RNAs is more sensitive.

Adenoviral Hepatitis

Posttransplantation adenoviral hepatitis mainly occurs in the pediatric population; presumably most adults have acquired protective immunity. Patients present with fever, respiratory distress, and diarrhea. The onset of the disease is usually between 1 and 10 weeks after transplantation.

The most characteristic findings are "pox-like" granulomas consisting mostly of macrophages, accompanied by geographic necrosis of the hepatocytes resembling HSV hepatitis, but less severe. Adenovirus inclusions are detected at the edge of necrotic areas or granulomas as intranuclear "blueberry-like" inclusions (Figure 4.9.5). Immunohistochemical stains may be used to confirm the diagnosis.

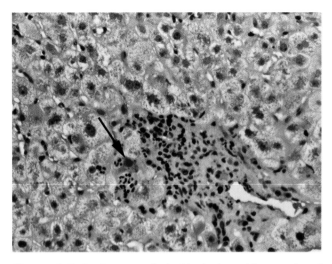

Figure 4.9.1 Cytomegaloviral inclusion with associated microabscess formation (arrow).

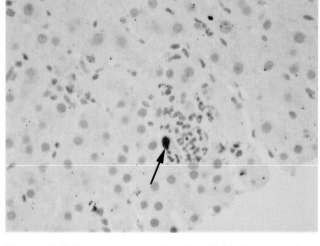

Figure 4.9.2 Immunostaining for CMV shows nuclear positivity (arrow).

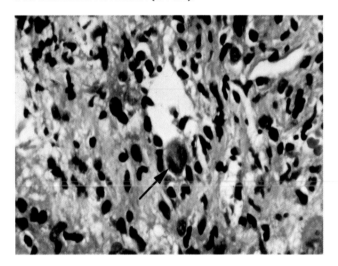

Figure 4.9.3 Cytomegaloviral inclusion affecting endothelial cell (arrow) can be obscured by accompanying inflammatory cells in the portal tract and mistaken for acute rejection.

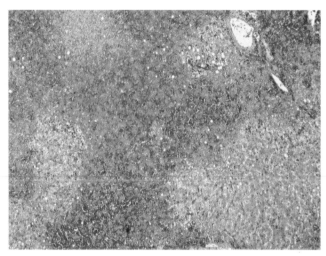

Figure 4.9.4 Severe herpes simplex hepatitis with submassive hepatic necrosis.

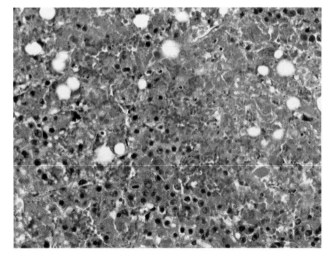

Figure 4.9.5 Adenovirus "blueberry" inclusions are noted at the edge of hemorrhagic necrosis.

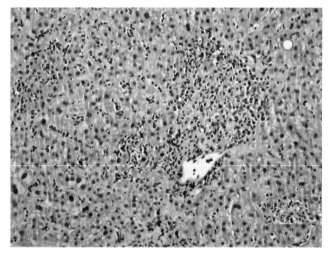

Figure 4.9.6 Atypical lymphocytes in the portal tract and sinusoids without significant hepatocellular damage in EBV hepatitis.

4.10 Posttransplant Lymphoproliferative Disorder

Posttransplant lymphoproliferative disorder (PTLD) represents a spectrum of disorders, which range from polyclonal expansion of B lymphocytes to full-fledged malignant lymphoma. It is a well-recognized complication of immunosuppression in transplant recipients, associated with active EBV infection, and can occur as early as 1 month after transplantation. The risk of developing PTLD is increased in unresolved or recurrent EBV syndromes and influenced by the duration of the immunosuppresion.

The clinical presentation is similar to that of EBV hepatitis. Depending on the extent of liver replacement by the lymphoproliferative disorder, the serum aminotransferase activities may be higher than in EBV hepatitis. Acute hepatic failure may complicate PTLD. The first-line treatment of PTLD includes reduction or withdrawal in immunosuppression with addition of antiviral agents such as acyclovir, regardless of the clinical or pathologic manifestation or clonality of the lesion. Patients failing to respond to withdrawal of immunosuppression may benefit from radiation or combination chemotherapy.

Pathologic Features

Posttransplant lymphoproliferative disorder is characterized by a spectrum of histologic changes ranging from benign proliferation of B lymphocytes to malignant B-cell lymphoma. Less commonly, PTLD may arise from T cells or NK cell. The involved portal tracts are enlarged and densely infiltrated by atypical lymphocytes with large nuclei and prominent nucleoli (Figures 4.10.1 and 4.10.2). The borders of the portal tracts are rounded and compress the surrounding hepatocytes. Infiltration by the same cells is seen within the sinusoids and sometimes within the central venules and portal veins, mimicking acute rejection. The presence of densely packed cells in the enlarged portal tracts helps to differentiate lymphoproliferative disease from EBV hepatitis, especially when the cells are monomorphic and distort the normal spatial arrangement of portal structures. When malignant lymphoma develops, neoplastic infiltrates in the portal tracts expand even farther and may coalesce with tumor nodules from adjacent portal tracts (Figures 4.10.3 and 4.10.4). Necrosis of tumor cells is often seen. The liver parenchyma shows cholestasis and ischemic necrosis.

In patients with suspected PTLD, immunophenotyping should be performed, including immunostains for CD20, κ and λ light chains, and EBV antigens. In situ hybridization for EBV RNA is confirmatory. Immunophenotyping of lymphocytes reveals predominantly or exclusively B cells in lymphoproliferative disease, whereas in EBV hepatitis, both B- and T-cell populations are seen.

Differential Diagnosis

The differential diagnosis of PTLD includes most posttransplant disorders featuring prominent portal inflammation, such as acute rejection, recurrent chronic viral hepatitis, and acute hepatitis (Figures 4.10.5 and 4.10.6).

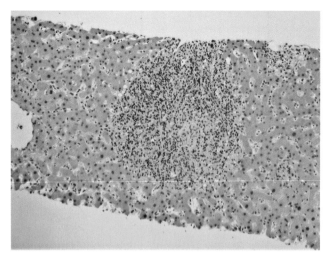

Figure 4.10.1 Posttransplant lymphoproliferative disorder with expansion of portal tract and sinusoidal infiltration by atypical lymphocytic infiltrate.

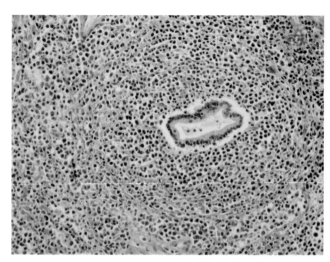

Figure 4.10.2 Posttransplant lymphoproliferative disorder with densely packed atypical lymphocytic infiltrate with large nuclei in the portal tract surrounding preserved bile duct.

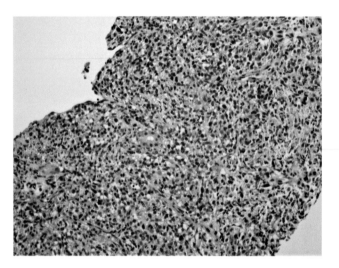

Figure 4.10.3 Large cell lymphoma obliterating portal structures and liver parenchyma.

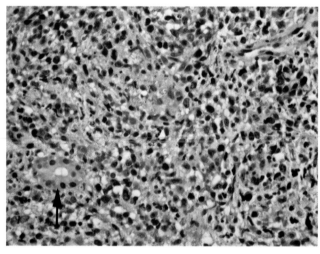

Figure 4.10.4 Densely packed large cell lymphoma surrounding a bile duct (arrow).

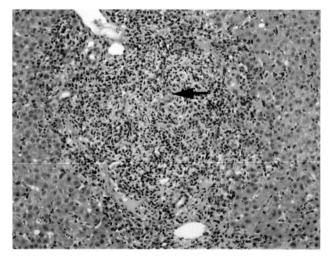

Figure 4.10.5 Acute rejection with bile duct damage (arrow) and mixed inflammatory infiltrate including immunoblasts, plasma cells, lymphocytes, and eosinophils in the portal tract.

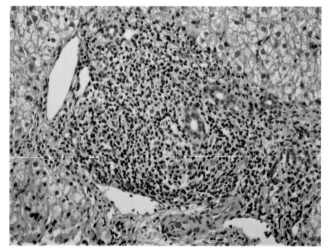

Figure 4.10.6 Recurrent chronic hepatitis C with dense mature lymphocytes in the portal tract. Bile ducts and portal vein branches are spared from damage and endotheliitis.

Table 4.10.1 WHO Post Transplant Lymphoproliferative Disorder Classification

Category	Type	Histopathologic Features	Clonality	Comments
Early lesions	Infectious mononucleosis-like Reactive plasmacytic hyperplasia	Architectural preservation of the involved tissue; plasma cells and lymphocytes; scattered immunoblasts; mild atypia	Polyclonal B cells, plasma cells and T cells. EBV-positive	Usual regression with reduced immunosupression
Polymorphic PTLD	Polymorphic B-cell hyperplasia Polymorphic B-cell lymphoma	Destruction of underlying architecture; full range of B-cell maturation; atypical immunoblasts; mitoses; may have necrosis	Majority are monoclonal, rarely polyclonal. Mixture of B and T lymphocytes, surface and cytoplasmic Ig polytypic or monotypic. Most cases EBV positive	Variable regression with reduced immunosuppresion
Monomorphic PTLD	B-cell neoplasms: diffuse large B-cell lymphoma, Burkitt or Burkitt-like lymphoma, plasma cell myeloma, plasmacytoma-like lesions	Morphological lymphoma and classified according to lymphoma classification. Most morphologically like diffuse B-cell lymphoma, other types are less common	Monoclonal Ig genes in B-cell PTLD. EBV-positive cases also have clonal EBV	Regresion is possible but uncommon if compared to early lesions and polymorphic PTLD
	T-cell neoplasms: peripheral T-cell lymphoma, other types	Monomophic T-cell PTLD includes most or all types of T-cell neoplasms	T-cell PTLD usually have clonal T-cell receptor; 25% with clonal EBV	
Hodgkin lymphoma and Hodgkin lymphoma-like	Classic Hodgkin lymphoma Hodgkin lymphoma-like	Reed Sternberg cells in appropriate background		Diagnosis requires appropriate morphologic and immunophenotypic features

Adapted from Harris NL, Swerdlow SH, Frizzera G, Knowles DM. Post-transplant lymphoproliferative disorders. In: Jaffe ES, Harris NL, Stein H, Vardiman JW, eds. *World Health Organization Classification of Tumours. Pathology and Genetics of Tumours of Haematopoietic and Lymphoid Tissues.* Lyon: IARC Press; 2001:264-269.

4.11 Bone Marrow Transplantation

After bone marrow transplantation, there are a variety of hepatic disorders that can occur, such as veno-occlusive disease (VOD), nodular regenerative hyperplasia, opportunistic infections, and acute and chronic graft-versus-host disease (GVHD), as well as acute viral hepatitis and drug-induced hepatitis.

Acute Graft-Versus-Host Disease

Acute GVHD occurs as early as 1 to 3 weeks after transplantation with peak onset at 30 to 50 days and no longer than 120 days. Acute GVHD involves the skin, the gastrointestinal tract, and the liver, resulting in skin rash or exfoliative erythroderma, diarrhea, elevation of serum bilirubin levels, and alkaline phosphatase and aminotransferase activities. With progression, coagulopathy, hepatic failure, ascites, and encephalopathy may develop.

Acute GVHD may show similarities to, but less severe than, acute allograft rejection. The changes include mild portal inflammation, bile duct damage, and in a small subset of patients, endotheliitis of portal vein branches and central venules. Bile duct damage is due to direct attack of donor lymphocytes to bile duct epithelium, which results in cytoplasmic vacuolization, nuclear pleomorphism, loss of nuclei, and detached biliary epithelium (Figure 4.11.1). Residual bile duct cells may appear squamoid. Hepatocanalicular cholestasis, hepatocellular damage, apoptosis, and lobular lymphocytic inflammation are not prominent but can often occur. The inflammatory infiltrate in the portal tracts consists predominantly of lymphocytes and may include neutrophils, eosinophils, and plasma cells. Because patients with acute GVHD are usually pancytopenic, the degree of bile duct and portal tract inflammation may be minimal despite significant damage to the bile ducts.

Chronic GVHD

Chronic GVHD develops 3 to 12 months after bone marrow transplantation. Graft-versus-host disease, including hepatic dysfunction, may be reversed by immunosuppressive therapy. Chronic GVHD involves the skin, gastrointestinal tract, salivary glands, lungs, musculoskeletal system, and liver. Patients with liver involvement are jaundiced and exhibit elevations of bilirubin levels and alkaline phosphatase and aminotransferase activities. Morbidity and mortality are high in chronic GVHD with multiple organ involvement.

In chronic GVHD, centrilobular cholestasis is invariably present, associated with hepatocellular ballooning and dropout. Portal tracts show mild portal fibrosis, mild lymphocytic inflammation, and variable degrees of damage, lymphocyte infiltration, and eventual loss of small bile ducts. The affected bile ducts are generally of small caliber, which appear atrophic with eosinophilic cytoplasm and large dark nuclei (senescence) (Figure 4.11.2). Endotheliitis is rarely seen. Bile duct loss may lead to vanishing bile duct syndrome and overt cirrhosis.

Veno-occlusive Disease

Veno-occlusive disease is the complication of cytoreductive therapy due to toxic injury to the sinusoidal endothelium. Veno-occlusive disease usually occurs within 100 days after bone marrow transplantation and at the same time frame with GVHD. Patients present with jaundice, tender hepatomegaly, and ascites, with elevation of serum aminotransferase activities.

Acute VOD is characterized by centrilobular congestion, hepatocyte necrosis, and accumulation of hemosiderin-laden macrophages (Figures 4.11.3 and 4.11.4). The hepatic venules exhibit intimal edema but without thrombosis. Proliferation of perisinusoidal lining cells and deposition of extracellular matrix occur subsequent to the acute injury, resulting in obliteration of sinusoidal spaces, hence giving an alternative name to this disorder, "sinusoidal obstruction syndrome." Subacute and chronic VOD are characterized by progressive centrilobular collagen deposition, which leads to occlusion of hepatic venules and dense perivenular fibrosis radiating out into the remainder of the parenchyma (Figure 4.11.5). The scar tissue contains hemosiderin-laden macrophages.

Opportunistic Infection

Liver biopsy after bone marrow transplantation is often performed to rule out hepatic involvement by systemic opportunistic fungal or viral infections.

Cytomegaloviral infection is the most common viral infection. Cytomegaloviral inclusion can be seen in hepatocytes, bile ducts, sinusoidal lining cells and vascular endothelial cells (Figure 4.11.6). Immunohistochemical staining for CMV is useful to confirm the presence of antigens, particularly in cases where there are suggestive inflammatory lesions but no inclusions have been identified.

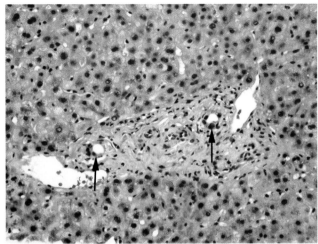

Figure 4.11.1 Graft-versus-host disease with bile duct damage (arrows) resulting in nuclear pleomorphism and squamoid appearance. The brown pigment/discoloration of the hepatic parenchyma is due to secondary iron overload.

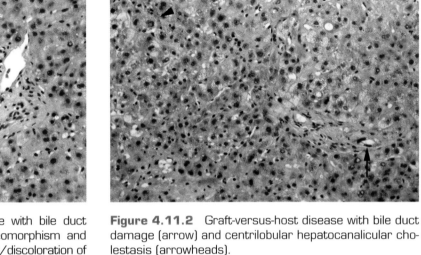

Figure 4.11.2 Graft-versus-host disease with bile duct damage (arrow) and centrilobular hepatocanalicular cholestasis (arrowheads).

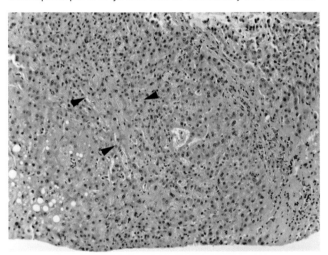

Figure 4.11.3 Acute veno-occlusive disease with centrilobular congestion and hepatocyte atrophy (arrows).

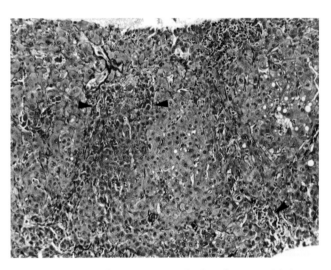

Figure 4.11.4 Acute veno-occlusive disease with hepatocyte dropout and collection of hemosiderin-laden macrophages (arrows) (trichrome stain).

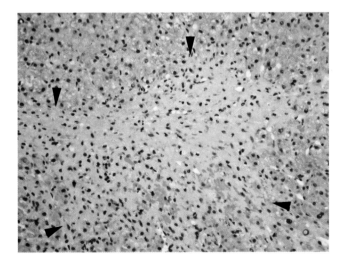

Figure 4.11.5 Subacute VOD with congestion, centrilobular collagen deposition, occlusion of the hepatic venule, and fibrosis radiating out into the remainder of the parenchyma (arrowheads).

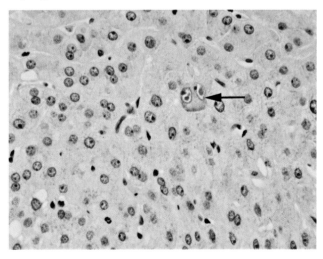

Figure 4.11.6 Cytomegaloviral inclusion (arrow) in hepatocyte of patient after bone marrow transplantation.

Table 4.11.1 Pathologic Findings After Bone Marrow Transplantation

Days After BMT	Common Findings	Less Common Findings
0-30 d	Veno-occlusive disease	Graft-versus-host-disease
	Drug-induced toxicity	Opportunistic infections
	Cholestasis related to sepsis	
30-100 d	Acute graft-versus-host disease	Recurrent lymphoma/leukemia
	Veno-occlusive disease	Total parenteral nutrition
	Opportunistic infections	Viral hepatitis
	Drug-induced toxicity	Nodular regenerative hyperplasia
>100 d	Chronic graft-versus-host-disease	Opportunistic infections
	Viral hepatitis	Recurrent lymphoma/leukemia
	Drug-induced toxicity	EBV-associated lymphoma

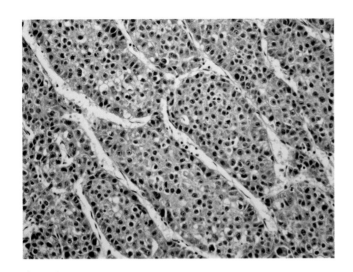

CHAPTER 5

FOCAL LESIONS AND NEOPLASTIC DISEASES

5.1 Hepatic Granulomas

Hepatic granulomas are always part of a systemic disease, particularly sarcoidosis, infectious disease (tuberculosis, viral and fungal infections), schistosomiasis, primary biliary cirrhosis, and drug reactions. The incidence of hepatic involvement ranges from 50% to 90%. Therefore, the importance of hepatic granuloma lies in the opportunity to diagnose the underlying disease. The prognosis and treatment of hepatic granuloma depends on the underlying disease.

Hepatic granuloma is often asymptomatic. Some patients may have low-grade fever and nonspecific constitutional symptoms, but overt features of hepatic involvement are rare.

Hepatic granulomas have a common histologic pattern consisting of nodular accumulations of inflammatory cells, most importantly epithelioid macrophages as well as lymphocytes, capillaries, and fibroblasts. The histologic alterations described below may be helpful in the differential diagnosis of hepatic granulomas. Many other less common causes must also be considered. Step sections of the liver biopsy specimen, as well as special stains and cultures for microorganisms, should be performed in all specimens of patients suspected of harboring hepatic granulomas. The complete diagnostic workup must include a detailed clinical history and careful biochemical, serologic, and microbiologic screening. In spite of these measures, the cause of hepatic granulomas cannot be established in up to 25% of patients.

Sarcoidosis

Sarcoid granulomas are seen in the liver in up to 90% of cases. They are located more frequently in portal tracts than in hepatic lobules. Characteristically, they are multiple large noncaseating granulomas with eosinophils and multinucleated giant cells, which may contain Schaumann bodies, asteroid bodies, or calcium oxalate crystals. They often coalesce to form conglomerates of several granulomas (Figure 5.1.1). Special stains show abundant reticulin fibers but no microorganisms. Frequently, the granulomas undergo fibrosis with formation of concentric layers of dense hyalinized collagen, which eventually develop into nodular fibrous scars in the liver. Thus, different stages of the evolution of sarcoid granulomas may be observed in a liver biopsy specimen. The remainder of the liver shows mild nonspecific reactive inflammatory changes. Occasionally, isolated multinucleated giant cells may be found in the hepatic sinusoids of patients with sarcoidosis, even in the absence of granulomas. Biliary cirrhosis, portal hypertension, cholestatic syndrome with primary biliary cirrhosis-like picture, and Budd-Chiari syndrome are rare complications of hepatic sarcoidosis.

Tuberculosis

Tuberculous granulomas are seen in more than 25% of patients with tuberculosis. Typically, the granulomas are located in portal tracts and parenchyma and are all at the same stage of development (Figure 5.1.2). Langhans giant cells, central necrosis, and caseation may be absent, especially in small tuberculous granulomas. Special stain for acid-fast bacilli is not sensitive enough to detect the usually small amount of microorganisms present in tuberculous granulomas; therefore, a negative special stain does not exclude tuberculosis as the cause of the granulomatous disease. Submitting fresh tissue for culture is necessary when suspicion of tuberculosis is high. The remainder of the liver often shows lymphocytic infiltration of sinusoids and portal tracts, activation of sinusoidal lining cells, and scattered focal hepatocyte necroses. Reticulum staining demonstrates destruction of reticulum fibers within the granulomas. In AIDS patients with tuberculosis, hepatic granulomas are poorly formed or entirely absent. Acid-fast staining, however, reveals acid-fast bacilli in Kupffer cells and portal macrophages, particularly in patients infected with *Mycobacterium avium-intracellulare*. In these instances, small clusters of macrophages are seen stuffed with the organisms, often in the absence of other inflammatory cells. Therefore, special stains for mycobacterium should be performed on all liver biopsy specimens of patients with AIDS. *Mycobacterium avium-intracellulare* are periodic acid–Schiff (PAS) positive after diastase digestion. Fungi should be demonstrated by diastase-resistant PAS staining or silver staining.

Fibrin Ring Granulomas

Fibrin ring granuloma is characterized by a central lipid droplet surrounded by fibrin and inflammatory cells (Figure 5.1.3). The fibrin ring is better visualized by special stain for fibrin or on trichrome stain. The granulomas are predominantly in the lobule. The pathogenesis is unclear, and they are commonly observed in association with Q fever. Q fever is a zoonotic disease caused by *Coxiella burnetii*. Cattle, sheep, and goats are the primary reservoirs of *C. burnetii*. Infection of humans usually occurs by inhalation of these organisms from air that contains airborne barnyard dust contaminated by dried placental material, birth fluids, and excreta of infected herd animals.

Fibrin ring granulomas have also been described in other processes, such as cytomegalovirus and Epstein-Barr virus infections, visceral leishmaniasis, allopurinol toxicity, hepatitis A, and systemic lupus erythematosus.

Schistosomiasis

In chronic schistosomiasis unshed schistosoma eggs, which are highly antigenic and can induce an intense granulomatous response and fibrosis, migrate through the bowel wall to the portal circulation and lodged in the portal tracts.

Granulomas are found primarily in portal tracts and consist of accumulation of epithelioid cells, eosinophils, multinucleated giant cells, and fibrosis (Figure 5.1.4). Multiple sections may be needed to find the ova and identify the lateral spine of *Schistosoma mansoni* and the spherical ova of *Schistosoma japonicum*. Acid-fast staining may demonstrate fragmented egg shells. Kupffer cells and portal macrophages may contain very fine, brown to black, iron-negative pigment (Figure 1.9.6). Portal fibrosis with phlebosclerosis of portal vein branches (Symmers clay pipe-stem fibrosis) is often present, resulting in portal hypertension.

Drug Reaction–Related Granulomas

Drug reactions may result in noncaseating granulomas, particularly sulfonamides, allopurinol, carbamazepine, quinine, and phenylbutazone. The granulomas are located in portal tracts or hepatic lobules. Granuloma can be single or multiple, may contain eosinophils and giant cells, and may be accompanied by acute hepatitis or cholestatic hepatitis (Figure 5.1.5). Although eosinophils are often seen in drug-induced injury, the absence of eosinophil in granuloma or in the surrounding liver parenchyma does not exclude drug-induced-injury.

Lipogranulomas

Lipogranulomas do not represent true granulomas because epithelioid cells are usually not present. They are often seen in livers with steatosis or in patients ingesting mineral oil and are located in portal tracts and adjacent to the central venules. They consist of focal accumulations of fat droplets, lipid-laden macrophages, scattered lymphocytes, and occasional eosinophils, accompanied by focal fibrosis (Figure 5.1.6). They are of little diagnostic or prognostic significance and should not be confused with hepatic granulomatous disease.

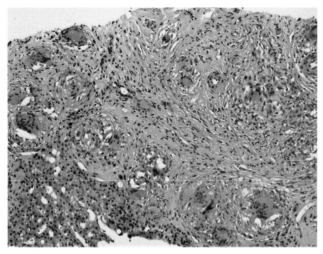

Figure 5.1.1 Coalescing sarcoid granulomas with multinucleated giant cells and associated fibrosis.

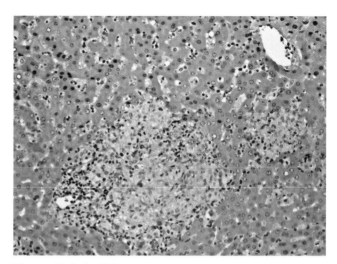

Figure 5.1.2 Ill bordered tuberculous granulomas accompanied by lymphocytic infiltration in sinusoids and activation of sinusoidal lining cells.

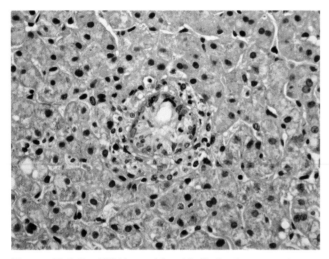

Figure 5.1.3 EBV hepatitis with fibrin ring granuloma.

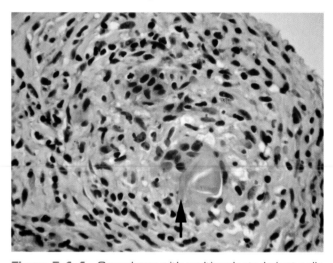

Figure 5.1.4 Granuloma with multinucleated giant cells and ovum of *Schistosoma* (arrow).

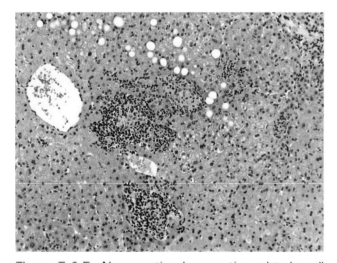

Figure 5.1.5 Noncaseating drug reaction–related small granulomas with lymphocytic cuff.

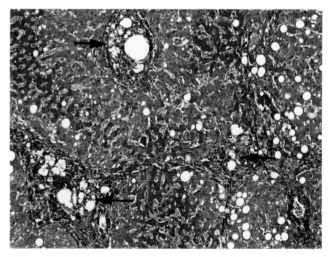

Figure 5.1.6 Lipogranulomas contain fat droplets and are associated with localized fibrosis (trichrome stain).

Table 5.1.1 Differential Diagnoses of Common Hepatic Granulomas

Conditions	Granuloma Characteristics	Location	Fibrosis	Other Findings
Sarcoidosis	Noncaseating coalescing multiple epithelioid granulomas, occasional multinucleated giant cells with Schaumann bodies, asteroid bodies or calcium oxalate crystals.	More in portal tracts than in lobules	Yes	Different stages of granuloma evolution.
Tuberculosis	Caseating granulomas with Langhans giant cells. Central necrosis and caseation may be absent. Special stains for acid-fast bacilli are positive in less than 10% of cases. In AIDS patients, granulomas are poorly formed or absent.	Portal tracts and lobules	No	Granulomas at the same stage of development. In AIDS patients, Kupffer cells and portal macrophages may be filled with acid-fast bacilli.
Drug reactions	Noncaseating granulomas.	Portal tracts and lobules	No	Often accompanied by lobular or cholestatic hepatitis. Eosinophils may be present.
Primary biliary cirrhosis	Poorly defined noncaseating granulomas. Giant cells are usually absent.	Predominantly in portal tracts, around damaged bile ducts	No	Granulomas are more frequent in early stage of PBC.
Schistosomiasis	Granulomas with eosinophils, multinucleated giant cells, and fibrosis. Ova may be present.	Portal tracts and often associated with portal fibrosis	Yes	Kupffer cells and portal macrophages may contain fine, brown to black, iron-negative pigment. Portal vein branches maybe occluded.
Lipogranuloma	Fat globules, macrophages, and associated fibrosis.	Portal tracts and perivenular	Yes	Little clinical significance. Not to be mistaken as epithelioid granulomas.
Hepatitis C-associated microgranuloma	Noncaseating small round/compact solitary epithelioid granulomas. No multinucleated giant cell or rim of chronic inflammatory cells.	Lobules	No	No diagnostic or prognostic significance. More often in patient receiving pegylated interferon.

5.2   Ductular Proliferative Lesions

Ductular proliferative lesions are commonly encountered during frozen section examination. Coupled with inherent frozen section artifact, they can be difficult to interpret. Ductular proliferative lesions in general can be divided into localized and diffuse lesions. Localized lesions include biliary hamartoma and bile duct adenoma, whereas diffuse lesions include ductular reaction and congenital hepatic fibrosis.

Bile Duct Adenoma

Bile duct adenoma is a benign neoplasm of intrahepatic bile ducts, also known as peribiliary gland hamartoma. It is asymptomatic and usually found incidentally at surgery or autopsy. It is unrelated to fibropolycystic disease of the liver. The importance in recognizing bile duct adenoma lies in the differentiation from metastatic adenocarcinoma and from its malignant counterparts cholangiolocarcinoma and cholangiocarcinoma (CC).

Bile duct adenoma is a well-circumscribed, but non-encapsulated subcapsular nodule that is composed of small, irregular branching of bile duct structures in a fibrous stroma (Figure 5.2.1). The ductal components are usually tubular, lined by regular, cuboidal bile duct epithelial cells without nuclear dysplasia, polyploidy, or mitoses (Figure 5.2.2). Their nuclei are lighter than those of bile ducts, and the cytoplasm may contain α-1-antitrypsin-like globules. In contrast to microhamartomas, the bile duct structures are rarely dilated or cystic and do not contain bile in their lumens. Collagen fibers surround the tubular structures. Densely hyalinized areas are usually seen in the center, and loose stroma at the periphery (Figure 5.2.3). Dense lymphocytic rim is sometimes present at the periphery. Portal tracts usually remain intact within the nodule.

Biliary Microhamartoma

Biliary microhamartoma (von Meyenburg complex) is part of ductal plate malformation lesions and hence may be seen in combination with other forms of fibropolycystic disease of the liver. It is usually an incidental finding at surgery or autopsy.

Biliary microhamartomas are either solitary or multiple nodules of mature collagen containing dilated or elongated bile duct structures, lined by regular cuboidal epithelium with small dark nuclei (Figure 5.2.4). These channels may contain bile concretions. They are located adjacent to or within portal tracts. In comparison to bile duct adenoma, the bile duct structures in microhamartomas are larger, less numerous, and more separated from each other by abundant fibrous tissue than the tubular structures in bile duct adenoma.

Ductular Reaction

Ductular reaction is a unified term for the benign proliferation of ductular structures. Ductular structures may arise from the proliferation of preexisting cholangiocytes (proliferating bile ductules), progenitor cells (local and/or circulating cells probably bone marrow derived), or biliary metaplasia of hepatocytes. Ductular reaction occurs in large duct obstruction, in a variety of chronic liver disease, or as regenerative attempt after extensive hepatocellular loss, such as multiacinar, submassive, or massive hepatic necrosis (Figure 5.2.5).

In active proliferation, as seen in large duct obstruction, the ductular structures are accompanied by neutrophils, have small or no lumen, and may form a lattice network or back-to-back configuration, in the background of edematous stroma. In chronic conditions such as biliary cirrhosis, the neutrophils disappear, and the ductular structures have well-formed lumen and are separated from each other by fibrous stroma. In chronic liver disease, ductular reaction remains confined to portal tracts, along limiting plates, along fibrous septa, and in areas of collapse in cirrhosis. It consists of tubular or glandular structures formed by uniform, regularly arranged cuboidal cells on a basement membrane. The nuclei are evenly spaced and show little pleomorphism.

In liver with extensive hepatocellular loss, ductular reaction extends beyond the confines of portal tracts, occupies collapsed area, and demonstrates more abundant cytoplasm, larger nuclei, poorly defined lumen, and no basement membrane. These ductular structures have been referred to earlier as "neocholangioles" or ductular hepatocytes.

Ductular reaction can be so extensive as to raise the question of adenocarcinoma. Unlike the findings in adenocarcinoma, there is no increase in the nucleocytoplasmic ratio and no nuclear hyperchromasia or cellular anaplasia. Mucin is negative, but carcinoembryonic antigen (CEA) is positive, particularly on the luminal surface and to a much lesser degree in the cytoplasm. In contrast, adenocarcinoma tends to show both luminal and cytoplasmic CEA positivity. The glandular structures of adenocarcinoma are complex and invade the surrounding portal tracts and lobules, in the background of desmoplastic stroma (Figure 5.2.6).

162

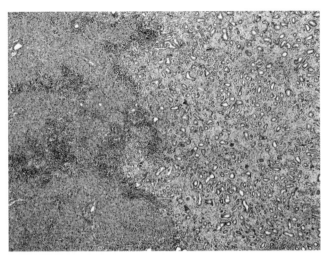

Figure 5.2.1 Bile duct adenoma composed of small irregular, but well-formed bile duct structures in fibrous stroma and with dense lymphocytic rim.

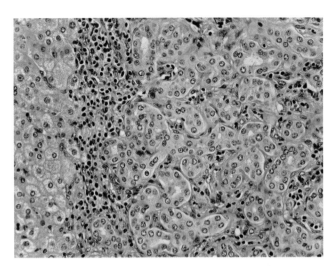

Figure 5.2.2 Tubular structures in bile duct adenoma.

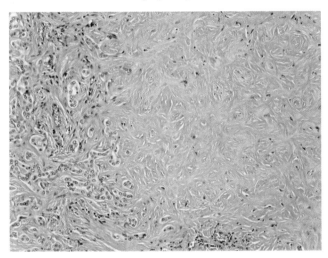

Figure 5.2.3 Dense hyalinized fibrous stroma at the center of bile duct adenoma.

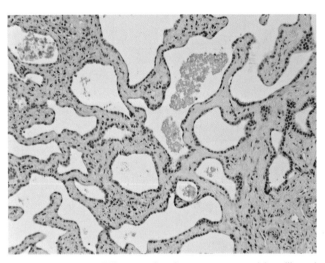

Figure 5.2.4 Biliary microhamartoma with dilated and irregular glands containing inspissated bile (von Meyenburg complex).

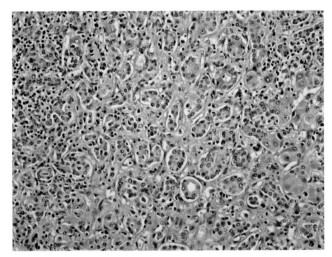

Figure 5.2.5 Ductular reaction after submassive hepatic necrosis. The ductular structures are located in the lobules and have more eosinophilic and abundant cytoplasm than proliferating bile ductules.

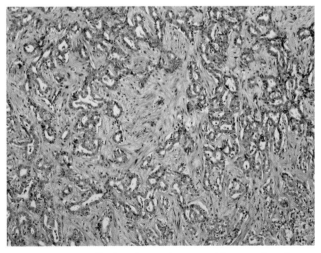

Figure 5.2.6 Cholangiocarcinoma with complex ductular structures in desmoplastic stroma.

Table 5.2.1 Differential Diagnosis of Ductular Proliferative Lesions

Histologic Features	Ductular Reaction	Biliary Hamartoma	Bile Duct Adenoma	Cholangiocarcinoma	Metastatic Adenocarcinoma
Ductular pattern	Small, narrow or no lumen, at edge of portal tracts or in fibrous stroma	Dilated and irregular lumen with bile concretion, in fibrous stroma	Packed, no or very narrow lumen, rarely with mucous concretion	Single cells or irregular glands with various differentiation and shape	Irregular glands with various differentiation and shape
Cytological features	Flat to cuboidal, open chromatin	Flat to cuboidal, small hyperchromatic nuclei	Cuboidal, may contain mucin or eosinophilic globules.	Pleomorphic cuboidal to low columnar, high nuclear cytoplasmic ratio	Pleomorphic cuboidal to columnar, high nuclear cytoplasmic ratio
Mitoses	Present, normal	None	Rare	Common, atypical	Common, atypical
Portal tract in lesion	Always present	Often present	Often present	Generally absent, only at periphery of lesion	Generally absent, only at periphery of lesion
Stroma	Edematous to fibrotic stroma	Fibrous collagenized stroma	Dense fibrosis in center. Loose stroma at the periphery	Desmoplastic stroma, often densely fibrotic	Desmoplastic stroma
Inflammation	Neutrophils	Lymphocytic, mild	Lymphocytic rim	Mild at periphery	Mild at periphery
Cytokeratin 7	+	+	+	+	+ (pancreas, lung, breast), – (colon)
Cytokeratin 20	–	–	–	–	+ (colon, some pancreas), – (lung, breast)
p53	–	–	–	+	+
CEA, monoclonal	+ (luminal)	+ (luminal)	+ (luminal)	+ (luminal & cytoplasmic)	+ (luminal and cytoplasmic)
Smad4	+	+	+	+/–	+/– (cholangio- and pancreatic carcinoma may be –)
Organ specific antibody	–	–	–	–	CDX-2 + (colon), TTF-1 + (lung), GCDFP15 + (breast), ER/PR + (gynecologic tract and breast), PSA + (prostate)

+, positive; –, negative

5.3 Cysts of the Liver

Cysts are increasingly being diagnosed by improved methods of imaging of the liver and biliary tree. Small cysts rarely cause symptoms, and their findings are invariably incidental, whereas larger cysts may displace or compress adjacent structures and therefore symptomatic.

Simple Biliary Cyst

Simple biliary cyst is a unilocular cyst lined by a single layer of biliary epithelium and surrounded by dense fibrous stroma (Figure 5.3.1). Simple biliary cyst can be single or multiple and occurs at all ages, but most simple biliary cysts occur in patients more than 40 years old, and the prevalence increases with age. When multiple, they often represent a component of autosomal dominant adult polycystic disease. Simple biliary cysts have no malignant potential.

The cyst is usually subcapsular and is not connected to the biliary tree. The content is serous or mucoid yellow clear fluid, blood stained if traumatized, or purulent if infected. Macrophages containing hemosiderin, cholesterol, or cellular debris may be present in the wall. Biliary microhamartomas (von Meyenburg complexes) are often found adjacent to simple biliary cysts (Figure 5.3.2). Repeated hemorrhage or infection may cause cyst wall thickening or mural nodule formation.

Peribiliary Cyst

Peribiliary cysts are retention cysts of peribiliary glands of the hepatic hilum and large portal tracts. Synonyms include multiple hepatic hilar cysts and periductal hepatic cysts. They arise from preexisting hepatobiliary diseases such as advanced chronic liver diseases, cirrhosis, portal hypertension, or congenital diseases. Although most patients with peribiliary cysts are asymptomatic, large peribiliary cysts can compress the biliary tree, causing stenosis, proximal dilatation, cholangitis, and jaundice.

Multiple cysts are located along the bile ducts of the hepatic hilar region or along large intrahepatic bile ducts. They are round to ovoid and vary in size from 0.2 to 2.0 cm in diameter. The cysts are not connected to bile ducts, and their content is clear colorless fluid. The cysts are lined by a single layer of flattened or cuboidal epithelial cells without atypia, surrounded by fibrous wall, containing scattered peribiliary glands (Figure 5.3.3).

Ciliated Foregut Cyst

Ciliated foregut cyst is a benign, solitary, unilocular cyst lined by pseudostratified ciliated columnar epithelium, sub-epithelial connective tissue, and smooth muscle layer (Figure 5.3.4). Ciliated foregut cysts arise from the embryonic foregut with bronchial differentiation. Ciliated foregut cysts occur more frequently in men and in the medial segment of the left hepatic lobe. Complete excision of the cyst is curative.

Biliary Cystadenoma and Cystadenocarcinoma

Biliary cystadenoma is a solitary, unilocular, or multilocular cyst, lined by mucinous epithelium with underlying "ovarian-like" stroma (Figure 5.3.5). Biliary cystadenocarcinoma is the malignant counterpart of biliary cystadenoma (Figure 5.3.6).

Most patients with cystadenoma or cystadenocarcinoma are females. Patients may present with abdominal mass and/or pain. Rarely, a patient may present with recurrent jaundice. It is often located in the right lobe. Imaging studies of cystadenoma usually disclose a solitary, multiloculated, cystic structure, which on angiography is avascular and displaces the surrounding vessels. Thickening of internal septation and the presence of mural nodule should raise the suspicion of cystadenocarcinoma.

Cystadenoma/carcinoma can measure up to 28 cm. They are globoid with bosselated surface, depending on the complexity of internal septation and the number of cysts. Stretched vessels can be seen on the surface. The content of the cysts vary from clear thin to thick mucoid fluid. Dark blood-tinged fluid or necrotic material may be found in traumatized cyst or cystadenocarcinoma, whereas purulent mucoid material is often seen in infected cyst. Mural nodules are common in cystadenocarcinoma.

The epithelial lining varies from a single layer of columnar, cuboidal, or flattened mucinous epithelium in cystadenoma, to pleomorphic malignant cells with tubulopapillary growth pattern that may invade the stroma and capsule in cystadenocarcinoma. Areas of transition from benign epithelial lining to malignant cells may be found. The underlying dense fibrous, hyalinized, or cellular "ovarian-like" stroma is characteristic of these lesions, often requiring extensive sampling to demonstrate its presence. The cellular "ovarian-like" stroma is positive for estrogen and progesterone receptors by immunostaining and is seen only in female patients.

The treatment for biliary cystadenoma/carcinoma is complete excision. Incomplete excision may lead to recurrence.

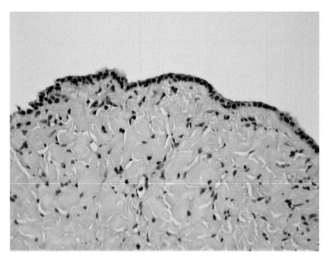

Figure 5.3.1 Simple biliary cyst lined by a single layer of biliary epithelium and surrounded by fibrous stroma.

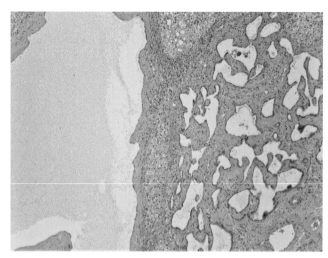

Figure 5.3.2 Biliary cyst in polycystic liver (left field) accompanied by biliary microhamartoma (right field).

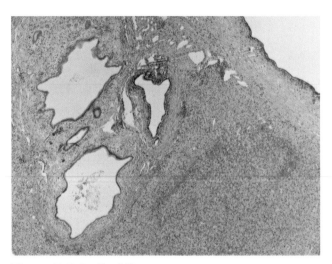

Figure 5.3.3 Peribiliary cysts.

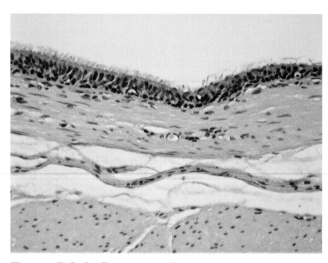

Figure 5.3.4 Pseudostratified ciliated columnar epithelium, subepithelial fibrous tissue and smooth muscle layer in ciliated foregut cyst.

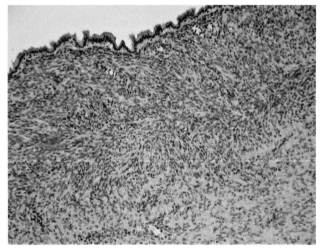

Figure 5.3.5 Mucinous epithelium with underlying "ovarian-like" cellular stroma in biliary cystadenoma.

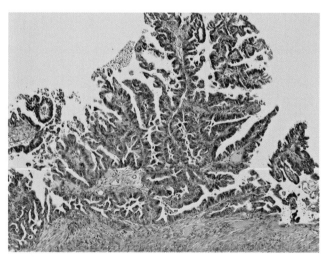

Figure 5.3.6 Biliary cystadenocarcinoma.

Table 5.3.1   **Cysts of the Liver**

Features	Simple Biliary Cyst	Peribiliary Cyst	Caroli Disease	Ciliated Foregut Cyst	Biliary Cystadenoma
Gross	Solitary or multiple unilocular cysts, parenchymal or subcapsular	Multiple unilocular cysts, in hepatic hilum	Multiple unilocular bile containing cysts, around biliary tree	Solitary unilocular cyst	Solitary uni- or multilocular cyst
Biliary tree connection	No	No	Yes	No	No
Epithelial lining	Cuboidal or low columnar epithelium	Flat or cuboidal epithelium	Cuboidal or columnar biliary epithelium	Low columnar ciliated epithelium	Cuboidal or columnar mucinous epithelium
Cyst wall stroma	Fibrous	Fibrous	Fibrous	Fibrous with smooth muscle layer	Fibrous with ovarian-type stroma in women
Cyst content	Clear serous fluid	Clear serous fluid	Bile, mucus or pus	Clear serous fluid	Thin to thick mucous, often blood tinged

5.4   Hepatic Abscess, Inflammatory Pseudotumor, and Hydatid Cysts

Hepatic Abscess

Hepatic abscesses are usually multiple and typically demonstrate central zone of necrosis and are commonly associated with cholangitis, colitis, diverticulitis, or appendicitis. Bacterial cholangitis can complicate biliary obstruction of any origin, including gallstones, strictures, neoplasm, parasites, and recurrent pyogenic cholangitis, and may follow endoscopic or surgical manipulation of bile ducts. Approximately 50% of hepatic abscesses yield positive culture results for bacterial organisms, which are often mixed in nature (eg, gram-negative enteric bacilli and gram-positive anaerobic cocci). Pyogenic hepatic abscess appears as destructive cavities, which vary in size, with purulent and necrotic content. Necrosis and intense neutrophilic infiltrate are seen at the center of the abscess with various degrees of inflammation, fibrosis, edema, and ductular reaction at the periphery (Figures 5.4.1 and 5.4.2).

Amoebic abscess is typically single in the dome of the right liver, containing red-brown thick necrotic material. It may be recognized by their content of amoebic trophozoites and cysts by PAS or silver stain, as well as abundant eosinophils in fibrous wall compressing adjacent liver parenchyma. After successful treatment, organizing amoebic abscesses may closely simulate inflammatory pseudotumor (IPT), and historical data may be crucial to their proper pathologic diagnosis.

Hepatic abscess should be differentiated from metastatic or largely necrotic primary tumors (Figure 5.4.3), which can be clinically indistinguishable and requires liver biopsy for confirmation.

Inflammatory Pseudotumor (Myofibroblastic Tumor)

Inflammatory pseudotumor/myofibroblastic tumor is a heterogenous group of benign to locally aggressive, inflammatory, fibrosing tumor composed of myofibroblasts, fibroblasts, and chronic inflammatory cells (Figure 5.4.4). The etiology of IPT of the liver remains unclear, although infection, abscess, biliary obstruction, chronic cholangitis, primary sclerosing cholangitis, primary biliary cirrhosis, Crohn disease, and IgG4-related diseases have all been suggested as possible causes. A variety of chromosomal changes, such as ALK-1 overexpression, dendritic cell clonal expression, and Epstein-Barr virus expression, have been detected in some lesions, which raises the possibility that IPT is a neoplastic process.

The most frequent clinical findings of IPT are fever, malaise, weight loss, and right upper quadrant pain. Most of the IPTs are solitary but can also be multifocal. Inflammatory pseudotumor of the liver is usually confined to the liver parenchyma. Imaging findings were variable because of the different degrees of fibrosis and cellularity and can be similar to metastatic tumors or intrahepatic CC.

Inflammatory pseudotumor is well demarcated and measures up to 25 cm, and the cut surface is white to tan, is nodular, and can be variegated. Infarction may be apparent, admixed with hemorrhage, myxoid, and fibrous scarring, producing a "geographic" gross appearance.

Different degrees of "maturation" are seen in large IPTs, which manifest in a diversity of microscopic findings, including densely collagenized stroma, fibroblastic/myofibroblastic and histiocytic proliferation, xanthogranulomatous reaction, and variable numbers of lymphocytes, eosinophils, and neutrophils. Typically, there are only small numbers of plasma cells. Periphlebitis and occlusive phlebitis are often seen in the periphery. IgG4-related IPT shows the abundance of IgG4-positive plasma cells rather than the usual fibrohistiocytic proliferation.

The prognosis of patients with hepatic IPT is generally excellent, and the lesion may spontaneously regress. IgG4-related IPT may benefit from steroid treatment.

Hydatid Cysts

Hydatid disease is a zoonosis caused by the larval stages of cestodes of the genus *Echinococcus*, most often *Echinococcus granulosus*. Hydatid or echinococcal cysts are typically single, unilocular, and spherical, with diameters ranging up to 35 cm and a predilection for the right lobe. The infection is often asymptomatic but may cause abdominal discomfort or mass, bile duct compression, secondary bacterial infection, rupture into the biliary tract with consequent cholangitis, or rupture into the peritoneal or pleural cavities. Leakage can result in urticaria or anaphylaxis.

Viable cyst contains scolices, surrounded by a hyalinized, white membrane of laminated, acellular PAS-positive material secreted by the parasite, and then encompassed by an outer peripheral zone of granulation tissue and fibrosis that merges into adjacent parenchyma (Figure 5.4.5). The inflammatory infiltrate in the wall of hydatic cyst consists predominantly of chronic inflammatory cells with prominent eosinophilic component and epithelioid histiocytes (Figure 5.4.6).

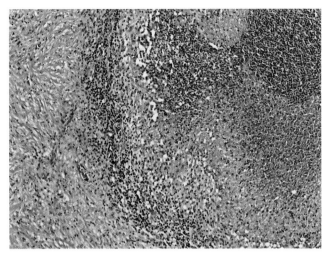

Figure 5.4.1 Central zone of necrosis with acute inflammatory infiltrate in hepatic abscess.

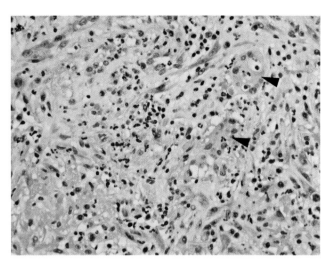

Figure 5.4.2 Hepatic abscess wall with neutrophilic infiltrate, edema and ductular reaction (arrowheads).

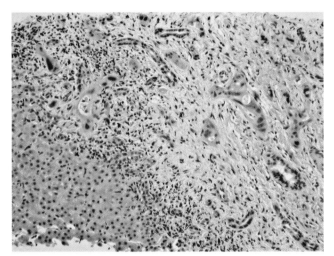

Figure 5.4.3 Biopsy from periphery of largely necrotic cholangiocarcinoma showing neoplastic glands.

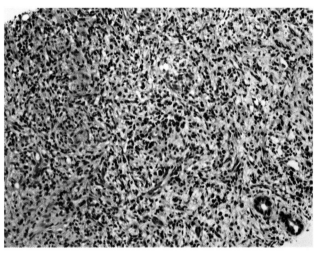

Figure 5.4.4 Inflammatory pseudotumor with mixed cellular infiltrate and granulomatous reaction.

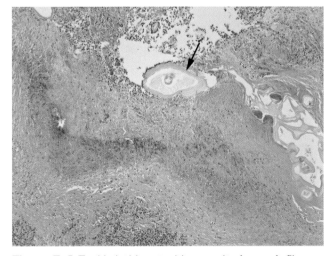

Figure 5.4.5 Hydatid cyst with parasite (arrow), fibrous wall and inflammation.

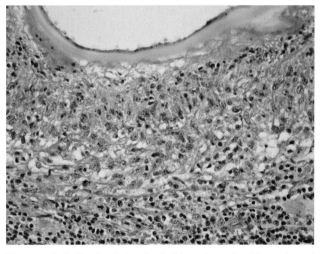

Figure 5.4.6 Acellular hydatid cyst wall with a rim of epithelioid histiocytes and eosinophils.

Table 5.4.1 Abscess, Inflammatory Pseudotumor, Parasitic Cysts of the Liver

Features	Abscess	Inflammatory Pseudotumor	Hydatid Cyst	Amoebic Cyst
Multiplicity	Usually multiple	Single or multiple	Usually single	Usually single
Gross	Necrotic, cystic lesion	Soft to rubbery solid lesion	Unilocular cystic lesion	Necrotic, cystic lesion
Content	Necrotic tissue, pus	None	Clear, watery fluid	Red brown, necrotic material
Microorganism	Bacteria or fungi	None	*Echinococcus* larvae with scolices	Amoebic trophozoites
Cellular infiltration	Neutrophils and macrophages	Lymphocytes, plasma cells, myofibroblasts	Eosinophils, epithelioid histiocytes	Eosinophils, macrophages

5.5 Benign Hepatocellular Tumors

Benign hepatocellular tumors in the noncirrhotic liver include focal nodular hyperplasia (FNH) and hepatocellular adenoma (HCA). In the last several years, there have been many studies confirming that FNH is a polyclonal lesion, whereas HCAs are monoclonal lesions with specific genetic mutations. Therefore, the latter are considered true neoplasm, requiring definitive treatment.

Focal Nodular Hyperplasia

Focal nodular hyperplasia is a circumscribed nodular lesion in the background of noncirrhotic liver parenchyma due to the localized increase of blood flow secondary to vascular malformation. It occurs at any age with slight female predominance. Most cases are discovered incidentally. Rarely, patients experience right upper quadrant pain and discomfort due to large mass.

Focal nodular hyperplasia shows central stellate scar and fibrous septa containing abnormal vessels with fibromuscular thickening of the walls (Figure 5.5.1). The fibrous septa contain scattered inflammatory cells and proliferating bile ductules, separating parenchymal nodules (Figures 5.5.3 and 5.5.4). Well developed bile ducts are absent. The nodules are formed by normal appearance hepatocytes arranged in 2-cell thick plates. The cells contain increased amounts of glycogen and occasionally fat, which give the tumor a lighter color than the surrounding liver. Rhodanine stain often demonstrate copper deposition in periseptal cells as the result of cholate stasis in the absence of bile ducts (Figure 5.5.5).

The normal surrounding liver and the absence of portal tracts or well-developed bile ducts within the nodule help in the differentiation FNH from cirrhosis, particularly biliary cirrhosis with paucity of intrahepatic bile ducts, which sometimes can be difficult in a small needle biopsy specimen. When FNH are found in multiple numbers, the diagnosis of inflammatory/telangiectatic HCA should be considered.

Hepatocellular Adenoma

Hepatocellular adenoma is a benign monoclonal proliferation of hepatocytes in an otherwise normal liver. It has a strong association with oral contraceptive steroids. The risk for its development depends on the duration of use and the dose of steroids. It is also associated with androgen-anabolic steroids and glycogenosis types I and III. Hepatocellular adenoma presents with right upper quadrant mass, pain, or acute intraperitoneal hemorrhage. Malignant transformation, although very rare, has been described; therefore, complete excision should be assured.

Hepatocellular adenoma can be solitary or multiple, such as in adenomatosis (>10 adenomas). It is soft, rarely encapsulated, and can measure up to 20 cm in diameter. On cut sections, the tumor is light-tan to yellow with interspersed dark red or brown areas of hemorrhage and infarction. Abnormal and dilated blood vessels may be present at the periphery of the tumor.

Hepatocellular adenoma consists of normal-looking or hyperplastic hepatocytes without dysplasia (Figures 5.5.6 and 5.5.7). The cells have regular nuclei with inconspicuous nucleoli and abundant pale cytoplasm because of the increased fat and glycogen content (Figures 5.5.8). Bile may rarely accumulate in the canaliculi formed by tumor cells. The tumor cells are arranged in sheets or irregular thickened trabeculae with compressed sinusoids and with little reticulum and fibrous stroma. Areas of hemorrhage, blood cysts similar to those of peliosis, and infarction may be seen (Figure 5.5.9). Abnormal veins or arteries are prominent. Portal tracts, bile ducts, and ductular reaction are absent. On rare occasions, brown-pigmented HCA can be encountered (Figure 5.5.10).

In recent years, there have been studies in refining the classification of HCA variants based on molecular studies into HCA with HNF1α mutation, HCA with β-catenin mutation, inflammatory/telangiectatic HCA, and unclassified HCA. Inflammatory/telangiectatic HCA had been sometimes referred to as telangiectatic FNH, occurring in multiple FNH syndrome. Although many of the conventional features of HCA are present in each of the different molecular pathways, each of the molecular alteration translates to additional specific morphologic features and clinical association described below.

Hepatocellular Adenoma With HNF1α Mutation

HNF1α mutation is found in up to 40% of HCAs and is associated with HCAs that demonstrate marked steatosis or glycogen content, no cytologic atypia, and no inflammatory infiltrates. Patients with germline mutation are younger with or without diabetes (maturity onset diabetes of the young 3-MODY3) and frequently have family history of liver adenomatosis.

Hepatocellular Adenoma With β-Catenin Mutation

β-Catenin mutated adenomas represent less than 10% adenomas and occur more frequently in males. β-catenin mutation leads to activation of Wnt/β-catenin pathway. They are characterized by cytologic atypia and pseudoglandular structures/acinar pattern; therefore, they are more frequently interpreted as borderline lesion between HCA and hepatocellular carcinoma (hence the term *atypical adenoma* is often used), have a higher risk of malignant transformation, and are often difficult to distinguish from well differentiated hepatocellular carcinoma (Figure 5.5.11). Immunohistochemical stains show overexpression of β-catenin and glutamine synthetase.

Hepatocellular Adenoma, Inflammatory/Telangiectatic Type

Inflammatory/telangiectatic HCA represents approximately 40% of HCAs. There are no specific genetic abnormalities, but inflammatory HCA is associated with increased inflammatory markers, such as serum amyloid A and C-reactive protein, which can be demonstrated immunohistochemically. Inflammatory/telangiectatic HCAs more often occur in overweight and insulin-resistant patients.

The histologic features range from chronically inflamed to peliotic and telangiectatic changes with sinusoidal dilatation filled with red blood cells (Figures 5.5.12 and 5.5.13). Portal-tract–like structures containing arteries surrounded by ductular reaction with associated lymphocytic and neutrophilic infiltrate are found throughout the tumor (Figure 5.5.14). Thin-walled ectatic vessels, often draining directly to sinusoids, and clustered small ectatic vessels are common; hence previously this lesion has been referred as teleangiectatic FNH. Steatosis is often present, may be severe, and localized, with dense lymphocytic infiltrate and occasional ballooning degeneration (Figures 5.5.15 and 5.5.16).

Hepatocellular Adenoma, Unclassified

Unclassified HCA represents approximately 10% of HCAs that do not express any of the above-mentioned phenotypic markers. The gross morphology and histologic features are those of conventional HCA.

Immunohistochemical Stains

Serum amyloid A, C-reactive protein, glutamine synthetase, β-catenin, CK 7 and Ki67 are often used in differentiating benign hepatocellular tumors, particularly in differentiating FNH from conventional HCA or in differentiating FNH from inflammatory HCA or for prognostication of HCA. It should noted that ductular structures are present only in FNH and inflammatory HCA and not in other types of HCA. Focal nodular hyperplasia shows positivity for CK7 in the ductules, map-like staining pattern for glutamine synthetase and negative for serum amyloid A. Inflammatory hepatocellular adenoma shows positive staining for serum amyloid A and C-reactive protein because of the inflammatory nature of the lesion, and occasional CK7 staining in ductular structures (Figures 5.5.17 and 5.5.18). Conventional hepatocellular adenoma shows diffuse or patchy (not map-like) positivity for glutamine synthetase, and negative for CK7 and serum amyloid A. High rate of Ki67, diffuse strong positivity for glutamine synthetase, and nuclear positivity for β-catenin are seen in hepatocellular adenoma with β-catenin mutation and high risk of transformation to hepatocellular carcinoma.

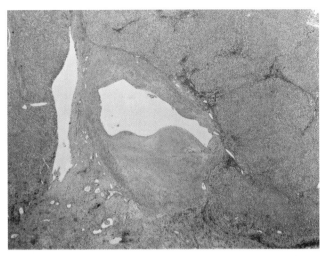

Figure 5.5.1 Large blood vessel with eccentric fibromuscular thickening in focal nodular hyperplasia.

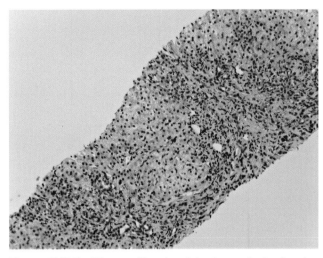

Figure 5.5.2 Biopsy of focal nodular hyperplasia showing nodular liver parenchyma separated by fibrous bands containing bile ductules in the absence of normal portal tract.

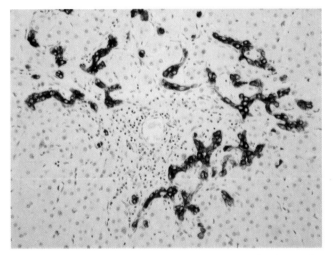

Figure 5.5.3 CK7 immunostain in focal nodular hyperplasia demonstrating bile ductules without normal bile duct.

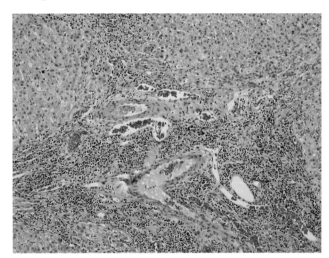

Figure 5.5.4 Large dystrophic blood vessels and marked lymphocytic infiltrate in fibrous bands of focal nodular hyperplasia.

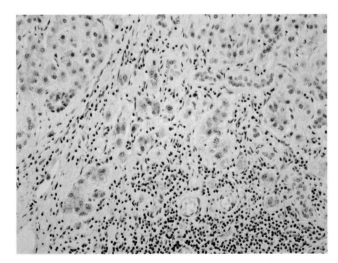

Figure 5.5.5 Rhodanine stain for copper shows copper deposition in hepatocytes at periphery of nodules in focal nodular hyperplasia.

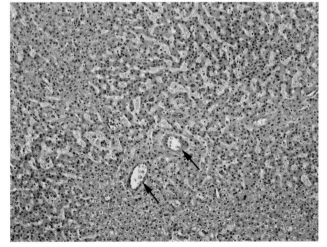

Figure 5.5.6 Hepatocellular adenoma with hyperpastic hepatocytes, sinusoidal dilatation, and abnormal tortuous artery (arrows).

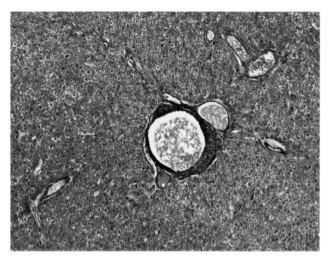

Figure 5.5.7 Hepatocellular adenoma shows large un-paired arteries without fibrous bands (trichrome stain).

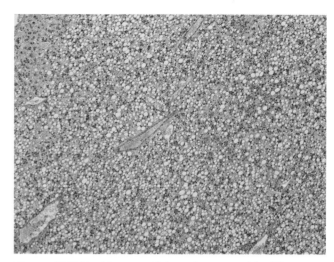

Figure 5.5.8 Hepatocellular adenoma with diffuse steatosis and unpaired arteries.

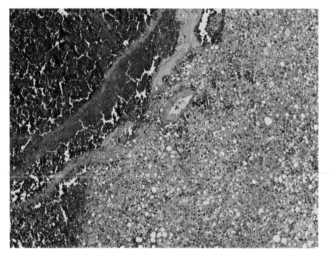

Figure 5.5.9 Hepatocellular adenoma with hemorrhage.

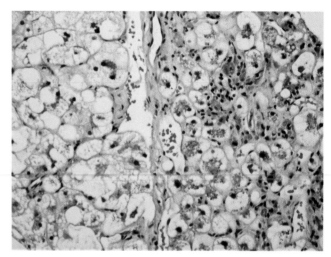

Figure 5.5.10 Pigmented hepatocellular adenoma with Dubin-Johnson-like pigments.

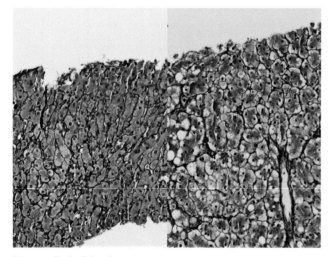

Figure 5.5.11 Reticulin stain shows thickening and distortion of hepatocyte plates in hepatocellular carcinoma (right) arising from hepatocellular adenoma (left), a rare and difficult diagnosis.

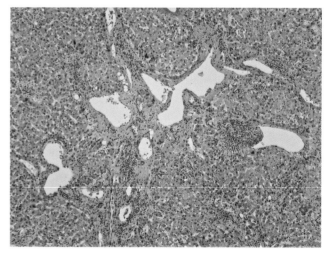

Figure 5.5.12 Inflammatory hepatocellular adenoma with dilated thin-walled ectatic vessels and chronic inflammatory infiltrate.

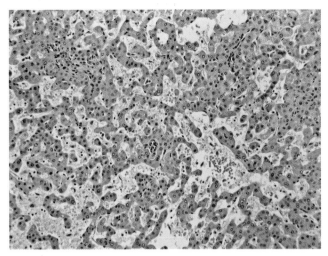

Figure 5.5.13 Dilated sinusoids in telangiectatic hepatocellular adenoma.

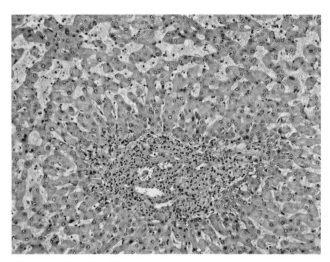

Figure 5.5.14 Portal tract-like structure containing arteries, ductular reaction, lymphocytes, and occasional plasma cells and neutrophils. There is no true bile duct in telangiectatic hepatocellular adenoma.

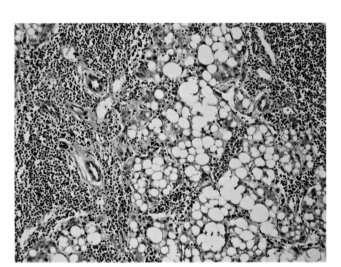

Figure 5.5.15 Marked lymphocytic infiltration, steatosis, and presence of unpaired arteries in inflammatory hepatocellular adenoma.

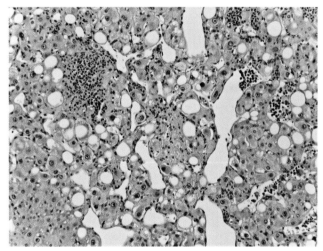

Figure 5.5.16 Dilated sinusoids, steatosis, ballooning degeneration and chronic inflammatory infiltrate in inflammatory hepatocellular adenoma.

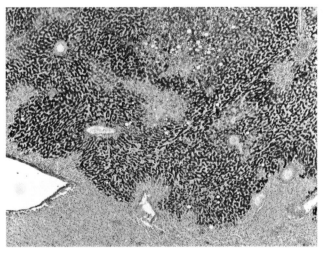

Figure 5.5.17 C-reactive protein immunostain is positive in inflammatory hepatocellular adenoma.

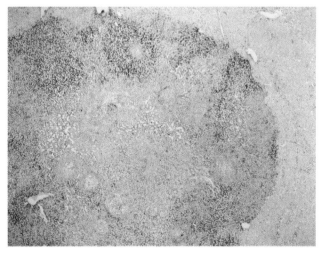

Figure 5.5.18 Serum amyloid A immunostain is positive in inflammatory hepatocellular adenoma.

Table 5.5.1 Differential Diagnoses of Benign Hepatocellular Tumors

Features	Focal Nodular Hyperplasia	Inflammatory/ Telangiectatic Hepatocellular Adenoma	Conventional Hepatocellular Adenoma	Hepatocellular Carcinoma
Gross appearance	Nodular, bulging, paler and firmer than surrounding liver	Soft, congested or hemorrhagic, unencapsulated	Soft, congested or hemorrhagic nodule, unencapsulated.	Nodular lesion, bile stained. Larger lesion with variegated appearance, necrosis and hemorrhage
Central scar	+ (in most cases)	–	–	–/+ (only in fibrolamellar carcinoma)
Fibrous bands	+ (numerous and thick)	+ (occassional and thin)	–	+/–
Hemorrhage and infarction	–	+/–	+/–	+/–
Hepatocytes	Normal to mildly hyperplastic, large cell change, feathery degeneration	Normal, hyperplastic, focal atypia, feathery degeneration	Hyperplastic, monomorphic, atypical hepatocytes in β-catenin–mutated lesion	High nuclear cytoplasmic ratio, pleomorphic nuclei
Trabecular thickness	1–2 cells	1–3 cells	1–3 cells	>3 cells
Mitoses	None	Rare	Rare	Common
Steatosis	+/– (rare, focal)	+/– (focal, can be severe & circumscribed)	+ (common, focal or diffuse)	+/–
Ductular reaction (CK7 +)	++	+	–	–
Thick dystrophic vessels	+	+/–	–	–
Thin walled ectatic vessels	+/– (focal)	+ (numerous)	–	+/–
Sinusoidal ectasia	+/– (mild, focal)	+ (prominent feature)	+ (focal)	+/–
CD34+ sinusoidal cells	+ (around fibrous septa)	+ (around portal tract-like structures)	+ (around unpaired arteries)	+ (diffuse)
Lymphocytic infiltrate	+ (in fibrous septa)	+ (often abundant)	–	+/–
Pseudogland/acinar	–	+/–	+/–	+ (common)

++ indicates almost always present; +, usually present; +/–, occasionally present; –, usually absent.

5.6 Nodules in Cirrhosis

Nodules in cirrhotic liver include large regenerative nodule, low-grade dysplastic nodule (LGDN) and high-grade dysplastic nodule (HGDN), and early HCC. Dysplastic nodules are considered to be preneoplastic lesions, supported by accumulation of evidence favoring the existence of a sequence of events in dysplastic nodules preceding the emergence of HCC. The evolution of dysplastic nodules into early carcinoma includes induction of an arterial blood supply and stromal invasion.

Cytologically, dysplasia in hepatocarcinogenesis takes the form of small cell change, which is recognized as hepatocyte with decreased cytoplasmic volume, cytoplasmic basophilia, mild nuclear pleomorphism and hyperchromasia, and increased nuclear cytoplasmic ratio (Figure 5.6.1). A cluster of hepatocytes with small cell change measuring less than 1 mm in diameter is referred to as dysplastic focus (Figure 5.6.1). Dysplastic focus is often iron-free in liver with hemochromatosis.

Unlike small cell change, large cell change is not directly related to hepatocarcinogenesis, but it is more prevalent in cirrhotic livers with HCC and has been reported to be an important independent risk factor for the subsequent development of HCC (Figure 5.6.2).

Large Regenerative Nodule

Large regenerative nodules, previously known as macroregenerative nodules or adenomatous hyperplasia, are found in cirrhotic liver or liver after submassive hepatic necrosis. They represent nodules of regenerating hepatocytes that stand out from the surrounding liver parenchyma (larger than 5 mm in diameter), and the majority is less than 1.5 cm. They are usually multiple large nodules occupying a large portion of the liver, as seen in "macronodular" cirrhosis. The importance of these lesions lies in the growing evidence that they may progress into dysplastic nodule and small HCCs.

Large regenerative nodules lack cytologic atypia or architectural atypia. Portal tracts and hepatocytes with oncocytic and large cell change are often present (Figures 5.6.3 and 5.6.4).

Dysplastic Nodules

Dysplastic nodules are considered preneoplastic lesions and are classified as LGDNs and HGDNs based on cytologic and architectural atypia on microscopic examination. Dysplastic nodules bulge and differ from the surrounding liver parenchyma.

In LGDN, the hepatocytes rarely show clonal population and show minimal nuclear atypia and slight increase in nuclear cytoplasmic ratio (Figures 5.6.5 and 5.6.6). Mitotic figures are absent. Large cell change is often present. Without obvious clonal population, the distinction between LGDN and large regenerative nodule is difficult and does not carry any practical consequences as long as the nodules lack features of HGDN.

High-grade dysplastic nodule shows cytologic and/or architectural atypia but is insufficient for the diagnosis of HCC. Small cell change and architectural atypia, such as thick plates (up to 3 cells thick) and occasional pseudoglandular structures, are common (Figure 5.6.7). Expansile subnodules with marked atypia are referred to as nodule-in-nodule lesions (Figure 5.6.8). In needle biopsies, the differential diagnosis between HGDN and well-differentiated HCC may be difficult or impossible.

The vascular supply of dysplastic nodules is altered, particularly in HGDN, where unpaired arteries can occasionally be found, and increase of sinusoidal capillarization can be demonstrated on CD31 or CD34 immunostain.

Small HCC

Small HCCs up to 2 cm in diameter are classified into distinctly nodular type and vaguely nodular type (Figures 5.6.10 and 5.6.11). Distinctly nodular HCCs (progressed HCCs) are mostly moderately differentiated, lacks portal tracts, and show evidence of microvascular invasion. Vaguely nodular HCC (also known as early HCC) is well differentiated, lacks fibrous capsule, and contains portal tracts. The tumor cells grow around preexisting portal tracts and/or invade the portal tracts (stromal invasion) (Figure 5.6.12).

Vaguely nodular HCC or early HCC retains the basic architecture of the background cirrhotic liver, and the neoplastic cells grow in and replace the nonneoplastic liver cords. It consists of small neoplastic cells (reminiscent of small cell change), arranged in irregular, thin trabeculae with pseudoglandular structures or fatty change. Most vaguely nodular HCCs are well differentiated HCC. Most of these nodules are clinically hypovascular because of the insufficient development of unpaired tumor arteries and incomplete sinusoidal capillarization.

Distinctly nodular HCC or progressed HCC is biologically more advanced and usually of higher grade with typical HCC features and contains well-developed unpaired tumor arteries, which facilitate their detection by contrast-enhanced imaging methods.

Small nodules with nodule-in-nodule appearance are either HGDN with subnodule of HCC or well-differentiated HCC with a subnodule of moderately differentiated HCC. The former is commonly hypovascular, but the latter is usually detected as hypovascular nodule containing a hypervascular focus on contrast images.

Stromal invasion, as a criterion of carcinoma, is easier to identify in distinctly nodular HCC but is obscure in vaguely nodular type. The absence of CK7-positive ductular reaction is a feature of areas of stromal invasion in small HCC and can be helpful in distinguishing small HCCs from dysplastic nodules, minimally invasive HCCs of the vaguely nodular type, and overtly invasive HCCs of the distinctly nodular type.

A combination of glypican 3, heat shock protein 70, and glutamine synthetase immunostaining may aid the distinction between HGDNs and HCCs. At least 2 diffusely positive staining out of the 3 markers are seen in early or well-differentiated HCC.

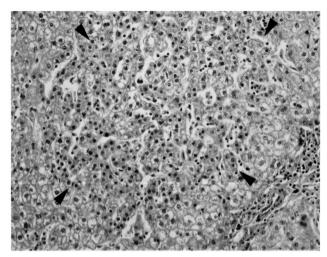

Figure 5.6.1 Dysplastic focus consisting of small cell change (arrows) with darker nuclei and higher nuclear to cytoplasmic ratio than the surrounding cirrhotic liver parenchyma.

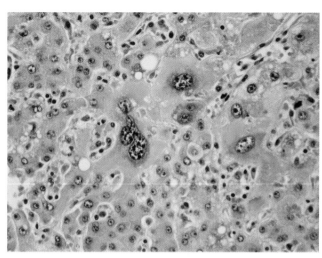

Figure 5.6.2 Hepatocytes with large cell change have abundant eosinophilic cytoplasm, hyperchromatic large single or double nuclei but without increase in nuclear/cytoplasmic ratio.

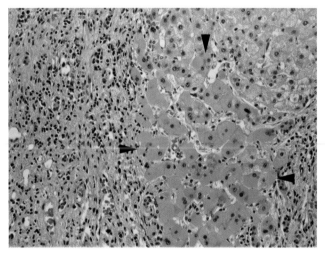

Figure 5.6.3 Hepatocytes with oncocytic change (arrowheads) in cirrhosis.

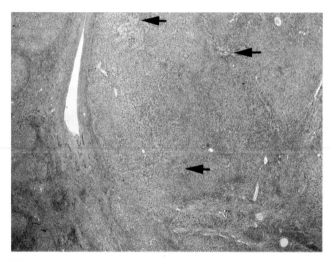

Figure 5.6.4 Large regenerative nodule with few portal tracts (arrows).

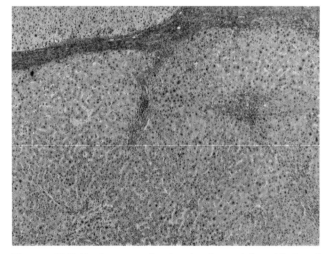

Figure 5.6.5 Low grade dysplastic nodule with focal small and large cell change and a portal tract.

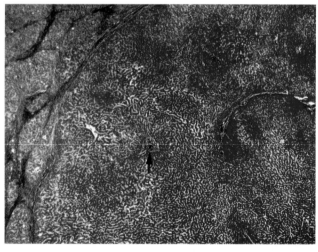

Figure 5.6.6 Well circumscribed low grade dysplastic nodule with rare portal tracts (arrow) (trichrome stain).

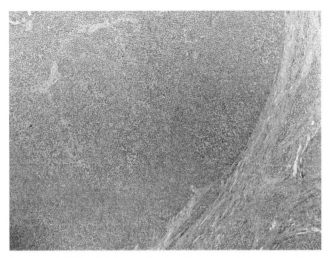

Figure 5.6.7 High grade dysplastic nodule with diffuse small cell change.

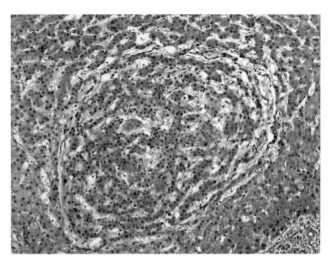

Figure 5.6.8 Nodule within nodule of HGDN with well-differentiated HCC.

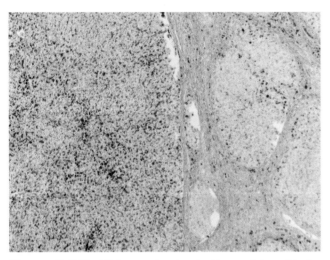

Figure 5.6.9 High grade dysplastic nodule with increased iron content in patient with hereditary hemochromatosis.

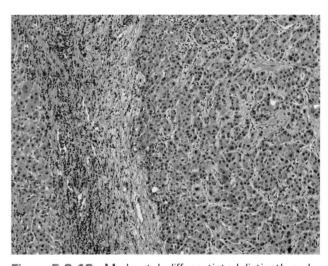

Figure 5.6.10 Moderately differentiated distinctly nodular small hepatocellular carcinoma with fibrous capsule.

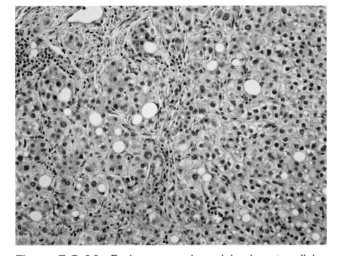

Figure 5.6.11 Early or vaquely nodular hepatocellular carcinoma.

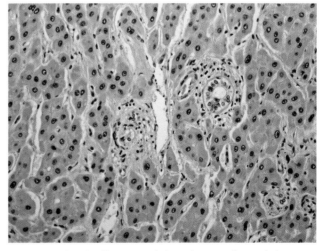

Figure 5.6.12 Entrapped portal tracts in early hepatocellular carcinoma as a consequence of stomal invasion. Tumor cells are present between portal vein branch and the bile duct.

Table 5.6.1 Differential Diagnoses of Nodules in Cirrhosis

Features	Large Regenerative Nodule	Low-Grade Dysplastic Nodule	High-Grade Dysplastic Nodule	Early Hepatocellular Carcinoma
Hepatocyte size	Similar to cirrhotic nodules	Similar to cirrhotic nodules	Variable, close to normal size or smaller	Variable, smaller or larger cells
Small cell change	–	+/– (rare)	+ (focal or diffuse)	++
Large cell change	+/– (focal)	+/–	+/– (rare)	+/– (rare)
Oncocytic change	+/– (focal)	+/–	–	–
Mitoses	Rare	Rare	Few	Common
Cell plates >3 cells thick	–	–	+/–	+
Reticulin framework	Intact	Intact	Focal loss or decreased	Extensive loss
Increased iron deposits	+/–	+/–	+/–	–
Periphery of nodule	Well circumscribed	Well circumscribed	Well circumscribed	Indistinct borders
Stromal invasion	–	–	–	+/–
Portal or fibrous tissue zones	+	+	+/– (normal portal zones only in periphery of larger nodules)	+/–

++ indicate almost always present; +, usually present; +/–, occasionally present; –, usually absent.

5.7   Hepatocellular Carcinoma

Hepatocellular carcinoma (HCC) is the fifth most common cancer and the third cause of cancer-related deaths in the world. It is the most common cause of death in patients with cirrhosis. The incidence of HCC varies in different countries, depending on the prevalence of major causes, namely, chronic liver disease due to chronic viral hepatitis (hepatitis B and C) or other chronic liver disease (fatty liver disease, alcohol, hemochromatosis, and α-1-antitrypsin deficiency). It occurs more frequently in older than in young individuals and affects men more often than women at a ratio of 2:1 to 4:1.

Clinical Features

Patients complain of right upper quadrant mass or pain, with loss or rapid deterioration of liver function and symptoms related to the cirrhosis. Serum α-fetoprotein levels are elevated in one third to one half of the patients. Hepatocellular carcinoma typically exhibits hypervascularity on the arterial phase and "washout" during the venous phase of a contrast radiologic study (computed tomography [CT], magnetic resonance imaging, or contrast ultrasound) due to its arterial supply. Because of this typical radiologic appearance of HCC that is characteristic, biopsy is only required when the radiology appearance is atypical. It should be noted, however, that small or early HCC may be hypovascular, and contrast radiologic study and biopsy may not be reliable. Furthermore, fine-needle aspiration is not helpful in the diagnosis of very small lesions because it may be impossible to distinguish well-differentiated HCC from hepatocellular adenoma and from normal hepatocytes on fine-needle aspiration, where the architectural features of HCC such as thickened trabeculae are lost.

Pathologic Features

Hepatocellular carcinoma may form a large solitary mass with or without adjacent smaller satellite nodules, it may consist of multiple nodules scattered throughout the liver, or it may infiltrate the liver diffusely without forming nodules. Hepatocellular carcinoma is usually soft, tan to yellow, and sometimes bile stained and show areas of necrosis and hemorrhage. The surrounding liver is cirrhotic in 60% to 80% of cases. Invasion of small and/or large portal vein or hepatic vein branches may be seen. The pattern of microvascular invasion and the presence of satellites and macrovascular invasion correlate well with tumor recurrence post resection.

Hepatocellular carcinoma cells resemble hepatocytes in function, cytologic characteristics, and growth patterns. The cells show nuclear pleomorphism with high nuclear to cytoplasmic ratio. The cells may secrete bile and contain fat, glycogen, Mallory-Denk hyalins, hyalin globules, or fibrinogen. Typically, they are polygonal with granular, eosinophilic cytoplasm and arranged in multilayered trabeculae, papillae, solid sheets, or pseudoglandular structures. Characteristically, there is no intercellular stroma, and the malignant cells are lined directly by CD34- or CD31-positive endothelial cells. The presence of bile in canaliculi or cytoplasm of tumor cells and the presence of bile canaliculi highlighted by polyclonal CEA or CD10 immunostain are diagnostic. Clear, fatty, spindle cell, and giant cell variants may be observed. The surrounding liver is often cirrhotic and may show various dysplastic changes. Venous and capsular invasion are frequent (Figures 5.7.16 and 5.7.17). The tumor cells may contain α-fetoprotein or α-1-antitrypsin or fibrinogen demonstrable by immunohistochemical staining. It should be noted however that high serum α-fetoprotein level does not correlate with positive α-fetoprotein immunostaining; furthermore, α-fetoprotein immunostaining is positive in less than 40% of HCCs. Most well and moderately differentiated HCCs are positive for HepPar1, cytoplasmic TTF1, glutamine synthetase, glypican 3, and cytokeratins 8 and 18. CK19 staining in HCC is a surrogate marker of progenitor cell origin, and its positivity in HCC correlates with aggressive behavior and extrahepatic and lymph node metastasis (Figure 5.7.15).

The diagnosis of HCC in a small imaging-guided needle biopsy of a lesion in cirrhotic liver can be problematic. High nuclear cytoplasmic ratio, thick trabeculae and the presence of a sizeable artery in between these suspected cells are some of the features than can aid in the diagnosis of HCC. Hepatocellular carcinoma after chemoembolization often shows thickening of the capsule with large clusters of neoplastic cells separated by necrotic areas or dense fibrous septa. The remaining tumor sometimes resembles fibrolamellar carcinoma or cholangiocarcinoma with CK7- and CK19-positive glandular arrangements embedded in dense fibrocollagenous tissue, hence first diagnosis of fibrolamellar carcinoma or cholangiocarcinoma should not be made in this circumstance.

Differential Diagnosis

The main differential diagnoses of HCC include metastatic renal cell carcinoma, particularly when HCC exhibits clear cytoplasm due to its abundant glycogen or fat content, and adrenal cortical carcinoma, when it arises from the right adrenal, and the distinction between a lesion subjacent to or in the liver is unclear. Angiomyolipoma of the liver is rare, but when it is predominantly composed of epithelioid cells, it can be difficult to distinguish from well-differentiated HCC. Metastatic carcinoid tumor can mimic HCC when the characteristic fine granular chromatin is not readily evident, such as in frozen section. Immunohistochemical staining is useful in most cases (see Table 5.7.1).

Fibrolamellar Carcinoma

Fibrolamellar carcinoma affects younger individuals, 5 to 35 years of age. In contrast to conventional HCC, it does not have male predominance but involves both sexes equally and has no association with cirrhosis or with chronic viral hepatitis. Patients present with abdominal mass or pain. Serum α-fetoprotein levels are normal.

Fibrolamellar carcinoma is usually a solitary, large, well-circumscribed tumor, which may be encapsulated. It contains gray-white fibrous bands that subdivide the tumor into smaller nodules resembling FNH. In contrast to HCC, it is more often found in the left lobe of the liver and is not associated with cirrhosis.

Fibrolamellar carcinoma consists of large polygonal cells with eosinophilic granular cytoplasm and large vesicular nuclei (Figure 5.7.18). The cytoplasmic granularity is due to abundant mitochondria. The cells are separated in groups by thin, parallel bands (lamellae) of hyaline, hypocellular fibrous tissue. Fibrinogen-containing tumor cells with PAS-diastase–negative "pale-inclusions" are often present.

Fibrolamellar carcinoma shows immunohistochemical profile similar to HCC, such as HepPar1, glypican 3, pCEA, and CD10 positivity, except for cytokeratin 7 and epithelial membrane antigen positivity that are seen in fibrolamellar carcinoma only, suggesting bile duct differentiation of this tumor.

Fibrolamellar carcinoma has better prognosis because the tumor is slow growing and in most cases completely resectable, and the surrounding liver is not cirrhotic.

Mixed HCC-CC

Mixed or combined hepatocellular carcinoma-cholangiocarcinoma (HCC-CC) is a tumor with histologic features of both hepatocellular and cholangiocarcinoma. It may represent collision of 2 different tumors or may result from malignant transformation of stem/progenitor cells and differentiation along 2 different cell lineages. It has clinical picture similar to that of HCC but must be separated particularly from the pseudoglandular type of HCC.

Staining for different cytokeratin polypeptides, monoclonal CEA, HepPar1, TTF-1, and EMA may be useful in the differential diagnosis. The hepatocellular component is positive for hepatocellular markers described above, whereas the cholangiocellular component is positive for cytokeratins 7 and 19, EMA, and monoclonal CEA.

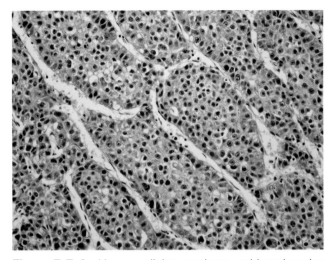

Figure 5.7.1 Hepatocellular carcinoma with trabecular pattern. The trabeculae are typically outlined by endothelial cells.

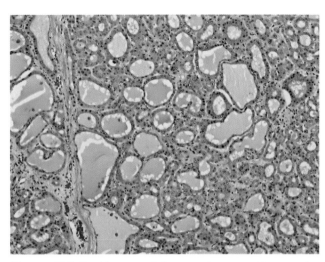

Figure 5.7.2 Hepatocellular carcinoma with pseudoglandular pattern.

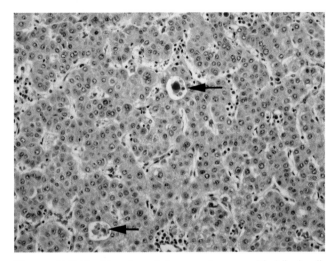

Figure 5.7.3 Hepatocellular carcinoma with bile in dilated bile canaliculi (arrows).

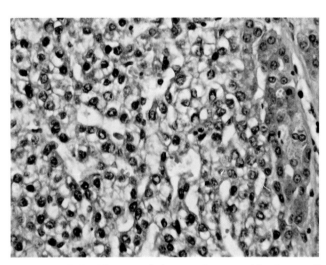

Figure 5.7.4 Hepatocellular carcinoma with clear cell features.

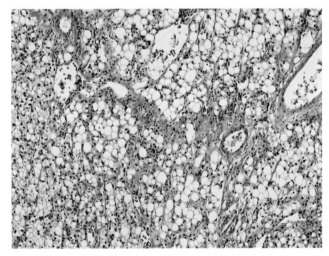

Figure 5.7.5 Hepatocellular carcinoma with macrovesicular steatosis.

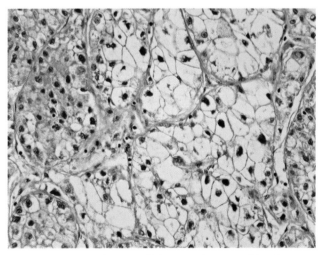

Figure 5.7.6 Hepatocellular carcinoma with glycogen content.

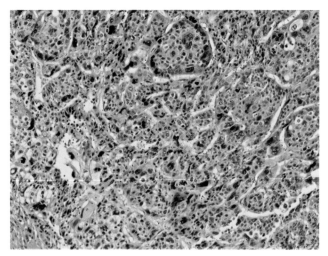

Figure 5.7.7 Poorly differentiated hepatocellular carcinoma with giant cell features.

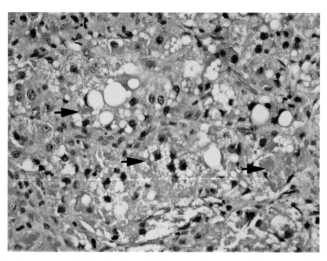

Figure 5.7.8 Hepatocellular carcinoma with steatosis and Mallory-Denk hyalins.

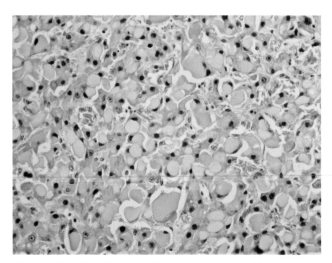

Figure 5.7.9 Hepatocellular carcinoma with intracytoplasmic fibrinogen "pale" inclusions.

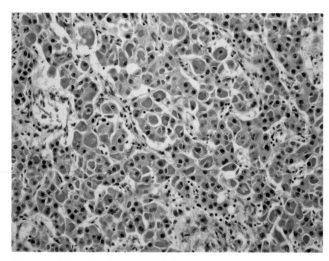

Figure 5.7.10 Hepatocellular carcinoma with intracytoplasmic eosinophilic inclusions.

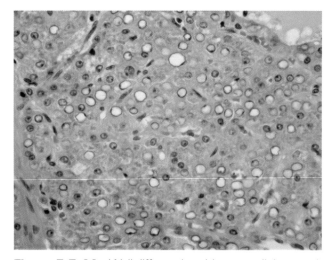

Figure 5.7.11 Well-differentiated hepatocellular carcinoma with glycogenated nuclei.

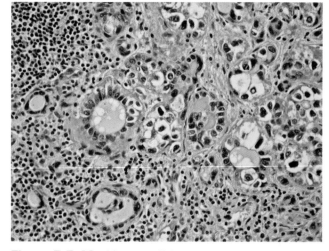

Figure 5.7.12 Hepatocellular carcinoma with pseudoglandular pattern and inflammatory stroma.

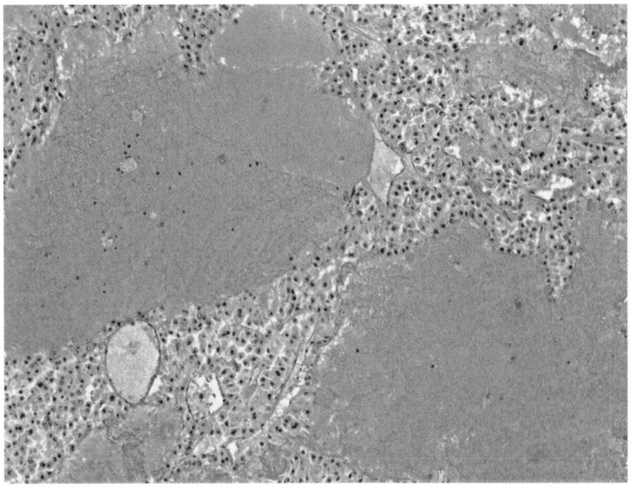

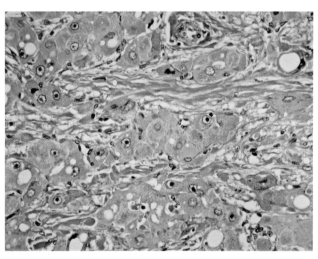

Figure 5.7.13 Peliotic hepatocellular carcinoma.

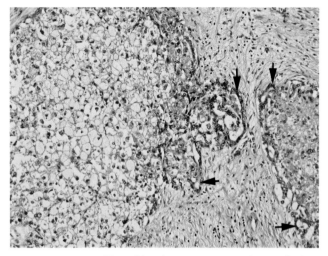

Figure 5.7.14 Transition between progenitor cells (arrows) and classical hepatocellular carcinoma.

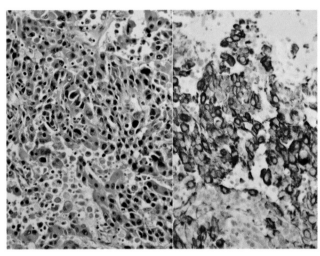

Figure 5.7.15 Aggressive, poorly differentiated hepatocellular carcinoma with CK19 immunostain positivity.

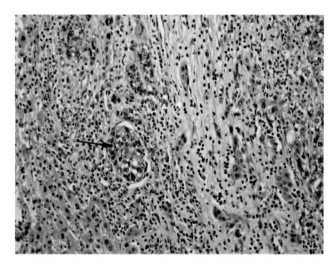

Figure 5.7.16 Hepatocellular carcinoma with microvascular invasion (arrow).

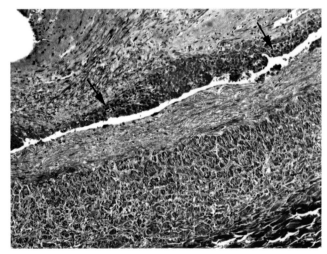

Figure 5.7.17 Hepatocellular carcinoma (arrows) in large branch of hepatic vein representing macrovascular invasion (trichrome stain).

Figure 5.7.18 Large polygonal cells separated by parallel bands of hyaline fibrous tissue in fibrolamellar carcinoma.

Table 5.7.1 Differential Diagnoses of Hepatocellular Carcinoma

Immunostains	Hepatocellular Carcinoma	Renal Cell Carcinoma	Adrenal Cortical Carcinoma	Carcinoid Tumor	Angiomyolipoma
Cytokeratin 7	−	+	−	+/−	−
Cytokeratin 8 or 18	+	−	−	−	−
Epithelial membrane antigen	−	+	−	+/−	−
HepPar1	+	−	−	−	−
Glypican-3	+	−	−	−	−
TTF-1	+ (cytoplasmic)	−	−	−	−
CEA polyclonal	+ (canalicular)	−	−	−	−
CD10	+ (canalicular)	+	−	−	−
HMB-45	−	−	−	−	+
Smooth muscle actin	−	−	−	−	+
Synaptophysin	−	−	+	+	−
Chromogranin	−	−	−	+	−
Inhibin	−	−	+	−	−
Calretinin	−	−	+	−	−
Melan-A	−	−	+	−	+

+ indicates commonly positive; −, negative.

5.8 Cholangiocarcinoma

Cholangiocarcinoma (CC) is an adenocarcinoma arising from bile duct epithelium. It is the second most common primary malignant tumor of the liver.

Cholangiocarcinoma may occur anywhere along the biliary tree from small bile ducts, bile ductules and remnants of ductal plate in the liver (intrahepatic cholangiocarcinoma) to large hilar and extrahepatic bile ducts (extrahepatic cholangiocarcinoma). Klatskin tumor is classified as extrahepatic cholangiocarcinoma. The arbitration between intrahepatic and extrahepatic CC is not just because of their difference in anatomic location, but also because of their distinct risk factors, clinical presentation, therapy, and epidemiology. Therefore, the term "cholangiocarcinoma" has been proposed exclusively for peripheral tumors and the term "bile duct carcinoma" for tumors arising from large bile ducts both at the hilum and along the extrahepatic biliary tree.

Extrahepatic cholangiocarcinoma represents 80% of all cholangiocarcinomas. The incidence rates of extrahepatic CC vary greatly among different areas of the world, related to distribution of risk factors. It affects older individuals with peak incidence in the sixth decade, slight male predilection, and rarely associated with cirrhosis. In Southeast Asia, the incidence is higher because of its association with liver fluke infestation (*Clonorchis sinensis* and *Opisthorchis viverrini*). Other predisposing conditions include primary sclerosing cholangitis, inflammatory bowel disease, hepatolithiasis, recurrent pyogenic cholangitis, choledochal cyst, fibrocystic disease of the liver, and Thorotrast exposure.

Intrahepatic cholangiocarcinoma accounts for less than 20% of cholangiocarcinomas. In the majority of intrahepatic CC cases no underlying liver disease is identified, but recent epidemiologic studies suggest chronic hepatitis C virus infection as a major risk factor for intrahepatic CC. It is, however, currently unclear how HCV is involved in cholangiocarcinogenesis.

Complete resection is the most effective treatment and the only treatment associated with prolonged disease-free survival, but CCs are often large or high stage at presentation, and recurrence after resection is common.

Clinical Features

Patients most commonly present with fever, malaise, and abdominal pain. Jaundice is present in one third of patients. There may be elevation of CEA or CA 19.9 serum levels, but α-fetoprotein levels are not elevated. Intrahepatic CC is hypovascular on angiography, quite large at the time of diagnosis and may be readily visualized on imaging studies. Extrahepatic CCs are more difficult to diagnose because they are usually infiltrative and not visible unless a large mass is formed and associated with biliary ductal dilatation. Biopsy combined with brushings for exfoliative cytology may lead to diagnosis, which largely depends on the amount of tissue obtained and the level of duct obstruction.

Pathologic Features

There are differences in gross morphology and microscopic features of intrahepatic CC and extrahepatic CC.

Intrahepatic CC is divided on the basis of morphologic appearance into mass forming, periductal infiltrating, and intraductal subtypes. Mass forming intrahepatic CCs are multilobulated, unencapsulated, firm, white-gray tumor, owing to extensive desmoplastic stroma. The periductal infiltrating subtype shows extensive infiltration along intrahepatic portal structures, while the intraductal subtype is confined within large bile ducts often with papillary architecture. The intraductal subtype is now referred as intraductal papillary neoplasm of bile duct. Extrahepatic CC typically forms ill-defined, infiltrating, firm lesion in the hepatic hilum or along extrahepatic bile duct.

Intrahepatic CCs are usualy well to moderately differentiated adenocarcinomas (Figures 5.8.1 to 5.8.6), classically consisting of small, well-differentiated uniform neoplastic glands, or larger elongated or tortuous glands composed of cuboidal neoplastic cells, or nests of cribiform structures (comedocarcinoma-like) made up of small cells with scant cytoplasm and dark nuclei. Intrahepatic CCs are often highly cellular at the periphery with hypocellular densely fibrotic center. The tumor cells insinuate the sinusoids and not the trabecular cords at the border of the lesion. Other non-classic microscopic types that can be encountered are trabecular type, hilar type, cholangiolocellular carcinoma and combined HCC-CC. Trabecular type of intrahepatic CC is characterized by polygonal cells with eosinophilic cytoplasm arranged in anastomosing trabeculae. Hilar type shows features resembling extrahepatic CC. Cholangiolocellular carcinoma is discussed later in this section, and combined HCC-CC is discussed in "Hepatocellular Carcinoma" because it is regarded to be closely related to HCC than intrahepatic CC.

Extrahepatic CCs characteristically show various sizes of irregular dilated glands with mucin production, pleomorphic cells and hyperchromatic nuclei, and occasional micropapillary structures (Figure 5.8.7). Extensive portal infiltration and perineural invasion are common. Biliary intraepithelial neoplasia can be found occasionally.

Tumor cells never excrete bile or α-fetoprotein but often produce mucin.

Almost all CCs show strong positivity for CK7 and CK19. Positivity for CK20 can be seen in up to 20% of cases. CEA staining is diffusely cytoplasmic in up to 75% of cases. Smad4 mutation can occur in approximately 50% of cases. P53 mutation is common.

Differential Diagnosis

The differential diagnoses of CC include biliary cystadenocarcinoma, metastatic adenocarcinoma, and epithelioid hemangioendothelioma.

Biliary cystadenocarcinoma represents the malignant counterpart of biliary cystadenoma, occurring in women and often in the right lobe. It is a large, multiloculated cystic lesion containing mucinous material that may be blood or bile stained. Multiloculated cystic lesion is not a feature of CC, but cystadenocarcinoma has to be distinguished from CC arising in a liver with fibropolycystic disease, in which the cystic structures are separated by dense fibrous tissue or liver parenchyma.

Unless metastatic adenocarcinomas express organ specific antigen, such as TTF-1, CK20, and CDX2; most immunohistochemical studies, including CEA, and various cytokeratins are not useful in separating CC from metastatic adenocarcinoma. Metastatic pancreatic adenocarcinomas are often difficult to distinguish from intrahepatic cholangiocarcinomas due to their histologic and immunophenotypic similarity. The presence of biliary intraepithelial neoplasia (BilIN) adjacent to tumor confirms CC.

Epithelioid hemangioendothelioma cells are positive for endothelial markers (factor VIII–related antigen, CD31, and CD34). Because of the "epithelioid" appearance and its pattern of growth, surrounded by dense fibrous or myxoid stroma and infiltrates the surrounding vessels or sinusoids, epithelioid hemangioendothelioma may be mistaken for CC. Intracellular vacuoles, often containing red blood cells, should be distinguished from signet ring cells of CC.

Cholangiolocellular Carcinoma

Cholangiolocellular carcinoma (CLC) is a subtype of intrahepatic CC, thought to originate from the ductules and/or canals of Hering, where hepatic progenitor cells (HPCs) are located. Hepatic progenitor cells can differentiate into hepatocytes and cholangiocytes and can, on their way to differentiation, give rise to tumors with a whole range of phenotypes with varying hepatocellular and cholangiocellular differentiation characteristics.

There are 2 or 3 different histological areas (CLC, HCC, and/or intrahepatic CC) within which CLC is the predominant component and composed of mixtures of small monotonous glands, antler-like anastomosing patterns with an abundant hyalinized and/or edematous fibrous stroma with lymphocytic infiltration (Figures 5.8.8 and 5.8.9). Tumor cells are cuboidal, smaller in size than normal hepatocytes, with scant eosinophilic cytoplasm, round or oval nuclei, and indistinct nucleoli. The CLC area is CK7, CK19, and NCAM (CD56) positive. The HCC area is usually located at the interface to the nonneoplastic liver parenchyma with trabecular growth pattern and shows canalicular staining for pCEA and CD10 and positive for HepPar1. The intrahepatic CC area is usually small with papillary and/or clear glandular formation, mucin production, abundant fibrous stroma, and positive for CK7, CK19, and cytoplasmic pCEA immunostaining. NCAM is useful in differentiating CLC from classical well differentiated intrahepatic CC, which commonly do not express this marker. It should be noted that bile ductules, ductular reaction and the majority of bile duct adenomas are also NCAM positive.

Although reportedly tumors showing HPC features have a worse prognosis with faster and more frequent recurrence after surgical treatment compared to tumors without HPC features, the biological behavior of CLC remains obscure.

Biliary Intraepithelial Neoplasia and Intraductal Papillary Neoplasm of Bile Duct

Both biliary intraepithelial neoplasia (BilIN) and intraductal papillary neoplasm of the bile duct (IPNB) are considered to be in situ lesions in the concept of multistep cholangio-carcinogenesis. The term *BilIN* applies to microscopic flat or low-papillary dysplastic epithelium, known previously as biliary dysplasia, atypical biliary epithelium, or carcinoma in situ (Figure 5.8.11). Biliary intraepithelial neoplasia occurs more often in hepatolithiasis, choledochal cysts, and primary sclerosing cholangitis. BilIN is classified into 3 grades based on the degree of cellular and structural atypia: BilIN-1, BilIN-2, and BilIN-3 (Table 5.8.1).

Intraductal papillary neoplasm of the bile duct is characterized by a markedly dilated and cystic biliary system and multifocal papillary dysplastic epithelial lesions with or without mucin production (Figure 5.8.12). This rare type of tumor resembles its counterpart, the intraductal papillary mucinous neoplasm of the pancreas. Several types of IPNB are recognized: pancreatobiliary, intestinal, gastric foveolar types, and the rare oncocytic type. The IPNB is associated with 2 types of invasive tumors: tubular carcinoma and mucinous carcinoma. Patient with invasive tubular carcinoma carries a worse prognosis than mucinous carcinoma or IPNB alone.

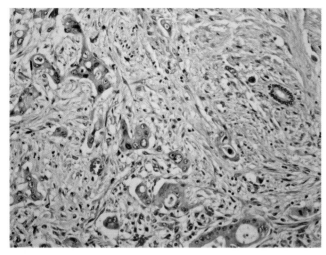

Figure 5.8.1 Intrahepatic cholangiocarcinoma with abundant desmoplastic stroma.

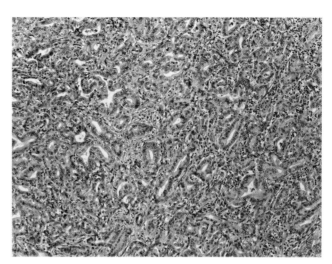

Figure 5.8.2 Intrahepatic cholangiocarcinoma with well differentiated glands.

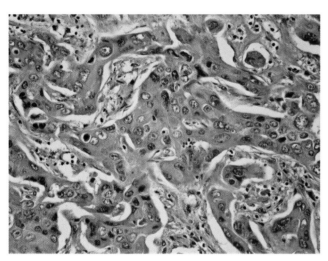

Figure 5.8.3 Intrahepatic cholangiocarcinoma with anastomosing glands.

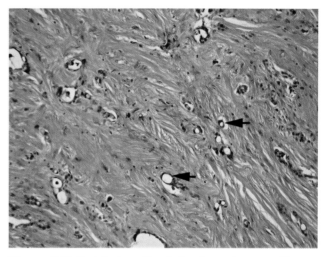

Figure 5.8.4 Intrahepatic cholangiocarcinoma with mucin-containing signet ring cells and dense desmoplastic stroma.

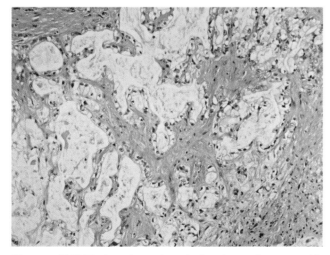

Figure 5.8.5 Intrahepatic cholangiocarcinoma with clear cell features.

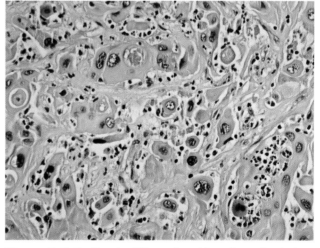

Figure 5.8.6 Poorly differentiated intrahepatic cholangiocarcinoma with giant cells, not to be mistaken as hepatocellular carcinoma.

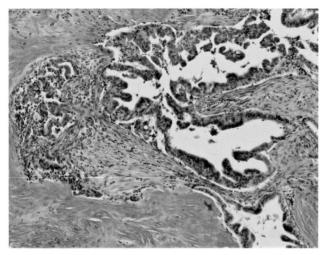

Figure 5.8.7 Hilar cholangiocarcinoma (Klatskin tumor) with perineural invasion.

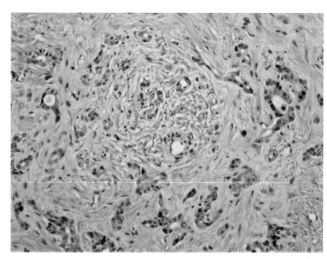

Figure 5.8.8 Cholangiolocellular carcinoma with small glands in fibrous stroma.

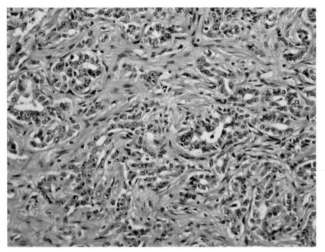

Figure 5.8.9 Cholangiolocellular carcinoma with small monotonous anastomosing glands.

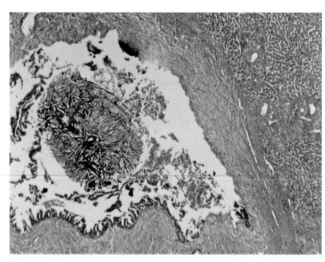

Figure 5.8.10 Hepatolithiasis with biliary intraepithelial neoplasia.

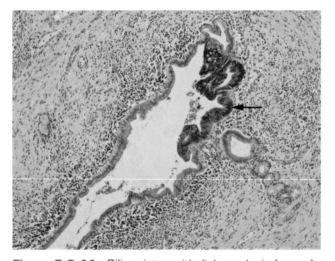

Figure 5.8.11 Biliary intraepithelial neoplasia (arrow).

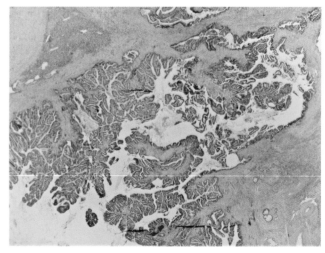

Figure 5.8.12 Intraductal papillary neoplasm of bile duct.

Table 5.8.1 Diagnostic Criteria of Biliary Intraepithelial Neoplasia (BilIN)

	Configuration	Cellularity	Cytology	Peribiliary Gland Involvement
Hyperplasia or regenerative change	Commonly flat. Micropapillary in hepatolithiasis or choledochal cyst	Slightly increased compared to normal	Round/oval slightly enlarged nuclei, smooth nuclear membrane, fine chromatin.	No
BilIN-1	Flat or micropapillary	Focal crowding or pseudostratification	Basally located uniform nuclei with subtle nuclear membrane irregularity, higher nuclear cytoplasmic ratio and nuclear elongation.	No
BilIN-2	Flat, pseudopapillary or micropapillary	Crowding and pseudostratification is common	Loss of cellular polarity, dysplastic nuclei (enlargement, hyperchromasia, irregular nuclear membrane). Some variations in nuclear sizes and shapes. Rare mitoses.	Sometimes
BilIN-3	Pseudopapillary or micropapillary, rarely flat	Generalized crowding with budding or cribriforming	Resemble carcinoma without invasion. Diffuse loss of polarity, hyperchromasia, abnormally large nuclei. Mitoses are observed.	Often

Adapted from Zen Y, et al. Biliary intraepithelial neoplasia: an international interobserver agreement study and proposal for diagnostic criteria. *Mod Pathol.* 2007;20(6):701–709.

5.9 Vascular Lesions

Cavernous Hemangioma

Cavernous hemangioma is the most common benign tumor of the liver and usually found incidentally during evaluation for metastatic disease, at surgery, or at autopsy. Cavernous hemangioma is usually a single and small lesion, but it may be multiple or very large and becomes clinically symptomatic. Symptoms include abdominal mass and pain due to thrombosis, infarction, or pressure on adjacent organs, but rupture is exceedingly rare. Vascular hum may be heard over the lesion. Consumption coagulopathy and microangiopathic hemolytic anemia may develop in patients with massive tumors. Imaging techniques are useful and sufficient for diagnosis in most cases. Needle biopsy using fine-needle under guidance is usually safe for intraparenchymal lesions. Resection is performed when giant cavernous hemangioma, severe abdominal pain, rapid expansion, or coagulopathy is present. Small cavernous hemangiomas (hemangioma-like vessels) are often seen in liver tissue adjacent to the main lesion. Recurrence of giant cavernous hemangioma after resection, which most probably develops from the rapid growth of these hemangioma-like vessels, has rarely been observed. Cavernous hemangioma consists of a communicating network of blood-filled or empty vascular spaces. The channels are separated by fibrous septa lined by flattened endothelial cells with scant cytoplasm (Figure 5.9.1). Areas of thrombosis, scarring, hyalinization, or calcification are often seen and may result in sclerosed hemangioma that is predominantly fibrotic with near-complete obliteration of the vascular spaces (Figures 5.9.2 and 5.9.3).

Peliosis Hepatis

Peliosis hepatis represents blood-filled cysts in the hepatic parenchyma that may complicate therapy with certain drugs, particularly anabolic steroids, high-dose oral contraceptive, or azathioprine in patients with solid organ transplants. It is also seen in systemic wasting diseases such as tuberculosis and immunocompromised patients. *Bartonella henselae* causes bacillary angiomatosis and peliosis in immunocompromised patients.

Symptoms and the liver enzyme profile are related to the underlying disease. Most cases of peliosis are detected incidentally, but rupture, intraperitoneal hemorrhage, and death have been reported. Peliosis may regress on stopping hormone or drug causing the lesion.

Peliosis hepatis consists of blood-filled cystic spaces, separated by cords of normal or compressed hepatocytes, distributed randomly in liver parenchyma (Figure 5.9.5). *Bartonella henselae* may be demonstrated by Warthin-Starry silver staining.

Epithelioid Hemangioendothelioma

Epithelioid hemangioendothelioma is a low-grade malignant vascular neoplasm. It affects middle-aged patients, and two thirds of them are women. Patient presents with abdominal pain, mass, weight loss, or malaise. Involvement of major hepatic vein may result in Budd-Chiari syndrome. Imaging studies show single or multiple masses that are avascular or calcified and may involve the entire liver. Treatment options include surgical resection for localized tumor or liver transplantation in patients with multifocal tumors.

Epithelioid hemangioendothelioma is typically a firm, gray tumor. It has a zonal pattern of cellularity; the periphery or the advancing front is more cellular than the central zone, which is hypocellular, sclerotic, or calcified; and the transition zone appears myxoid or cartilaginous. The underlying lobular architecture remains preserved with remnants of portal tracts (Figure 5.9.6). The tumor cells assume dendritic and epithelioid appearances. The dendritic cells are spindle or stellate shaped. The epithelioid cells resemble signet rings with vessel-like intracellular lumen, which may contain red blood cells (Figure 5.9.7).

Epithelioid hemangioendothelioma may be misdiagnosed as cholangiocarcinoma (CC) because of the epithelioid appearance, signet ring cells, and the sclerotic pattern of growth (Figure 5.9.8). It should be noted, however, that the lumens of CC do not contain red blood cells, and markers for endothelial cells such as factor VIII–related antigen, CD31, and CD34 antigens are not demonstrable in CC.

Angiosarcoma

Angiosarcoma is a high-grade malignant vascular neoplasm, and it is the most common sarcoma arising in the liver. It occurs in older patients and is more often in men. It can be caused by exposure to vinyl chloride, arsenic, anabolic steroids, radiation, and thorium dioxide (Figure 5.9.11). Patients typically present with abdominal pain, fatigue, jaundice, and weight loss. Rarely, patients present with Budd-Chiari syndrome. Hepatomegaly with or without splenomegaly and thrombocytopenia are common findings. Metastases occur frequently and rapidly to the spleen, lymph nodes, lung, bone, and adrenals. Liver failure and intra-abdominal bleeding are common causes of death.

Angiosarcoma forms numerous poorly defined variably sized nodules that are soft, spongy, hemorrhagic, and necrotic. The entire liver is frequently involved. The tumor is composed of pleomorphic spindle or epithelioid cells, often with bizarre or multinucleated forms (Figure 5.9.10). Mitoses are evident. Better-differentiated areas may show cavernous spaces that are lined by atypical endothelial cells. The tumor cells grow along and into sinusoids, peliotic areas, and branches of portal and hepatic veins.

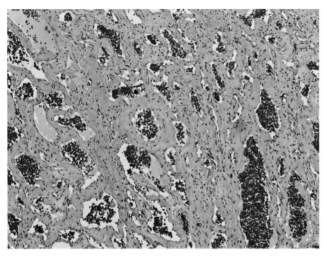

Figure 5.9.1 Cavernous hemangioma.

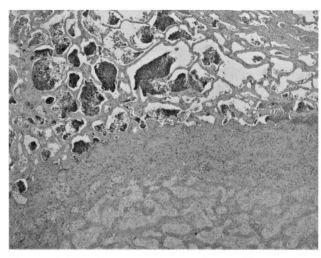

Figure 5.9.2 Cavernous hemangioma with organizing thrombus in the lower field.

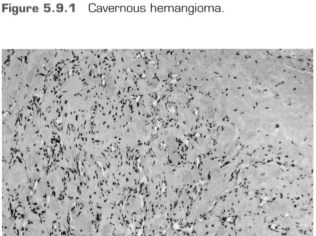

Figure 5.9.3 Sclerosed hemangioma.

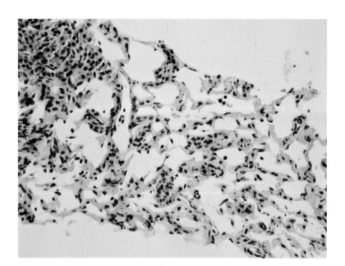

Figure 5.9.4 Lymphangioma with empty spaces separated by thin fibrous septa.

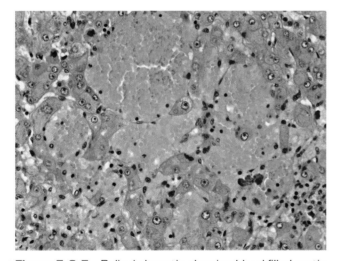

Figure 5.9.5 Peliosis hepatis showing blood-filled cystic spaces separated by cords of compressed hepatocytes.

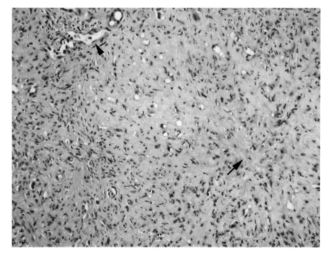

Figure 5.9.6 Epithelioid hemangioendothelioma with obliteration of portal tract (arrowhead) and central venule (arrow).

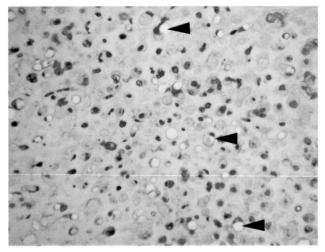

Figure 5.9.7 Epithelioid hemangioendothelioma with "lumina" (arrowheads).

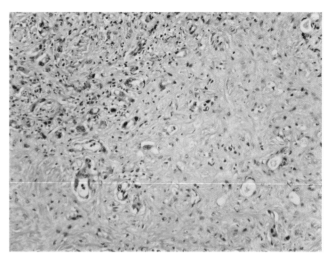

Figure 5.9.8 Epithelioid hemangioendothelioma with cholangiocarcinoma-like area.

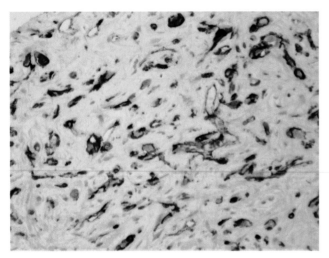

Figure 5.9.9 CD34 positivity in epithelioid hemangioen-dothelioma.

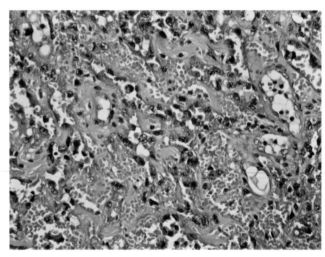

Figure 5.9.10 Angiosarcoma with vascular channels lined by pleomorphic cells.

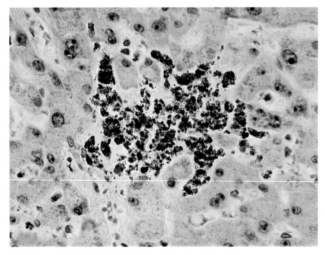

Figure 5.9.11 Thorium dioxide birefringent crystals can be found in association with angiosarcoma or chol-angiocarcinoma.

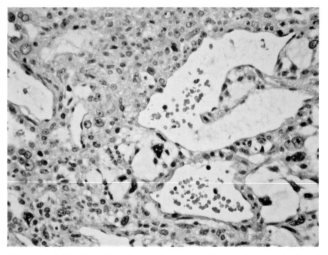

Figure 5.9.12 Angiomyolipoma with well vascularized area and pleomorphic perivascular epithelioid smooth muscle cells, but exceedingly rare mitoses.

Table 5.9.1 Differential Diagnosis of Vascular Lesions of the Liver

Diagnosis	Gross Features	Histologic Features	Others
Cavernous hemangioma	Soft, spongy, hemorrhagic. Focal area of fibrosis or scarring or calcification.	Blood-filled or empty spaces lined by endothelial cells (CD31, CD34, Factor VIII antigen positive) with scant cytoplasm, separated by fibrous septa. Thrombosis, hyalinization or calcification often present.	Thrombocytopenia and hypofibrinogenemia in massive tumors. Rupture and hemorrhage are rare.
Lymphangioma	Soft, spongy lesion containing clear or milky lymph.	Lymph-filled spaces lined by single layer of endothelial cells (CD31, CD34, factor VIII antigen and D2-40 positive) with occasional tufting. Scattered lymphocytes and thin delicate fibrous framework, no red blood cells.	Commonly associated with lymphangiomatosis in other organs.
Peliosis hepatis	Blood-filled cysts in the hepatic parenchyma.	Blood-filled cystic spaces, separated by cords of compressed hepatocytes. Extravasation of red blood cells into perisinusoidal spaces is common. Endothelial cell lining is not present.	Warthin-Starry stain may demonstrate *Bartonella henselae.* Associated with anabolic steroid use.
Angiomyolipoma	Soft, well-circumscribed, encapsulated, hemorrhagic yellow-tan.	Blood vessels, epithelioid perivascular cells, admixed with adipose tissue. Brown-pigment, hematopoietic elements and large atypical cells often present.	Perivascular epithelial cells are positive for HMB-45, S-100, and smooth muscle actin.
Hepatocellular adenoma, telangiectatic/ inflammatory type	Congested or hemorrhagic, unencapsulated, soft tan nodule. Focal fatty area may be present.	Benign hepatocytes separated by dilated and congested sinusoids. Scattered dilated dystrophic vessels, portal tract-like structures and thin fibrous septa containing ductular reaction. Steatosis is often seen.	Positive for serum amyloid A and C-reactive protein.
Epithelioid hemangioendothelioma	Firm, gray, well-circumscribed lesion. Obliteration of major vessels may be apparent.	Single or small clusters of epithelioid neoplastic cells, often arranged in ductular-like structure in densely fibrotic desmoplastic stroma. Periphery is more cellular and obliterates sinusoids and vascular structures of the liver.	Cells are positive for vascular markers.
Angiosarcoma	Multiple variegated, solid to hemorrhagic, necrotic lesion.	Pleomorphic spindle/epithelioid cells with hyperchromatic nuclei, mitoses and necrosis. Blood filled spaces throughout lesion.	Associated with thorotrast, vinyl chloride and arsenic exposure; anabolic steroid use.

5.10 Lipomatous Lesions

Focal Fatty Change

Focal fatty change or steatosis or metamorphosis is a localized area of fatty metamorphosis of hepatocytes. Although the exact pathogenesis is unknown, accumulation fat may be caused by the localized effect of vascular anomaly. It appears as a tumor with the density of fat by CT or ultrasound. It is usually asymptomatic and found incidentally. No treatment is required.

Focal fatty change shows diffuse macrovesicular fat droplets in hepatocytes (Figure 5.10.1). The lobular architecure, portal tracts, and central venules are intact. Lipogranulomas are often present.

Vaguely nodular (early) HCCs show preservation of portal tracts and may contain fat in 40% of them. The differentiation from focal fatty change may be difficult and relies on the identification of stromal invasion.

Angiomyolipoma

Angiomyolipoma of the liver is a rare tumor derived from perivascular epithelial cells, hence belonging to a group of tumors usually associated with tuberous sclerosis referred to as PEC-omas. Morphologically, hepatic angiomyolipoma is similar to the more commonly encountered angiomyolipoma of the kidney, but an association with tuberous sclerosis is less common. The tumor is asymptomatic and found incidentally. Rarely, it presents as right upper quadrant pain or mass. The tumor is a well-demarcated, radioluscent mass on CT and magnetic resonance imaging, a hyperechoic nodule with a sharp margin on ultrasound, and hypervascular on arteriography. A preoperative diagnosis of angiomyolipoma can be made when these characteristic findings on imaging studies are present. Fine-needle aspiration biopsy confirms the diagnosis. Angiomyolipoma never recurs after resection, and malignant transformation is exceedingly rare.

Angiomyolipoma is composed of varying proportions of blood vessels, smooth muscle, and mature adipose tissue. There are usually numerous thin-walled venous channels or sinuses and variable numbers of conspicuous thick-walled arteries and veins. Intimal proliferation, eccentric narrowing of the lumen of the vessels, and hyalinization of the wall and surrounding tissue may be present. The adipose tissue is composed of mature adipocytes in sheets or scattered throughout the tumor (Figures 5.10.2 and 5.10.3). The amount of fat component varies. The smooth muscle component is usually the most prominent feature. It consists of sheets and bundles of spindle and epithelioid cells (Figures 5.9.12 and 5.11.3). The epithelioid cells are polygonal or rounded. They have finely granular, eosinophilic cytoplasm and may closely resemble hepatocytes. Hematopoietic elements and chronic inflammatory cells are often present, and if hematopoietic elements are significant, the tumor may be referred to as angiomyomyelolipoma. Immunohistochemical stains are used to confirm the mesenchymal nature of the tumor. The entire tumor is negative for cytokeratin but positive for vimentin, HMB-45, S-100, and smooth muscle actin.

Myelolipoma

Myelolipoma is a benign tumor composed of an admixture of adipose tissue and hematopoietic elements in various proportions and more commonly occurring in the adrenal gland.

Pseudolipoma

Pseudolipoma (of Glisson capsule) is a benign degenerative lipomatous lesion at the surface of the liver. It is thought to arise from a detached piece of colonic fat (appendix epiploica) that undergoes necrosis and calcification and is covered by fibrous capsule. Microscopically, the lesion consists of degenerative mature adipose tissue with ghosts of fat cells without nuclei, areas of calcification, and surrounded by thick fibrous capsule.

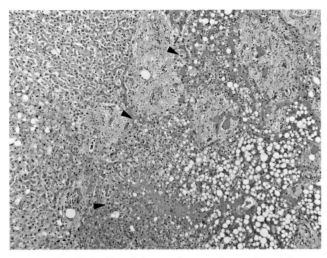

Figure 5.10.1 Focal fatty change (arrowheads) secondary to localized vascular anomaly.

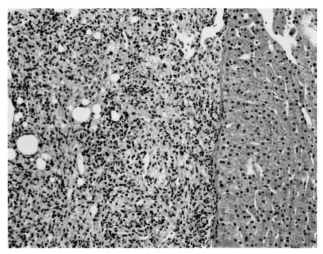

Figure 5.10.2 Angiomyolipoma, well circumscribed (left field) with adipocytes.

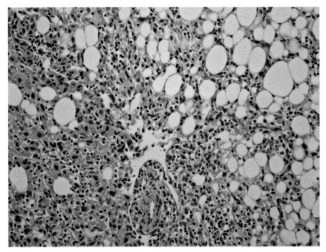

Figure 5.10.3 Angiomyolipoma with adipocytes and epitheliod smooth muscle cells.

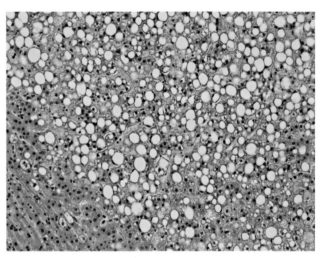

Figure 5.10.4 Hepatocellular adenoma with diffuse macrovesicular steatosis.

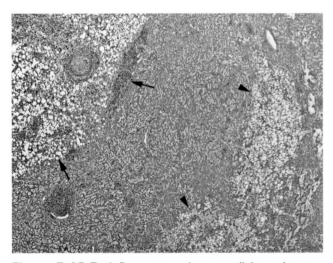

Figure 5.10.5 Inflammatory hepatocellular adenoma showing areas of steatosis with (arrows) and without (arrowheads) inflammation.

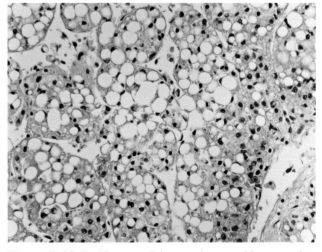

Figure 5.10.6 Hepatocellular carcinoma with steatosis.

Table 5.10.1 Differential Diagnosis of Lipomatous Lesions of the Liver

Diagnoses	Gross Features	Histologic Features	Others
Focal fatty change	Bright yellow unencapsulated lesion in a nonsteatotic liver parenchyma.	Hepatocytes with diffuse macrovesicular steatosis. Portal tracts are present. Lipogranulomas.	May represent changes adjacent to a space-occupying lesion.
Hepatocellular adenoma, conventional type	Yellow or congested unencapsulated soft nodular lesion. Focal hemorrhage.	Hepatocytes in 2–3 cell thickness, often with severe steatosis. Unpaired arteries. No portal tract in the lesion.	Patients with oral contraceptive, anabolic steroid use.
Hepatocellular adenoma, inflammatory/ telangiectatic type	Congested unencapsulated lesion with focal yellow discoloration.	Predominantly hepatocyte parenchyma with marked sinusoidal dilatation. Portal tract-like structures with ductular reaction. Focal area with severe macrovesicular steatosis and chronic inflammation.	Positive for serum amyloid A and C-reactive protein.
Angiomyolipoma, lipomatous	Nodular soft lesion, encapsulated with variegated appearance from yellow to brown tan with prominent vascularization.	Fat cells admixed with epithelioid smooth muscle cells. Prominent vascularization with hyalinized thick walled vessels. Brown melanin granules.	Perivascular epithelioid cells are positive for HMB-45.
Pseudolipoma	Yellow nodule surrounded by fibrous tissue, below the hepatic capsule.	Necrotic fat cells surrounded by fibrous capsule. Often shows calcification.	History of abdominal surgery.
Myelolipoma	Yellow soft and often hemorrhagic lesion.	Mature fat cells admixed with hematopoietic elements.	May represent focal change in angiomyolipoma.
Hepatocellular carcinoma	Yellow, hemorrhagic, focally necrotic or bile stained encapsulated or unencapsulated nodule.	Neoplastic cells in thick trabecular configuration with fat content or rarefied cytoplasm. Mallory-Denk hyalin often present.	Positive for HepPar1, Glypican-3, canalicular polyclonal CEA.
Metastatic renal cell carcinoma	Bright yellow, hemorrhagic well circumscribed lesion.	Neoplastic cells with clear cytoplasm, prominent nucleoli. Well vascularized.	Positive for EMA, CD10, vimentin, and renal cell carcinoma antigen.

5.11 Other Mesenchymal Tumors

The majority of primary spindle cell lesions of the liver represent either sarcomatoid hepatocellular carcinoma (HCC) or sarcomatoid cholangiocarcinoma (CC), or spindle cell neoplastic mimics such as inflammatory myofibroblastic tumor. Sarcomatoid HCC or CC is exceedingly more common than primary malignant mesenchymal tumors. Sarcomatoid HCC or CC often requires extensive sampling to demonstrate hepatocellular or cholangiocellular differentiation (Figures 5.11.5 and 5.11.6), which can be confirmed by immunohistochemical stains, such as HepPar1, glypican 3, polyclonal CEA, and CD10 for HCC; and EMA, monoclonal CEA, and CK7 for CC. The neoplastic spindle cells are markedly pleomorphic; occasional giant cells are not uncommon, accompanied by lymphocytic or neutrophilic inflammatory infiltrate. If metastatic carcinoma is being considered, it should be noted that metastatic poorly differentiated or sarcomatoid carcinomas often lose their organ-specific antigenicity; therefore, history of malignancy in other organ is often required.

Angiosarcoma is the most common type of primary malignant mesenchymal lesion. Other malignant mesenchymal tumors, such as fibrosarcoma, leiomyosarcoma, liposarcoma, and osteosarcoma, are rare. They more commonly represent metastases from extrahepatic sites or direct involvement of the liver from an adjacent organ. Nevertheless, a handful of reported cases of primary fibrosarcomas and leiomyosarcomas, and a few cases of liposarcoma and osteosarcoma exist in the literature. The morphologic features of these mesenchymal tumors are similar to their counterparts in the usual sites of origin. Comprehensive review of the patient medical and surgical histories, and imaging studies, are warranted to exclude extrahepatic site of origin.

Benign primary tumors have been reported rarely in the liver. Many of these are mesenchymal tumors, including solitary fibrous tumor, chondroma, fibroma, leiomyoma, lipoma, neurofibroma and schwannoma. Many of these tumors are solitary lesions and arise around the hepatic hilar region, most likely arising from hepatic hilar structures. Granular cell tumor may involve the biliary tract and cause large duct obstruction.

Metastatic sarcomas, such as gastrointestinal stromal tumor, fibrosarcoma, leiomyosarcoma, and liposarcoma, occur in the context of previously documented extrahepatic tumor and demonstrate markedly atypical spindle cells.

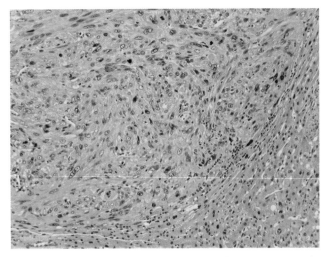

Figure 5.11.1 Metastatic uterine leiomyosarcoma in liver.

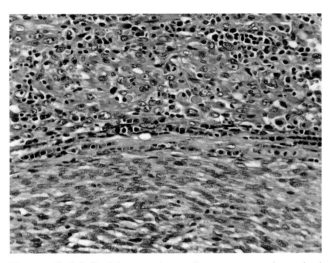

Figure 5.11.2 Metastatic malignant gastrointestinal stromal tumor.

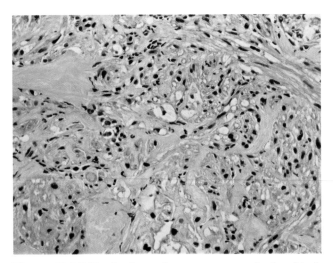

Figure 5.11.3 Angiomyolipoma composed of epithelioid smooth muscle cells.

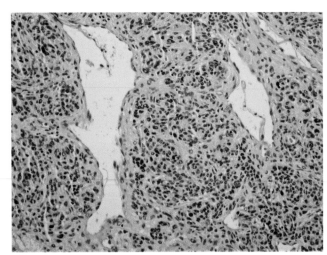

Figure 5.11.4 Solitary fibrous tumor composed of CD34-positive bland spindled cells and dilated angulated vessels.

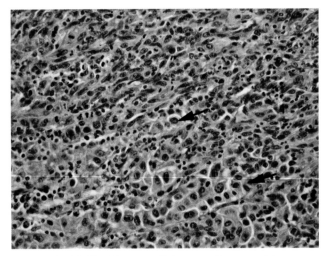

Figure 5.11.5 Hepatocellular carcinoma with sarcomatoid features. Arrows indicate hepatocellular differentiation.

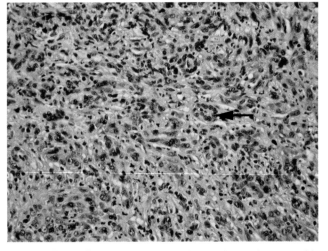

Figure 5.11.6 Sarcomatoid cholangiocarcinoma with rare glandular differentiation (arrow).

5.12 Lymphoma and Leukemia

Lymphoma is a malignant neoplasm derived from lymphoid cells. Lymphoma of the liver is often diagnosed as part of a workup of patients known to have lymphoma. Primary hepatic or hepatosplenic lymphomas are rare, representing less than 1% of extranodal non-Hodgkin lymphomas. Most are non-Hodgkin lymphomas of B-cell phenotype, most frequently diffuse large B-cell lymphoma. An increased incidence of primary hepatic lymphoma has been seen in chronic hepatitis B and hepatitis C viral infections, after transplantation, in acquired immunodeficiency syndrome, and in autoimmune conditions such as primary biliary cirrhosis.

Leukemia can accumulate in the liver in patients known to have leukemia. The liver abnormalities vary from mild elevation of liver function tests to acute liver failure.

Clinical Features

Lymphoma occurs in patients of all ages, with a slight male predominance. Patients may have fever, lymphadenopathy, hepatomegaly, splenomegaly, weight loss, elevations of aminotransferases, and jaundice. Rarely, patients with extensive liver involvement present with acute liver failure. Focal lesions may be shown by imaging techniques. In primary hepatic lymphoma, patients present with a liver mass or hepatomegaly without lymphadenopathy. There are no characteristic clinical findings that can be used to distinguish primary hepatic lymphomas from other malignancies in the liver. Table 5.12.1 lists various reported subtypes of hepatic lymphoma.

Most patients with low-grade lymphomas are asymptomatic, and the clinical course is indolent without extrahepatic involvement. In patients with high-grade, large cell lymphomas, the clinical course is usually aggressive.

Pathologic Features

Lymphoma may involve the liver as nodular lesions or diffusely. Intermediate- and high-grade primary hepatic lymphoma tends to form a solitary tumor mass or multiple masses without lymphadenopathy. A diffuse pattern is less common and may mimic hepatitis. This pattern is more common with low-grade, marginal zone, or other peripheral T-cell lymphomas.

In diffuse involvement of the liver, monomorphic appearance of the cellular infiltrate, irregular involvement of some but not all portal tracts, sinusoidal infiltration and compression of hepatocyte plates without hepatocyte necrosis (Figures 5.12.6 and 5.12.7), and partial necrosis of the infiltrate should raise the suspicion of lymphoma. Nonzonal sinusoidal dilatation is often present. In addition, poorly formed epithelioid granulomas or abscess-like infiltrate may be encountered in Hodgkin disease lymphomas (Figure 5.12.9).

Immunophenotyping should be performed to determine cell type and clonality of the infiltrate. A polymerase chain reaction study for gene rearrangement may be necessary.

Leukemic involvement of the liver typically diffuse with infiltration of the sinusoids by malignant cells, except for chronic lymphocytic leukemia (Figures 5.12.1 and 5.12.2) and acute lymphoblastic leukemia, which often involve the portal tract similar to lymphoma.

Amyloidosis may occur as the result of plasma cell dyscrasia/multiple myeloma, with deposition of amyloid that is positive with Congo red stain in perisinusoidal spaces and vascular wall (Figure 5.12.12). Extramedullary hematopoiesis in the liver can occur in patients with myelodysplastic syndrome and polycythemia vera (Figure 5.12.11).

Differential Diagnosis

Most primary hepatic lymphomas are high grade and are relatively easy to diagnose. Low-grade lymphoma or secondary liver involvement may be mistaken for chronic hepatitis, nonspecific reactive hepatitis, primary biliary cirrhosis, granulomatous inflammation, or inflammatory pseudotumor. Certain features, such as the monomorphic appearance of dense cellular infiltrates, partial necrosis of the infiltrate, cytologic characteristics, irregular involvement of some but not all portal tracts, and expansion of the portal infiltrates with compression of adjacent hepatocyes, are helpful in the diagnosis of lymphoma. In contrast to lymphoid follicles in hepatitis C, the density of lymphoma cells seems to be the same throughout small portal tracts (Figure 5.12.1).

Hepatosplenic T-cell lymphomas are commonly mistaken for a reactive or infectious process (Figure 5.12.8). When significant atypical lymphoid infiltrate in the sinusoids is accompanied by minimal hepatocellular injury, this type of lymphoma should be considered.

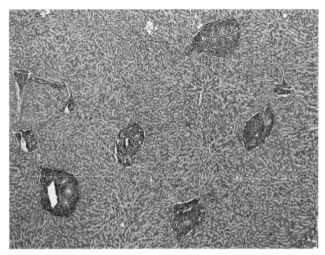

Figure 5.12.1 Small lymphocytic lymphoma involving portal tracts.

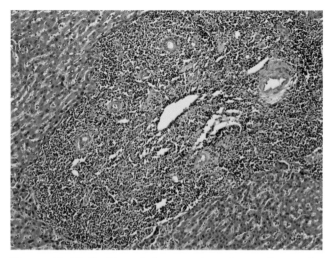

Figure 5.12.2 Rounded expansion of portal tract by monotonous cells of small lymphocytic lymphoma.

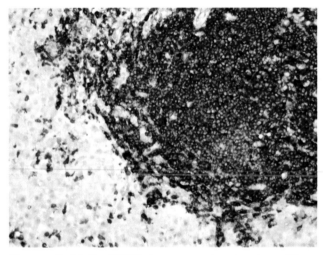

Figure 5.12.3 CD20 immunostain showing diffuse positivity for B cell lymphoma in portal tract and sinusoids.

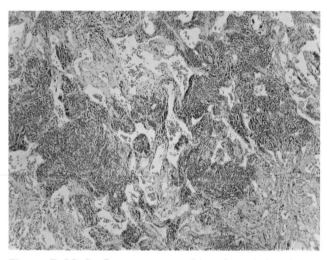

Figure 5.12.4 Concurrent small lymphocytic lymphoma and cavernous hemangioma.

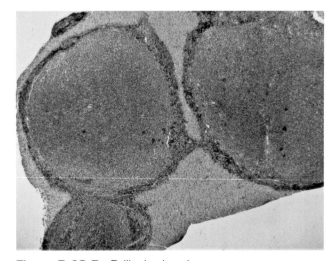

Figure 5.12.5 Follicular lymphoma.

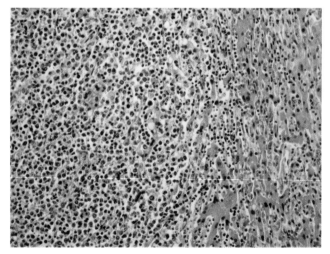

Figure 5.12.6 Expansion of portal tract by diffuse large lymphoma cells compressing the surrounding hepatocytes.

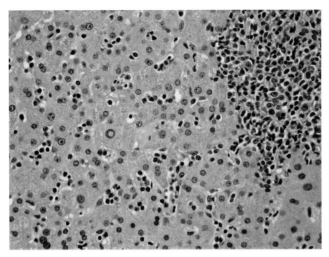

Figure 5.12.7 Infiltration of the sinusoids and the portal tract (right) by lymphoma cells without hepatocyte necrosis.

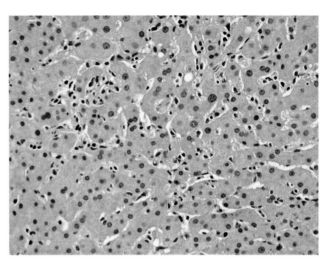

Figure 5.12.8 Hepatosplenic T-cell lymphoma with lymphoma cells in the sinusoids.

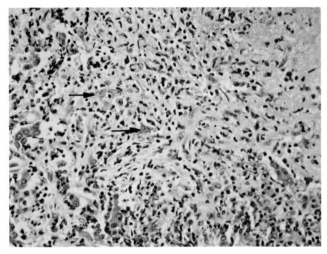

Figure 5.12.9 Hodgkin lymphoma with mixed inflammatory infiltrate, fibrosis and occasional Reed-Sternberg cells (arrows), can be mistaken for abscess or inflammatory lesion.

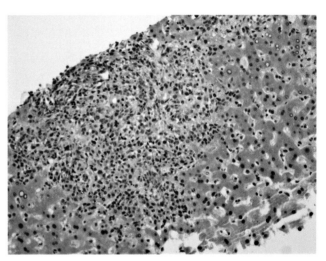

Figure 5.12.10 Acute monoblastic leukemia.

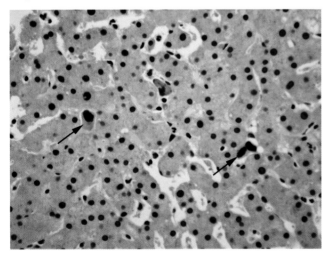

Figure 5.12.11 Extramedullary hematopoiesis in polycytemia vera with megakaryocytes (arrows).

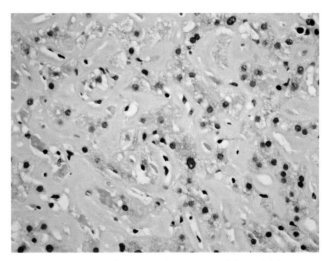

Figure 5.12.12 Amyloidosis in the perisinusoidal space, compressing the hepatocytes.

Table 5.12.1 Lymphomas in the Liver

Lymphomas	Usual Localization	Histologic Features	Immunophenotype	Comments
Diffuse large cell lymphoma	Solitary or multiple nodules	Diffuse large neoplastic cells with scant cytoplasm, vesicular nuclei and prominent nucleoli. Necrosis is common.	CD20+, CD22+, CD45+, surface Ig (SIg) +/−	The most common type of primary hepatic lymphoma.
Extranodal marginal zone B-cell lymphoma	Solitary or multiple nodules	Normal liver architecture with well differentiated lymphoid infiltrate, predominantly in portal tracts. Lymphoepithelial lesion involving bile ducts.	CD20+, CD43+, SIg+, CD5−, CD10−	Association with chronic hepatitis B, C and primary biliary cirrhosis.
Post transplant lymphoproliferative disorders (PTLD)	Diffuse	Ranging from atypical polymorphic lymphoplasmacytic portal infiltrate to monomorphic B-cell infiltrate. EBV positive.	EBV latent membrane protein and insitu hybridization for EBV DNA are positive.	Difficult to distinguish from recurrent chronic hepatitis or rejection in posttransplant patients.
T-cell rich B-cell lymphoma	Diffuse	Variant of diffuse large B cell lymphoma with few large neoplastic B-cell scattered among small T-cells and histiocytes.	CD20+, CD22+, CD45+, SIg+/−, CD15−, CD30−	May mimic chronic inflammatory diseases, including chronic hepatitis with interface hepatitis or Hodgkin disease.
Hepatosplenic (sinusoidal) T-cell lymphoma	Diffuse	Proliferation of gamma-delta T cells in hepatic sinusoids. Often mistaken for reactive hepatitis or infectious process.	CD3+, CD8+, CD5−	Occur in young adults with hepatosplenomegaly and thrombocytopenia.
Anaplastic large cell lymphoma	Multiple nodules	Diffuse large, pleomorphic cells with prominent nucleoli, horseshoe-shaped or multiple nuclei. Reed-Sternberg like cells may be seen.	CD30+, CD45+/−, EMA+/−	NPM/ALK oncogene rearrangement.
Follicular lymphoma	Multiple nodules	Proliferation of neoplastic B-cell with large atypical follicular formation.	CD10 +, CD20+, CD22+, SIg+, CD5−	Bcl-2 oncogene rearrangement with t(14;18) chromosome translocation.
Mantle cell lymphoma	Solitary nodule	Monotonous proliferation of round or cleaved small lymphocytes.	CD5+, CD20+, CD10−, CD23−, SIg+	Bcl-1/CyclinD1 rearrangement with t(11;14) chromosome translocation.
Lymphoplasmacytoid lymphoma	Solitary nodule	Monotonous proliferation of plasmacytoid lymphocytes. Immunoglobulin and nuclear inclusions may be seen.	CD20+, CD22+, CD5−, CD10−, CD23−, SIg+, cytoplasmic Ig+	Associated with Waldenstrom macroglobulinemia. Pax-5 rearrangement with t(9;14) chromosome translocation.

5.13 Metastatic Tumors

Metastatic tumor is the most common malignancy in the liver. Metastatic spread to the liver is usually hematogenous, but tumors can metastasize through peritoneal fluid or lymphatics. Most of the tumors are adenocarcinomas, and the most frequent primary sites are breast, lung, gastrointestinal tract, and pancreas carcinoma. Prostatic adenocarcinoma rarely metastasize to the liver. Other common tumor types include malignant melanoma, neuroendocrine tumors such as carcinoids, pancreatic endocrine neoplasm, and small cell neuroendocrine carcinomas, renal cell carcinoma, adrenal cortical carcinoma, and gastrointestinal stromal tumor.

The symptoms are due to enlarging hepatic mass, the primary tumor, or both. The liver may be enlarged or of normal size, and cirrhosis is usually absent. Serum CEA or CA19-9 levels may be elevated, but serum α-fetoprotein levels are not.

Metastatic tumors are single or multiple well-circumscribed nodules, often of about the same size. Except for malignant melanoma, the color is often lighter than that of the liver parenchyma, which only rarely shows cirrhosis. The consistency depends on the amount of fibrous stroma within the tumor and the extent of necrosis. Umbilication due to central necrosis is often seen in tumor nodules on the surface of the liver. Portal vein or bile duct invasion may be found.

Metastatic tumors may show histologic similarities to their primary lesions, but often, they are less differentiated and more anaplastic than the original tumors. Because of trabecular configuration and clear cell or eosinophilic/oncocytic cell appearance, metastatic renal cell and adrenal cortical carcinoma closely resemble hepatocellullar carcinoma (Figures 5.13.8 and 5.13.9). Metastatic pancreatic adenocarcinoma or adenocarcinoma from upper gastrointestinal tract may be indistinguishable morphologically and immunophenotypically from intrahepatic cholangiocarcinoma.

Special stains, such as mucicarmine for adenocarcinoma, and immunohistochemical studies to demonstrate cytokeratin intermediate filaments profile and organ-specific antigens are helpful in the search of the primary malignancy. Commonly used organ-specific antigens are CDX-2 for intestinal differentiation/origin (nuclear positivity), TTF-1 for pulmonary adenocarcinoma or small cell neuroendocrine carcinoma, estrogen or progesterone receptor for breast and female genital tract carcinoma, and PSA for protatic adenocarcinoma. HepPar1, cytoplasmic TTF-1, and glypican 3 are positive in hepatocellular carcinoma, and CK7 in cholangiocarcinoma.

In general, metastatic tumors in the liver pertain to poor prognosis. Isolated metastases from colorectal carcinomas usually grow slowly, and the patients may have longer survival after resection.

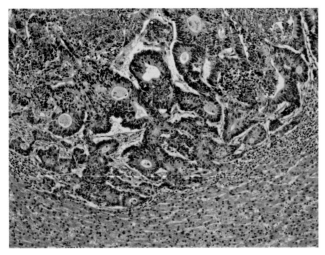

Figure 5.13.1 Metastatic colorectal adenocarcinoma with necrosis.

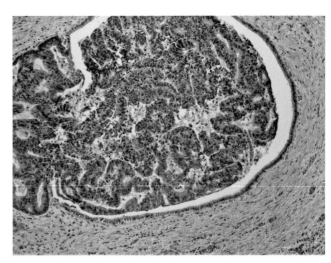

Figure 5.13.2 Metastatic colorectal adenocarcinoma involving bile duct, not to be mistaken as bile duct carcinoma. Bile duct epithelium is CK7+ and tumor is CK20+.

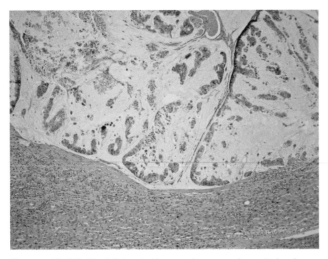

Figure 5.13.3 Metastatic mucinous colorectal adenocarcinoma.

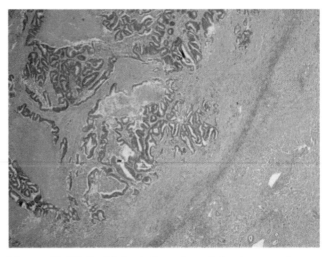

Figure 5.13.4 Metastatic colorectal adenocarcinoma with extensive necrosis and fibrosis after chemotherapy.

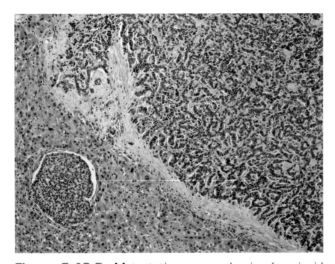

Figure 5.13.5 Metastatic neuroendocrine/carcinoid tumor.

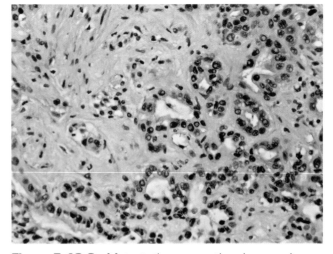

Figure 5.13.6 Metastatic pancreatic adenocarcinoma with desmoplastic stroma, difficult to differentiate from intrahepatic cholangiocarcinoma.

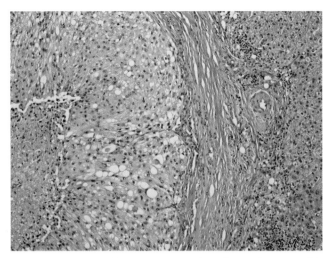

Figure 5.13.7 Metastatic renal cell carcinoma with necrosis.

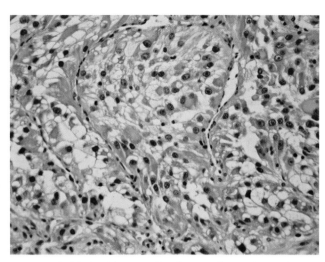

Figure 5.13.8 Metastatic clear cell renal carcinoma with trabecular pattern; mimicking hepatocellular carcinoma with clear cell features.

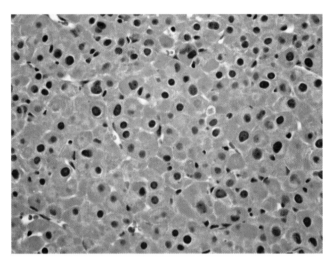

Figure 5.13.9 Metastatic adrenal cortical carcinoma with oncocytic features.

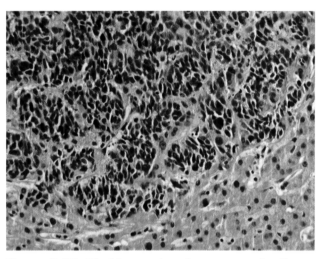

Figure 5.13.10 Metastatic pulmonary small cell neuroendocrine carcinoma.

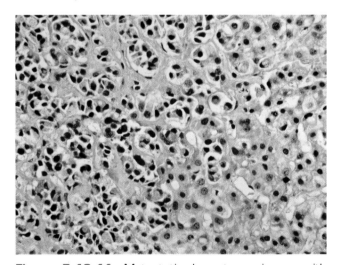

Figure 5.13.11 Metastatic breast carcinoma with lobular features.

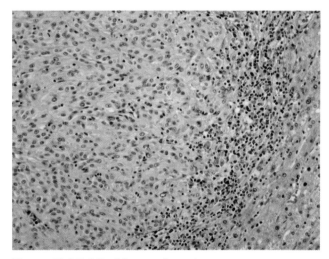

Figure 5.13.12 Metastatic melanoma.

Table 5.13.1 Immunohistochemical Stains of Various Metastatic Tumors

Tumor Type and Origin	Immunohistochemical Studies	Comments
Pulmonary adenocarcinoma	CK7+, CK20–, TTF-1+, CDX-2–.	Liver lesion in imaging studies.
Colorectal adenocarcinoma	CK7–, CK20+, CDX-2+, TTF-1–.	Large well-formed neoplastic glands with necrotic lumen.
Breast carcinoma	CK7+, CK20–, estrogen and progesterone receptor +/–, BRST Ag +/–.	Liver lesion on imaging studies. Occult primary may rarely occur.
Gastric adenocarcinoma	Variable cytokeratin positivity (CK7+, CK19+, CK20+).	Tumor cells are arranged in small tubular glands ranging from well to poorly differentiated.
Pancreatic adenocarcinoma	CK7+, CK19+, CK20+/–, loss of Smad 4 expression in up to 70%.	Often indistinguishable morphologically & immunophenotypically from intrahepatic cholangiocarcinoma or metastatic adenocarcinoma from the upper gastrointestinal tract.
Prostatic adenocarcinoma	CK7+, CK20+, PSA+	Small tubular glands
Gynecologic tract carcinoma	CK7+, CK20–, estrogen and progesterone receptor. +/–	Metastatic lesion may represent lymphovascular or peritoneal spread.
Melanoma	S100+, HMB45+, Melan-A+, CK–, EMA–.	Metastases may occur many years after the primary excised. Amelanotic melanoma may be mistaken for hepatocellular carcinoma.
Carcinoid/large cell neuroendocrine carcinoma	Synaptophysin+, chromogranin+, CD56+, variable cytokeratin positivity. Tumor from midgut and hindgut may show CDX-2 positivity.	Primary tumor may be small and is not evident at initial presentation. Liver may be extensively involved by multiple tumor nodules. Acinar formation or oncocytic features are difficult to differentiate from adenocarcinoma or hepatocellular carcinoma at frozen section.
Small cell neuroendocrine carcinoma	Synaptophysin+, chromogranin+, variable cytokeratin positivity often in punctate cytoplasmic staining, TTF-1+ in those from the lung and to less extent from other site.	Liver may be extensively involved while primary remain clinically occult.
Renal (clear) cell carcinoma	Vimentin+, EMA+, CK7+, CK20–, CD10+ membranous, renal cell carcinoma+	Clear cell variant of hepatocellular carcinoma may mimic metastatic renal cell carcinoma.
Adrenal cortical carcinoma	Inhibin+, synaptophysin+, melan-A+, calretinin+	Oncocytic/eosinophilic cytoplasm mimicking hepatocellular carcinoma
Gastrointestinal stromal tumor	Vimentin+, CD117+, CD34+, smooth muscle actin focal +/–, desmin- and S-100 protein–.	Primary tumor may be occult or asymptomatic.

5.14 Tumor-Associated Changes

Tumor-associated changes are seen in the liver of patients with primary or metastatic malignant neoplasms. These changes include changes in the vicinity of a space occupying lesion due to local compression, bile duct obstruction and venous outflow obstruction, focal fatty change or fatty sparing, and large bile duct obstruction. The severity of the changes depend on the size, the growth rate and the location (subcapsular) of the tumor.

Changes in the Vicinity of a Space-Occupying Lesion

It is diagnostically important to record these changes, particularly if the needle biopsy misses the tumor. The primary tumor may or may not be known, and liver biopsy is performed to determine the presence and origin of the metastases. The patients complain of malaise, weight loss, and right upper abdominal discomfort. The liver is enlarged, and the serum alkaline phosphatase and less commonly bilirubin and aminotransferase values are elevated.

Although the biopsy specimen does not include the neoplasm, a characteristic histologic triad is observed in the adjacent liver. These changes consist of edematous portal tracts infiltrated by a few scattered neutrophils (Figures 5.14.2 and 5.14.3). The bile ductules proliferate and are distorted with irregular epithelium and hyperchromatic nuclei. There is focal sinusoidal dilatation and congestion without zonal predilection (Figures 5.14.1 and 5.14.4). The liver cell plates are compressed and distorted with focal atrophy of hepatocytes. These histologic changes are the result of local obstruction of blood and bile flow by the expanding mass. The portal tract abnormalities are similar to the changes in large bile duct obstruction, but cholestasis is usually absent and only small portal tracts are involved.

The changes in the vicinity of a space-occupying lesion should lead to further diagnostic studies, particularly directed liver biopsy guided by an imaging method. The prognosis depends on the site, type, and stage of primary malignancy.

Fatty Change and Fatty Sparing

Fatty change or sparing often presents immediately adjacent to a space-occupying lesion. Fatty change occurs in the background of normal liver parenchyma, while fatty sparing occurs in the background of fatty liver. Additional features such as chronic inflammation, ductular reaction, and sinusoidal dilatation, which are caused by localized bile duct or vascular obstruction, are usually present as well and should lead to additional diagnostic biopsies.

Large Bile Duct Obstruction

Large bile duct obstruction is commonly caused by hepatic hilar tumor, common bile duct tumor, or pancreatic head tumor. When partial or intermittent, it is not accompanied by pain, fever, and/or jaundice. The liver is usually enlarged, and alkaline phosphatase activity is elevated. Liver biopsy is often done because of negative cholangiography or ultrasound studies.

Large bile duct obstruction can be distinguished from changes in the vicinity of the space-occupying lesion by the presence of widespread and more pronounced portal tract alterations and canalicular and cytoplasmic cholestasis in the absence of sinusoidal engorgement and compression of hepatocytes. The portal tracts exhibit edema, neutrophilic infiltration, and marked ductular reaction, particularly along the margins of the portal tracts (Figure 5.14.5).

Large bile duct obstruction should be treated by common bile duct stenting or surgical intervention. Prolonged large bile duct obstruction may lead to secondary sclerosing cholangitis and biliary cirrhosis (Figure 5.14.6). Its prognosis depends on the cause of obstruction.

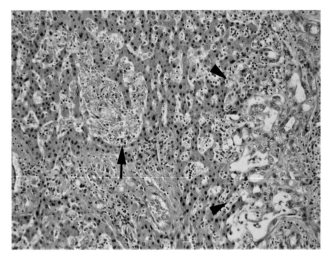

Figure 5.14.1 Liver parenchyma adjacent to cholangiocarcinoma (arrowheads) with sinusoidal dilatation (arrows).

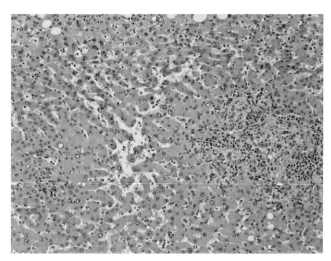

Figure 5.14.2 Changes in the vicinity of a space-occupying lesion include ductular reaction in the portal tract and sinusoidal dilatation.

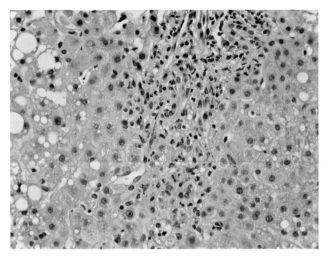

Figure 5.14.3 Ductular reaction accompanied by neutrophils and focal steatosis in the vicinity of a space-occupying lesion.

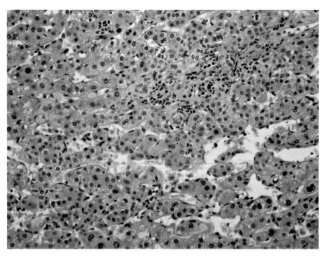

Figure 5.14.4 Sinusoidal dilatation in the vicinity of a space-occupying lesion.

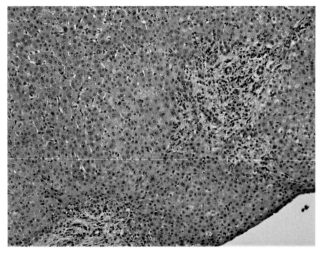

Figure 5.14.5 Portal edema, marginal ductular reaction and neutrophils in large bile duct obstruction secondary to hepatic hilar tumor.

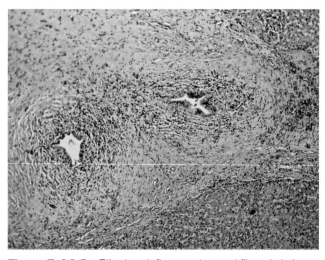

Figure 5.14.6 Bile duct inflammation and fibrosis in large bile duct obstruction secondary to hepatic hilar tumor.

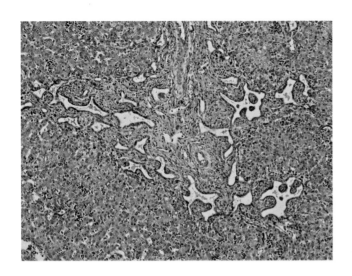

CHAPTER **6**

PEDIATRIC LIVER DISEASES

6.1 Pediatric Liver Biopsy

The most common indications for liver biopsy in the pediatric population are evaluation of cholestatic liver disease in infants; confirmation and assessment of the extent of liver injury, inflammation, and fibrosis in older children; and tumor diagnosis. In infants and young children, the diagnostic challenge is to distinguish surgically correctable obstructive disorders or developmental abnormalities, such as extrahepatic biliary atresia and choledochal cyst, from other causes of nonobstructive cholestatic disorders, including neonatal hepatitis, paucity of intrahepatic bile duct, ductal plate malformation, and hereditary and metabolic disorders (Table 6.1.1). In older children and adolescents, diagnosis of hereditary metabolic diseases (hemochromatosis, Wilson disease, and α-1-antitrypsin [AAT] deficiency), infectious diseases, and drug-induced injury is usually the reason for liver biopsies.

Although histologic examination remains important for diagnosis, genetic mutations linked to various disorders are increasingly identified; therefore, many of the pediatric liver diseases are ultimately confirmed or diagnosed by molecular diagnostic tests.

Handling and Processing of Pediatric Liver Biopsy Specimen

Because of the broad differential diagnosis of pediatric liver disease, which includes developmental anomalies, inherited disorders, and infectious diseases, the handling of pediatric liver biopsy specimen should at least include (1) a portion of the liver biopsy in formalin for routine histologic examination, (2) a portion for snap-frozen using liquid nitrogen to preserve mRNA for molecular studies, and (3) a small portion for electron microscopy. If glycogen storage disorder is suspected, alcohol fixation may be preferred over formalin fixation. For histologic examination, the specimen should be immediately immersed in formalin. Saline or other transport solution may distort tissue and should not be used.

Normal Pediatric Liver Histology

The lobular architecture, hepatocyte morphology, cytoplasmic content, and portal tract of liver in pediatric livers, particularly in infants and young children, differ from those of adults.

At birth, all but few hepatocytes are mononuclear. The hepatocytes are small, uniform, and arranged in 2-cell-thick plates that can be encountered well into the first 5 years of life, representing physiologic hyperplasia, which is morphologically similar to regenerative hepatocytes in adults (Figure 6.1.1). The hepatocytes normally contain hemosiderin and copper in the first few months of life, which gradually disappear and should be absent by 6 to 9 months of age. In older children and adolescents, copper deposition suggesting Wilson disease should not be overlooked.

Hepatocyte alterations, characteristic of various inherited metabolic diseases including storage diseases, may be inconspicuous in early infancy due to the required time for accumulation of abnormal substances and their effect on the hepatocytes. For example, a biopsy from an infant with AAT deficiency may not show diagnostic intracytoplasmic globules before 3 months of age.

Bile ducts should be present in most portal tracts at the same caliber as the hepatic artery. Ductal plate remnants can be found as a rim of biliary epithelium or ducts in portal tracts of immature livers (Figure 6.1.2). Dilated and anastomosing ductal plate remnants embedded in fibrous stroma suggest ductal plate malformation (Figure 6.1.3).

Hematopoietic elements, represented by clusters of erythroid precursor cells, are commonly present in liver biopsy specimens obtained during the first few months of life (Figures 6.1.4 and 6.1.5). Granulocytic extramedullary hematopoiesis can be seen in the portal tracts, whereas erythropoietic extramedullary hematopoiesis can be seen in the parenchyma (Figure 6.1.6).

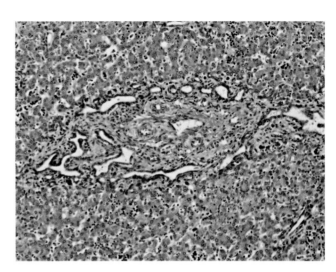

Figure 6.1.1 Extrahepatic biliary atresia with extensive marginal ductular reaction and small uniform hepatocytes that are arranged in 2-cell-thick plates, characteristic of pediatric liver parenchyma.

Figure 6.1.2 Ductal plate remnants encircling portal tract in a premature newborn (courtesy of Dr. Margret Magid).

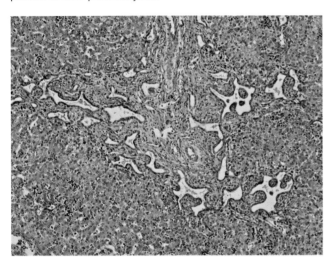

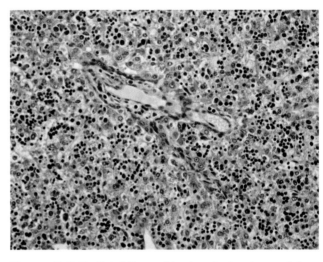

Figure 6.1.3 Abnormal dilated and anastomosing ductal plate remnants in ductal plate malformation.

Figure 6.1.4 Fetal liver with abundant extramedullary hematopoiesis.

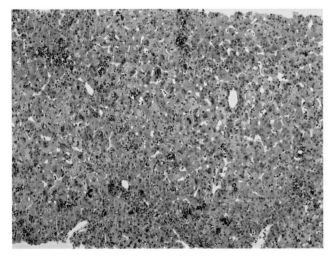

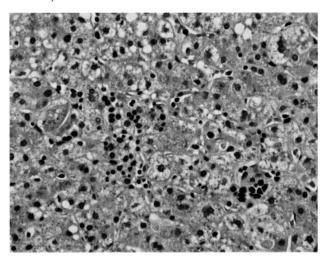

Figure 6.1.5 Dark clusters of round cells in the sinusoids representing extramedullary hematopoiesis in an infant.

Figure 6.1.6 Clusters of dark staining erythroid precursor cells representing extramedullary hematopoiesis.

Table 6.1.1 Etiology of Cholestatic Disease in Infants

Category		Abnormalities and Diseases
Developmental abnormalities of biliary tree	Large bile duct obstruction	Extrahepatic biliary atresia
		Choledochal cyst
		Biliary stricture
	Paucity of intrahepatic bile duct	Syndromic form—Allagille syndrome
		Nonsyndromic form
	Ductal plate malformation	Congenital hepatic fibrosis
		Caroli disease
Infection	Neonatal hepatitis	Cytomegalovirus
		Herpesvirus
		Hepatotropic viruses (HAV, HBV, HCV)
		Human immunodeficiency virus
		Parvovirus B19
		Paramyxovirus
		Enteric viruses (echoviruses, coxsackieviruses, adenoviruses)
		Rubella (congenital)
		Bacterial sepsis
		Listeriosis
		Toxoplasmosis
		Syphilis
Hereditary and metabolic disorders	α-1-Antitrypsin deficiency	
	Neonatal hemochromatosis	
	Hereditary disorders of bilirubin metabolism	Crigler-Najjar syndrome
		Gilbert syndrome
		Dubin-Johnson syndrome
	Hereditary disorders of bile formation or flow	Progressive familial intrahepatic cholestasis
		Defects in bile acid biosynthesis
	Disorders of amino acid metabolism	Tyrosinemia
	Disorders of carbohydrate metabolism	Galactosemia
		Glycogen storage disease
		Fructosemia
	Disorders of lipid metabolism	Niemann-Pick disease, types A and C
		Hunter disease, Hurler disease
		Cholesterol ester storage disease
		Wolman disease
		Gaucher disease
	Disorders of glycoprotein metabolism	
	Mitochondrial cytopathies	

6.2 Neonatal Hepatitis Syndrome

Neonatal hepatitis syndrome is a nonobstructive cholestatic hepatitis syndrome with many potential etiologies. An infant usually presents during the first few weeks or months of life with jaundice, acholic stools, and bilirubinemia. Aminotransferase activities are markedly elevated. It may be associated with inborn error of metabolism such as α-1-antitrypsin (AAT) deficiency, glycogen storage disease, and galactosemia. Serologic testing for hepatitis viruses, adenovirus, coxsackie viruses, or a TORCH screen may be positive, but in about 75% of patients, the cause remains unknown. The prognosis of neonatal hepatitis is variable depending on the underlying cause.

Pathologic Features

Neonatal hepatitis (also known as syncytial giant cell hepatitis) is a generic term for nonobstructive cholestasis due to a variety of causes listed above. All show a similar histologic pattern with diffuse hepatocellular damage, particularly swelling and multinucleation, cholestasis, and portal inflammation (Figure 6.2.1). Syncytial giant cells are enlarged hepatocytes with at least 4 nuclei that are often clustered in the center or periphery of the cell (Figure 6.2.2). The cytoplasm is rarefied and contains bile or lipofuscin pigment. Giant cells are probably the result of fusion of hepatocytes or very active regeneration in the young hepatocytes. It should be noted that giant cells are considered a nonspecific reactive change that is commonly present in infants with liver disease, regardless of the etiology.

Intralobular inflammation is often mild, but there may be hepatocyte necrosis and collapse with distortion of the reticulin framework causing lobular disarray, a helpful feature for distinction from intrahepatic paucity of bile ducts and large bile duct obstruction (Figure 6.2.5). Ductular reaction or portal fibrosis is not a prominent feature. Extramedullary hematopoiesis can be encountered during the first few months of life (Figure 6.2.3).

α-1-Antitrypsin deficiency should be ruled out by genetic testing and by periodic acid–Schiff (PAS) staining after diastase digestion, although the characteristic globules may not be seen until several months of age. Periportal macrovesicular steatosis in an infant with neonatal hepatitis is a clue to AAT deficiency. Immunohistochemical staining for AAT, and viruses such as hepatitis B virus and cytomegalovirus (CMV) (Figure 6.2.6), and electron microscopy, may be helpful. Paramyxovirus infection has been reported to be associated with syncytial giant cell hepatitis.

Differential Diagnosis

The main differential diagnosis of neonatal hepatitis syndrome is extrahepatic biliary atresia and paucity of intrahepatic bile duct. Neonatal hepatitis exhibits extensive lobular disarray and inflammation, accompanied by hepatocellular dropout. The portal tracts show no significant ductular reaction or edema such as seen in extrahepatic biliary atresia. Bile ducts can be inconspicuous but generally present. It should be noted, however, that giant cell transformation can also be seen in both extrahepatic biliary atresia and paucity of intrahepatic bile duct.

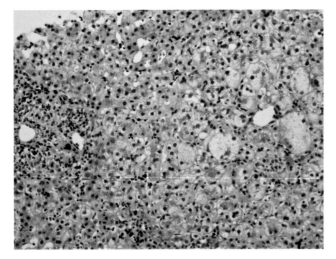

Figure 6.2.1 Neonatal hepatitis showing lobular disarray, portal and lobular inflammation, and multinucleated giant hepatocytes.

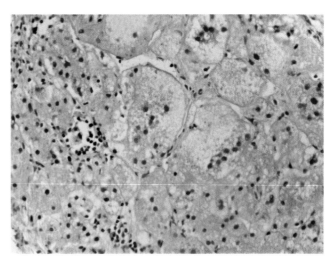

Figure 6.2.2 Multinucleated giant hepatocytes, lymphocytes, and cholestasis in neonatal hepatitis.

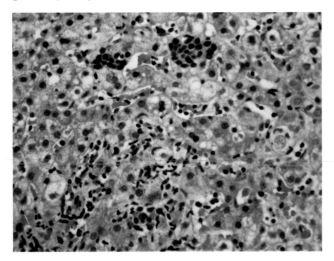

Figure 6.2.3 Neonatal hepatitis showing lobular lymphocytic inflammation (lower field) and extramedullary hematopoiesis (upper field).

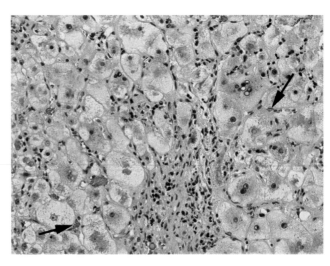

Figure 6.2.4 Neonatal hepatitis in a patient with sickle cell anemia (arrows).

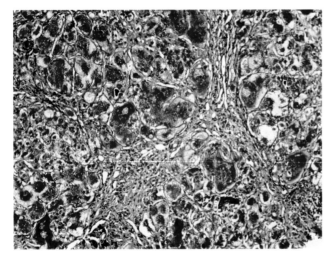

Figure 6.2.5 Neonatal hepatitis with submassive hepatic necrosis (trichrome stain).

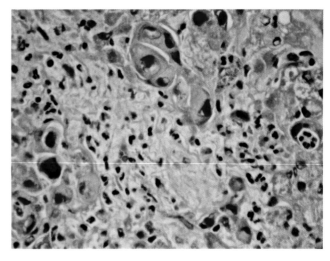

Figure 6.2.6 Neonatal hepatitis with multiple cytomegalovirus inclusions.

Table 6.2.1   Major Etiologies of Neonatal Hepatitis

Major Etiologies
α-1-Antitrypsin deficiency
Hepatitis viral infections
A, B or C
Miscellaneous viral infections
Cytomegalovirus
Rubella
Herpes simplex virus
Human herpes virus 6
Varicella
Coxsackievirus
Enteroviruses
Parvovirus B19
Paramyxovirus
Bacterial infection and sepsis
Disorders of amino acid metabolim
Tyrosinemia
Disorders of carbohydrate metabolism
Galactosemia
Fructosemia
Glycogen storage diseases
Disorders of lipid metabolism
Niemann-Pick disease
Idiopathic

6.3 Extrahepatic Biliary Atresia and Paucity of Intrahepatic Bile Duct

Extrahepatic Biliary Atresia and Large Bile Duct Obstruction

Large bile duct obstruction is usually due to extrahepatic biliary atresia, choledochal cyst (Figure 6.3.8), or other causes of biliary obstruction, such as neonatal sclerosing cholangitis.

Extrahepatic biliary atresia accounts for up to 30% of infants who present with cholestasis. Most cases are sporadic without any family history, and the pathogenesis is unknown. The infant becomes progressively jaundiced by the first week of life with dark urine and acholic stools. In extrahepatic biliary atresia, γ-glutamyltransferase activity and cholesterol levels are higher and aminotransferase activity is lower than in neonatal hepatitis. Biliary isotope scanning, ultrasonography, computed tomography scan, and cholangiogram are useful in evaluating the status of the biliary passages. The most important decision in the early postnatal period is whether or not cholestasis is due to extrahepatic biliary atresia. Percutaneous liver biopsy is often used to determine whether there is histologic evidence of large bile duct obstruction.

Large bile duct obstruction in an infant has histologic features similar to those of large bile duct obstruction in the adult. Portal tracts are expanded by edema, fibrosis, ductular reaction, and neutrophilic infiltration (Figure 6.3.1). Ductular reaction often containing inspissated bile is conspicuous (Figure 6.3.2). Hepatocanalicular cholestasis in the lobules is prominent. As the disease progresses, the inflammation of portal tracts becomes lymphocytic and scanty, and portal fibrosis increases with development of secondary biliary cirrhosis (Figures 6.3.3 to 6.3.6). Extramedullary hematopoiesis may be present depending on the infant's age. Diffuse ductular reaction and early fibrosis are helpful in the distinction from neonatal hepatitis and paucity of intrahepatic bile ducts. In contrast to the findings in neonatal hepatitis, giant cells are focal and often periportal, and there is no hepatocyte necrosis and collapse. If large bile duct obstruction persists, intrahepatic bile ducts and ductules may disappear, and distinction from paucity of intrahepatic bile ducts is difficult.

The prognosis of large bile duct obstruction depends on the success of surgical intervention. Early diagnosis is crucial. Optimally, the Kasai portoesterostomy operation is performed for extrahepatic biliary atresia by 2 months of age, but liver transplantation often becomes necessary.

Paucity of Intrahepatic Bile Duct

Paucity of intrahepatic bile ducts (intrahepatic biliary atresia) usually causes jaundice within 3 days of birth, but it may be delayed for months or years. The nonsyndromic form is not associated with systemic abnormalities and may be related to known causes such as AAT deficiency, cystic fibrosis, Down syndrome, abnormal bile salt metabolism, or viral infection such as reovirus type 3, rubella, or CMV. CMV is the most important among congenital infections. Clinically, paucity of intrahepatic bile duct is indistinguishable from neonatal hepatitis, but serum γ-glutamyltransferase and cholesterol levels are very high.

The syndromic form (arteriohepatic dysplasia or Allagile syndrome) is associated with extrahepatic manifestations, such as abnormal facies, skeletal changes (butterfly vertebral bodies), and ocular and/or cardiac abnormalities, particularly pulmonic stenosis. In contrast to the nonsyndromic form, it is inherited in autosomal dominant fashion with variable expression and penetrance. Mutation in *JAG1* gene, or rarely in *Notch2* gene, has been identified in patients with Allagile syndrome.

The prognosis of paucity of intrahepatic bile ducts depends on the underlying cause. The syndromic form often improves with time, and neither cirrhosis nor portal hypertension ensues. Children with severe nonsyndromic paucity of intrahepatic bile ducts usually die by 5 years of age due to biliary cirrhosis, and liver transplantation should be considered.

Paucity of intrahepatic bile ducts is characterized by loss of interlobular bile ducts (Figures 6.3.7 to 6.3.10). The diagnosis depends on establishing the bile duct-to-portal tract ratio (normal ≥0.9). For this purpose, the bile ducts are counted in at least 6 portal tracts with hepatic artery branches that usually accompany bile ducts. A ratio less than 0.5 duct per portal tract indicates paucity. Early in the disease, there may be interlobular bile duct damage with lymphocytic infiltration, periductal fibrosis, and mild ductular reaction. Other histologic features include canalicular cholestasis, focal giant cell formation, and hepatocellular necrosis. This stage is difficult to distinguish from neonatal hepatitis, but intralobular inflammation is usually absent or mild. Later, inflammation of portal tracts is replaced by fibrosis, sometimes with progression to secondary biliary cirrhosis. In contrast to extrahepatic biliary atresia, ductopenia is evident from the beginning, and ductular reaction is focal or absent. Hepatic copper levels are increased. The distinction of the syndromic form from the nonsyndromic form of paucity of intrahepatic bile ducts is based on clinical findings. Once a diagnosis of paucity of intrahepatic bile ducts has been made, associated diseases should be ruled out, particularly AAT deficiency, progressive familial intrahepatic cholestasis, cystic fibrosis, and viral infections.

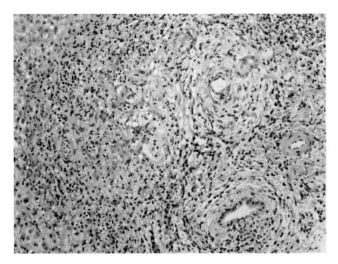

Figure 6.3.1 Portal edema, inflammation, ductular reaction, and bile duct damage in a 1-month-old infant with extrahepatic biliary atresia.

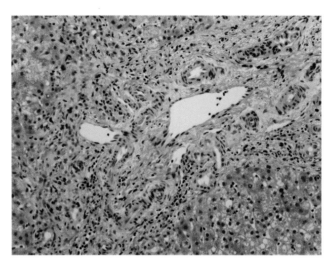

Figure 6.3.2 Portal fibrosis and ductular reaction with progression of extrahepatic biliary atresia.

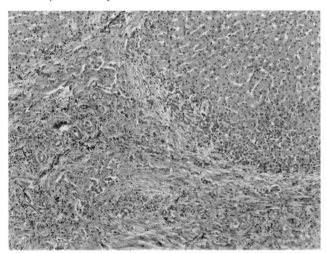

Figure 6.3.3 Portal fibrosis followed by bridging fibrosis and nodule formation in extrahepatic biliary atresia.

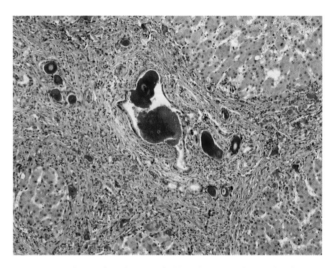

Figure 6.3.4 Inspissated bile in extrahepatic biliary atresia.

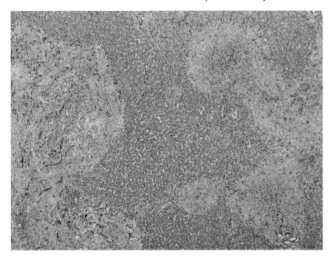

Figure 6.3.5 Biliary-type cirrhosis in extrahepatic biliary atresia.

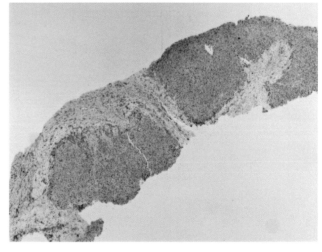

Figure 6.3.6 Biopsy with extrahepatic biliary atresia after Kasai operation showing biliary-type cirrhosis.

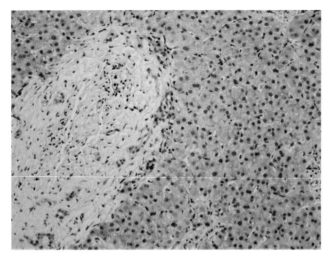

Figure 6.3.7 Densely fibrotic portal tract with absence of interlobular bile duct in extrahepatic biliary atresia.

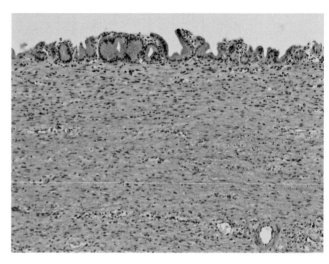

Figure 6.3.8 Choledochal cyst lined by biliary epithelium.

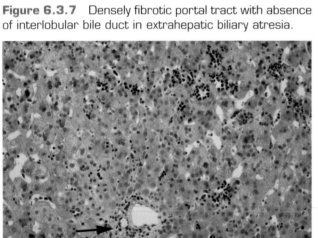

Figure 6.3.9 Absence of intrahepatic bile duct in the portal tract (arrow) of patient with paucity of intrahepatic bile duct. There is no portal tract fibrosis, ductular reaction, or significant lobular inflammation and disarray. Dark clusters of cells represent extramedullary hematopoiesis.

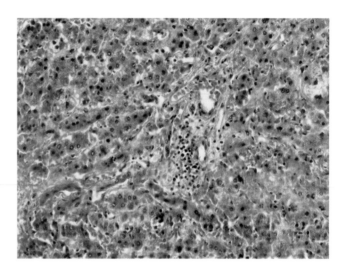

Figure 6.3.10 Paucity of intrahepatic bile duct showing absence of bile duct in the portal tract without portal fibrosis, inflammation, and ductular reaction.

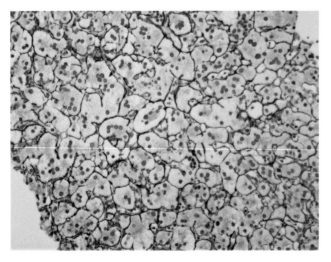

Figure 6.3.11 Preservation of lobular architecture in paucity of intrahepatic bile duct.

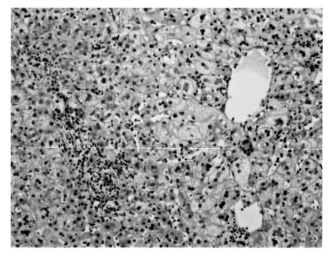

Figure 6.3.12 Neonatal hepatitis showing portal and lobular inflammation, extramedullary hematopoiesis, and lobular disarray.

Table 6.3.1 Differential Diagnosis of Cholestatic Syndromes

	Neonatal Hepatitis	Extrahepatic Biliary Atresia	Paucity of Intrahepatic Bile Duct
Clinical features	Variable, usually jaundice and severely ill	Normal at birth, but progressive jaundice soon after	Normal at birth, but progressive jaundice after, may be delayed for months or years
Imaging studies	Normal	Abnormal cholangiography, biliary scintigraphy of extrahepatic bile duct	Extrahepatic bile duct is normal
Portal changes	Expanded with inflammation and edema, no fibrosis	Expanded with ductular reaction and edema, followed by fibrosis	None to mild fibrosis
Portal inflammation	Variable, lymphoplasmacellular, neutrophils, can be prominent	Mild, neutrophils	Minimal, lymphocytes
Intrahepatic bile duct	Present	Present in the beginning with damage, atrophy and eventually loss	Absent or loss >50%
Ductular reaction	Mild	Prominent with ductular cholestasis	Mild or none
Lobular inflammation	Variable, mild to severe	Absent	Absent or minimal
Lobular architectural disarray	Prominent	Mild	Mild
Syncytial giant cell hepatocytes	Prominent	Can occur	Can occur
Hepatocyte necrosis	Variable, can be severe	Minimal	Minimal
Cholestasis	Hepatocanalicular	Hepatocanalicular and ductular	Hepatocanalicular

6.4 Fatty Liver Disease

Nonalcoholic fatty liver disease (NAFLD) has become the most common cause of chronic liver disease in children and adolescents in conjunction with the increased incidence of obesity and insulin resistance. The incidence in the general population is 2% but increases to 50% in obese children. If undiagnosed, nonalcoholic steatohepatitis (NASH) may progress silently and result in cirrhosis, portal hypertension, and liver-related death in early adulthood. Diagnosis of NASH requires a liver biopsy.

Nonalcoholic fatty liver disease occurs as early as 2 years old but more often after age of 8 years, and the typical age at presentation is 12 years. Children with NAFLD are commonly asymptomatic, and clinical evaluation is typically initiated with obesity, vague abdominal pain, hepatomegaly, and elevated serum aminotransferase activities. Acanthosis nigricans is seen in up to 50% of children with NAFLD.

The prognosis of children with NAFLD is related to the severity of the liver histology. Advanced fibrosis in liver biopsy can be seen in up to 10% of children with NAFLD. Cirrhosis secondary to pediatric NAFLD has been reported; some required liver transplantation in adolescents. As with any form of chronic liver disease, children with NAFLD may develop hepatocellular carcinoma in adulthood.

Pathologic Features

Studies of pediatric NAFLD have described patterns of inflammation and fibrosis that differ from those reported in adults with NAFLD. Based on these studies, there are 2 different forms of NASH in pediatric NAFLD, type 1 and type 2. Type 1 is similar to NASH described in adults, characterized by steatosis, ballooning degeneration, and perisinusoidal fibrosis, in the absence of portal features (Figure 6.4.2). Type 2 is the predominant form of NASH in children, characterized by steatosis, portal inflammation, and portal fibrosis, in the absence of ballooning degeneration and/or perisinusoidal fibrosis (Figures 6.4.3 and 6.4.4).

Overlap of type 1 and type 2 NASH occurs but is uncommon. Boys are significantly more likely to have type 2 NASH and less likely to have type 1 NASH than girls. Children with type 2 NASH have a greater severity of obesity and advanced liver fibrosis than those with type 1 NASH. Type 1 NASH is more common in Caucasian children, whereas type 2 NASH is more common in children of Asian, Native American, and Hispanic ethnicity.

Differential Diagnosis

The differential diagnoses of NAFLD in the pediatric population include autoimmune hepatitis and glycogenic hepatopathy. Autoimmune hepatitis is supported by autoimmune markers and histologically different with abundant plasmacellular infiltrate, panlobular hepatitis, interface hepatitis, periportal hepatocyte rosettes, and often with perivenular and bridging necrosis. Glycogenic hepatopathy occurs in adolescents and young adults with uncontrolled type I diabetes mellitus, characterized by diffuse accumulation of glycogen in hepatocytes, similar to those seen in patients with glycogenosis, accompanied by minimal steatosis, minimal inflammation, hepatocytes with glycogenated nuclei, and occasional giant mitochondria (Figure 6.4.5).

Reye syndrome is one of the differential diagnoses if a biopsy of severely steatotic liver is not accompanied by sufficient clinical information. It occurs in children and adolescents up to 15 years old and rarely in adults. Intractable vomiting is followed by encephalopathy after 3 to 7 days of viral-type illness, which often has been treated with salycylates. Reye syndrome is characterized by diffuse microvesicular steatosis without significant inflammation, cholestasis, or hepatocellular necrosis (Figure 6.4.6). Electron microscopy reveals degeneration of mitochondria, fat globules, and no glycogen in the hepatocytes.

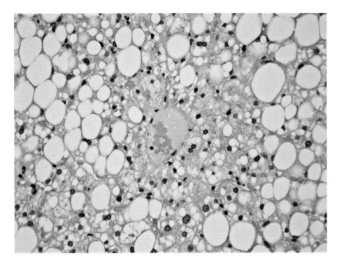

Figure 6.4.1 Macrovesicular steatosis, rare ballooned hepatocytes, and minimal lobular inflammation in NASH.

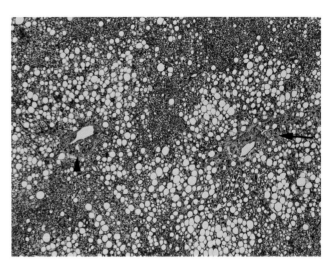

Figure 6.4.2 Type 1 NASH with perisinusoidal fibrosis (arrow) and absence of portal inflammation and fibrosis (arrowhead) (trichrome stain).

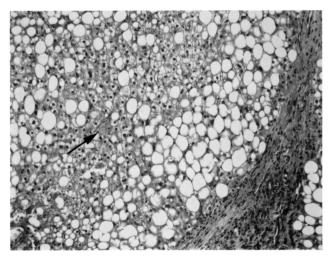

Figure 6.4.3 Type 2 NASH with steatosis, portal inflammation, and fibrosis and absence of perisinusoidal fibrosis (arrow, central venule) (trichrome stain).

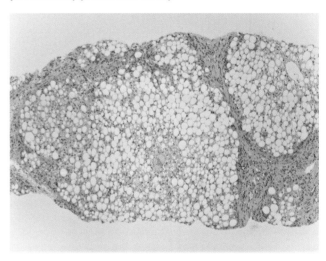

Figure 6.4.4 Cirrhosis due to NASH in an adolescent.

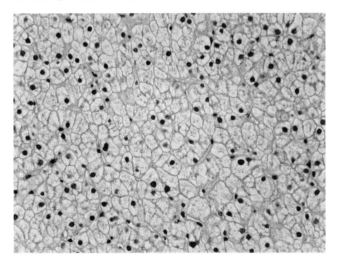

Figure 6.4.5 Diffuse accumulation of glycogen producing swollen pale staining hepatocytes in glycogenic hepatopathy.

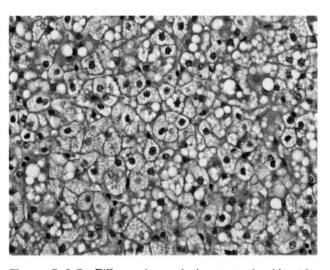

Figure 6.4.6 Diffuse microvesicular steatosis without inflammation or hepatocellular necrosis in Reye syndrome.

Table 6.4.1 Nonalcoholic Steatohepatitis Types, Histopathologic Features, and Variations

	Type 1	Type 2
Steatosis	+	+
Ballooning degeneration	+	−
Perisinusoidal fibrosis	+/−	−
Portal inflammation	−	+/−
Portal fibrosis	−	+/−

Adapted from Schwimmer JB, et al. Histopathology of pediatric nonalcoholic fatty liver disease. *Hepatology.* 2005;42:641-649.

6.5 Total Parenteral Nutrition–Induced Cholestatic Liver Disease

Total parenteral nutrition (TPN)–induced cholestatic liver disease predominates in infants, particularly premature infants, whereas older children and adults develop steatosis and steatohepatitis. Typically, the premature infant who receives prolonged TPN with little or no enteric feeding develops insidious jaundice after 2 to 3 weeks. Contributing factors include necrotizing enterocolitis, major surgery, sepsis, and hypoxia. Direct bilirubin levels and aminotransferase activities are increased.

Total parenteral nutrition–induced cholestatic liver disease progresses as long as the infant receives exclusive parenteral nutrition and persists for variable periods after discontinuation. Treatment should focus primarily on prevention by decreased or shortened use of TPN if possible and early introduction to enteral feedings, even in small amounts.

Pathologic Features

Total parenteral nutrition–induced cholestatic liver disease shows a variety of histologic changes. The major component is often severe hepatocanalicular cholestasis, particularly in centrilobular areas without significant inflammation (Figure 6.5.1). The hepatocytes undergo feathery degeneration (Figure 6.5.2). Giant cell transformation of hepatocytes may occur but is uncommon (Figure 6.5.3). Typically, hyperplastic ceroid containing Kupffer cells accumulate in the sinusoids. In contrast to the findings in cholestatic hepatitis, hepatocellular damage is inconspicuous, although centrilobular hepatocyte injury may develop due to cholestasis. Portal tracts exhibit ductular reaction and neutrophilic infiltration simulating obstructive liver disease. Ductular cholestasis may be observed. After prolonged TPN, progressive portal fibrosis develops, which can lead to cirrhosis in less than 3 months (Figure 6.5.4). Macrovesicular steatosis with or without steatohepatitis is common in older children.

Differential Diagnosis

The main differential diagnosis of TPN-induced cholestatic liver disease is cholestatic hepatitis and sepsis.

Cholestatic hepatitis in children is caused by acute viral hepatitis, particularly hepatitis A virus, and drug-induced cholestasis or drug-induced cholestatic hepatitis. The young patient presents with fatigue and malaise, rapid onset of painless jaundice, increased bilirubin levels, and elevated aminotransferase activities. Cholestastic hepatitis shows the characteristic changes of acute hepatitis, including panlobular disarray, increased cellularity, degenerative and regenerative changes of hepatocytes, and canalicular and cytoplasmic cholestasis (Figure 6.5.6). In contrast to TPN-induced cholestatic liver disease, diffuse hepatocellular damage and inflammatory infiltrate throughout the lobule are found. The portal tracts are expanded by inflammatory cells, predominantly lymphocytes and macrophages. In hepatitis A, plasma cells and periportal necrosis may be prominent, whereas fibrosis of portal tracts and ductular reaction are inconspicuous.

Hepatocanalicular cholestasis and ductular reaction are common features of sepsis similar to TPN-induced cholestatic liver disease, but in addition to these features, sepsis also shows more remarkable degree of ductular cholestasis with dense "bile concretions" at the interface area (Figure 6.5.5). Occasional neutrophilic clusters may be seen in the sinusoids and form microabscesses. Centrilobular coagulative necrosis may be observed in patients with septic shock.

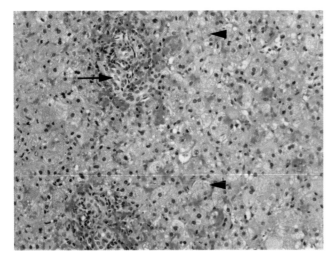

Figure 6.5.1 Total parenteral nutrition–induced cholestatic liver disease showing hepatocellular cholestasis (arrowheads) and ductular cholestasis (arrow).

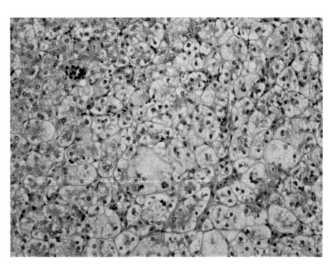

Figure 6.5.2 Feathery degeneration and giant cell hepatocytes in TPN-induced cholestatic liver disease.

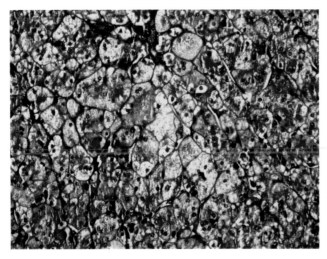

Figure 6.5.3 Giant cell hepatocytes in TPN-induced cholestatic liver disease (trichrome stain).

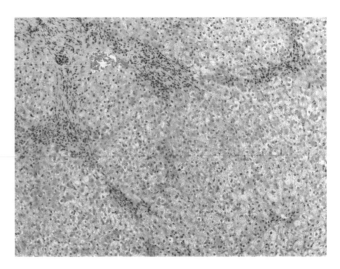

Figure 6.5.4 Portal-to-portal bridging fibrosis in TPN-induced cholestatic liver disease.

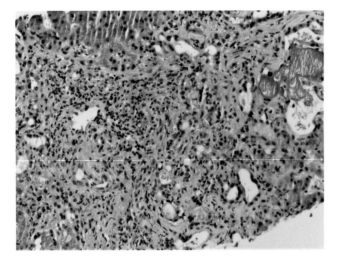

Figure 6.5.5 Severe ductular cholestasis with bile concretion in sepsis.

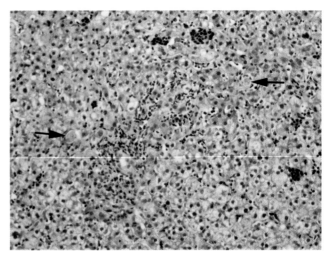

Figure 6.5.6 Neonatal hepatitis with portal and lobular inflammation, extramedullary hematopoiesis, and apoptotic hepatocytes (arrows).

Table 6.5.1   Differential Diagnosis of TPN-Induced Cholestatic Liver Disease

	TPN-Induced	Cholestatic Hepatitis	Sepsis
Portal inflammation	+/–	+	+/–
Ductular reaction	++	+/–	++
Ductular cholestasis	+/–	–	++
Acute cholangitis	–	–	+/–
Lobular inflammation	–	+	–
Lobular architectural disarray	–	++	–
Syncytial giant cell hepatocytes	+	++	+/–
Hepatocyte injury	+/–	+	–
Steatosis	+	–	–
Hepatocanalicular cholestasis	++	+	++

++ indicates almost always present; +, usually present; +/–, occasionally present; –, usually absent.

6.6 Congenital Hepatic Fibrosis

Congenital hepatic fibrosis occurs both in sporadic form and in familial form with autosomal recessive inheritance. It is often associated with autosomal recessive polycystic renal disease and supported by recent molecular studies that suggest congenital hepatic fibrosis represents a broadened spectrum of autosomal recessive polycystic renal disease. The kidney disease may manifest in early life, whereas the liver disease is diagnosed between the ages of 3 and 10 years or even later. The patients present with portal hypertension and its complications, such as esophageal variceal bleeding, splenomegaly, and a large firm liver rather than liver failure. The biochemical liver profile is usually normal. Congenital hepatic fibrosis should be suspected in children with unexpected clinical symptoms of portal hypertension even though it is exceedingly rare.

Pathologic Features

Congenital hepatic fibrosis is characterized by broad and narrow bands of dense fibrous tissue, surrounding small and large islands of normal hepatocytes (Figures 6.6.1 and 6.6.2). The parenchymal islands vary in shape like a mosaic and maintain a normal vascular relationship with central venules. The hepatocytes are arranged in regular plates rather than regenerative 2-cell-thick plates forming true nodules as in cirrhosis and do not exhibit cholestasis, necrosis, or inflammation. The fibrous bands contain elongated, narrow, or dilated biliary channels, representing abnormal ductal plate remnants that may contain inspissated bile (Figure 6.6.3). Portal tracts are incorporated in the fibrous bands and may contain normal interlobular bile ducts in the center. The mature fibrous tissue contains few inflammatory cells, and portal vein branches are hypoplastic (Figure 6.6.1). Inflammation, ductular reaction, cholestasis, and/or cholangitis should raise the possibility of associated Caroli disease or choledochal cyst.

Differential Diagnosis

The main differential diagnoses of congenital hepatic fibrosis in pediatric patients are cirrhosis and prolonged large bile duct obstruction.

Cirrhosis in infants and children has many different causes, including neonatal hepatitis (hepatitis B and C and chronic rubella), autoimmune hepatitis, biliary disorders, Wilson disease, AAT deficiency, and other inborn errors of metabolism. Cirrhosis is characterized by fibrous septa surrounding regenerative nodules. In contrast to the findings in congenital hepatic fibrosis and prolonged bile duct obstruction, the parenchyma is nodular and consists of regenerating hepatocytes in 2-cell-thick plates. The normal architecture is lost, and central venules are incorporated into the fibrous septa. The latter contains inflammatory cells and ductular reaction rather than malformed biliary channels.

Prolonged large bile duct obstruction is usually due to extrahepatic biliary atresia, choledochal cyst, primary sclerosing cholangitis, or other less common causes of biliary obstruction. As in congenital hepatic fibrosis and in contrast to the findings in cirrhosis, hepatocytes do not regenerate and central venules are preserved. Broad perilobular fibrous septa, linking adjacent portal tracts, are formed, resulting in irregularly shaped parenchymal islands in mosaic pattern. In contrast to the findings in congenital hepatic fibrosis, however, cholestasis and marginal ductular reaction are observed, often accompanied by neutrophils and, in long-standing cases, by lymphocytes.

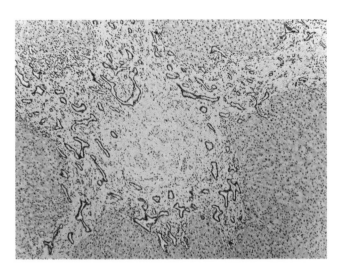

Figure 6.6.1 Congenital hepatic fibrosis showing numerous anastomosing ductal plate remnants, encircling a portal tract with its hepatic arteries, but no visible portal vein due to hypoplasia.

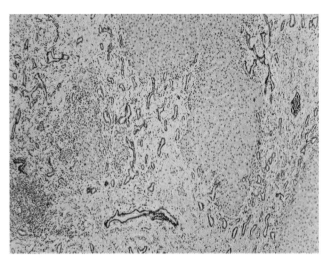

Figure 6.6.2 Congenital hepatic fibrosis showing mature dense fibrous bands containing ductal plate remnants, separating parenchymal islands composed of normal hepatocytes.

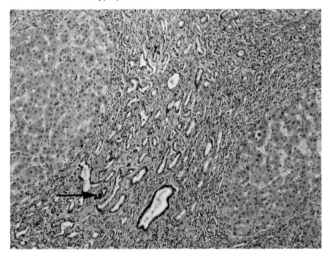

Figure 6.6.3 Ductal plate remnants with inspissated bile (arrow) in congenital hepatic fibrosis.

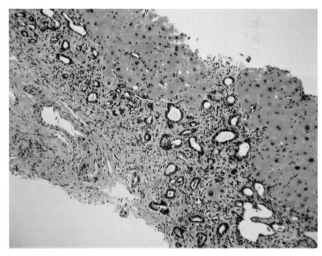

Figure 6.6.4 Biopsy of patient with congenital hepatic fibrosis showing numerous ductal plate remnants in mature fibrous bands.

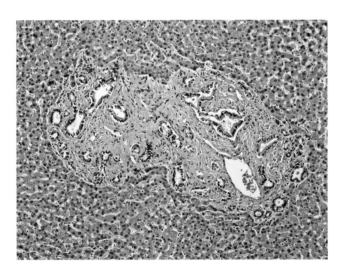

Figure 6.6.5 Milder form of congenital hepatic fibrosis with portal fibrosis and fewer ductal plate remnants, which can be undiagnosed until adulthood.

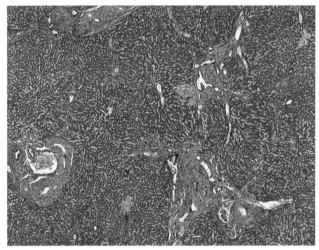

Figure 6.6.6 Milder form of congenital hepatic fibrosis lacking thick mature bridging fibrous bands (trichrome stain).

Table 6.6.1 Differential Diagnosis of Congenital Hepatic Fibrosis

	Congenital Hepatic Fibrosis	Cirrhosis	Prolonged Large Bile Duct Obstruction
Thick mature fibrous bands	++	+	+/−
Portal edema	−	−	+/−
Ductular reaction	−	+/−	++
Ductal plate remnants	++	−	−
Parenchymal inflammation	−	+/−	−
Giant cell hepatocytes	−	+/−	+/−
Hepatocanalicular cholestasis	−	+/−	+/−
Ductular cholestasis	+/−	−	−

++ indicates almost always present; +, usually present; +/−, occasionally present; −, usually absent.

6.7 Progressive Familial Intrahepatic Cholestasis

Progressive familial intrahepatic cholestasis (PFIC) is a heterogenous group of rare autosomal recessive diseases caused by defect in biliary protein involved in formation and flow of bile in the liver. It is characterized by intrahepatic cholestasis usually occurring in childhood and progresses to fibrosis and end-stage liver disease as early as in the first decades of life.

PFIC1 (also known as Byler disease) and PFIC2 (previously referred as "Byler syndrome") are caused by impaired bile salt secretion due, respectively, to defects in *ATP8B1* encoding the FIC1 protein and in *ABCB11* encoding the bile salt export pump protein (BSEP). Defects in *ABCB4* gene, encoding the multidrug-resistant 3 protein (MDR3), impair biliary phospholipid secretion resulting in PFIC3. Other cholestatic liver diseases attributed to MDR3 deficiency are adult biliary cirrhosis, low phospholipids cholelithiasis, intrahepatic cholestasis of pregnancy, transient neonatal cholestasis, and drug-induced cholestasis. Milder forms of intrahepatic cholestasis without fibrosis, involving PFIC1 gene referred to as benign recurrent intrahepatic cholestasis, are discussed in Chapter 2.

FIC1 deficiency, formerly referred to as PFIC1, and BSEP deficiency, formerly referred to as PFIC2, usually appear in the first months of life, whereas onset of MDR3 deficiency, formerly referred to as PFIC3, may also occur later in infancy, in childhood, or even during young adulthood. Additional genetic abnormalities are likely to be discovered, as approximately 30% of patients with a PFIC phenotype have no mutations in any of the known genes associated with these disorders.

The main clinical manifestations include cholestasis, pruritus, and jaundice during the first months or year of life. Intractable pruritus out of proportion to the level of jaundice is an important feature. Diarrhea, fat malabsorption, and failure to thrive are common. Serum γ-glutamyltransferase is low or normal in FIC1 deficiency and BSEP deficiency. In BSEP deficiency, but not in FIC1 deficiency, serum aminotransferase activities are elevated to at least 5 times normal values. Progression to cirrhosis and end-stage liver disease occurs at a variable rate. The BSEP deficiency progresses to cirrhosis faster than FIC1 deficiency, often before 2 years old. Patients with BSEP deficiency are at risk for hepatocellular carcinoma and cholangiocarcinoma. In contrast to FIC1 deficiency and BSEP deficiency, patients with MDR3 deficiency progress slowly to biliary cirrhosis with or without overt cholestatic jaundice and less pruritus.

Pathologic Features

Liver biopsy in early FIC1 deficiency shows canalicular and ductular cholestasis and minimal inflammation (Figure 6.7.1), which progresses to micronodular or biliary-type cirrhosis in late stages (Figures 6.7.2 to 6.7.5). Paucity of interlobular bile ducts has been occasionally reported, and other features of cholestasis, such as hepatocellular ballooning, hepatocyte rosetting, and giant cell transformation, may be seen.

In BSEP deficiency, neonatal hepatitis with giant cell formation may be the predominant histologic feature. Fibrosis occurs earlier in the disease progression with bridging portal-to-central fibrosis and eventually biliary cirrhosis.

The liver in MDR3 deficiency exhibits extensive ductular reaction, portal inflammation, and fibrosis, which may be confused with large bile duct obstruction. Later liver biopsies show biliary cirrhosis with preserved bile ducts, preserved bile duct epithelium, and no significant periductal fibrosis.

Immunohistochemical staining for BSEP and MDR3 may show no protein expression in BSEP deficiency and MDR3 deficiency, respectively. BSEP and MDR3 expression is normal in FIC1 deficiency. No specific immunohistochemical stain is available for FIC1. CD10 is not normally expressed before 24 months of life; therefore, it cannot be used for FIC1 diagnosis in younger children, but absence or reduced CD10 immunostaing can be seen as in benign recurrent intrahepatic cholestasis that occurs later in life. Characteristic coarse or granular "Byler" bile is seen in dilated bile canaliculi in FIC1 deficiency, while in BSEP deficiency bile is amorphous or finely filamentous.

Differential Diagnosis

The main differential diagnoses of PFIC are neonatal hepatitis and large bile duct obstruction or extrahepatic bile duct atresia. In particular, BSEP deficiency may resemble neonatal hepatitis, and MDR3 deficiency may resemble large bile duct obstruction or extrahepatic bile duct atresia.

The distinguishing feature of neonatal hepatitis from PFIC, if present, is significant lobular necroinflammation and portal inflammation, whereas large bile duct obstruction or extrahepatic biliary atresia usually has a higher degree of portal edema and ductular reaction (Figure 6.7.6).

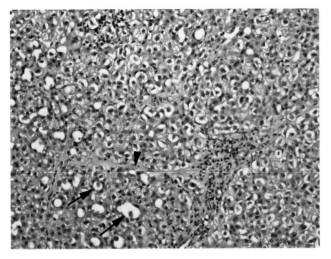

Figure 6.7.1 FIC1 deficiency at initial presentation showing hepatocellular and canalicular cholestasis (arrows), mild hepatocyte ballooning, and fibrous septum formation (arrowhead).

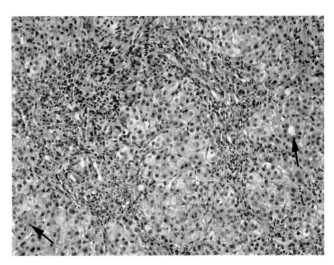

Figure 6.7.2 Biliary cirrhosis in late-stage FIC1 deficiency. Foci of hepatocyte rosettes are noted (arrows).

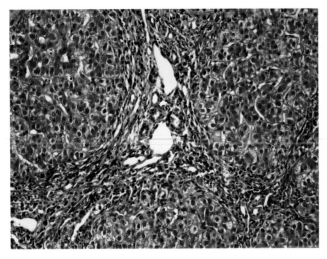

Figure 6.7.3 Portal-to-portal bridging fibrosis in FIC1 deficiency (trichrome stain).

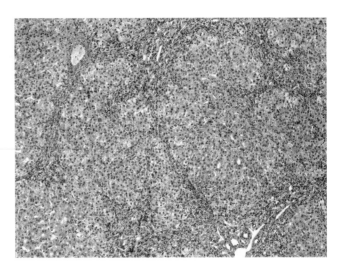

Figure 6.7.4 Parenchymal micronodules are separated by portal-to-portal and portal-to-central bridging fibrous bands containing ductular reaction in FIC1 deficiency.

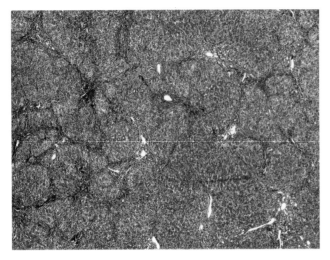

Figure 6.7.5 Micronodular biliary cirrhosis in late-stage FIC1 deficiency (trichrome stain).

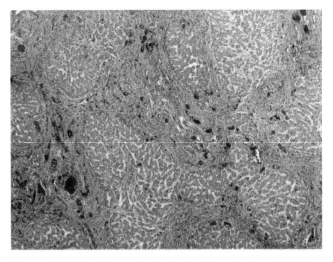

Figure 6.7.6 Biliary cirrhosis due to extrahepatic biliary atresia with bile concretions in the thick fibrous bands.

Table 6.7.1   Features of Different Types of Progressive Familial Intrahepatic Cholestasis*

	PFIC1 (FIC1 deficiency)	PFIC2 (BSEP deficiency)	PFIC3 (MDR3 deficiency)
Clinical features			
Onset	Birth-9 mo	Birth-6 mo	1 mo-20 y
Other symptoms	Pancreatitis, diarrhea	Cholelithiasis	Cholelithiasis
GGT	Normal/low	Normal/low	High
ALT	Mildly elevated	>5 times normal	>5 times normal
Serum bile acid	High	High	High
High serum cholesterol	+/−	+	−
Pathologic features			
Hepatocanalicular cholestasis	+	+	+
Ductular cholestasis	−	−	+/−
Ductular reaction	+/−	+	+
Giant cell neonatal hepatitis	−	+	−
Paucity of bile ducts	+/−	+	−

GGT indicates γ-glutamyltransferase; ALT, alanine aminotransferase; +, usually present; +/−, occasionally present; −, usually absent.

*Adapted from Morotti RA, et al. Progressive Familial Intrahepatic Cholestasis (PFIC) Type 1, 2 and 3: A Review of the Liver Pathologic Findings. *Semin Liver Dis* 2011;31(1):3-10.

6.8 Hereditary and Metabolic Liver Disorder

Hereditary and metabolic disorders usually present in infancy or childhood with general symptoms such as failure to thrive, growth retardation, muscle weakness, and/or hepatosplenomegaly rather than specific symptoms reflecting liver injury. A history of familial liver disease is often, but not always, present. More specific symptoms attributable to involvement of other organs may predominate. The routine liver profile reveals nonspecific abnormalities. Several metabolic disorders present with cholestasis in the newborn.

Hereditary and metabolic liver disorders lead to progressive dysfunction of the involved organs, but the natural history can often be modified by treatment. α-1-Antitrypsin deficiency, cystic fibrosis, Gaucher disease, glycogenosis type IV, lipidoses, galactosemia, and tyrosinemia may progress to cirrhosis and sometimes hepatocellular carcinoma. Liver transplantation is often successful, as long as other organ involvement is mild.

Early diagnosis followed by genetic counseling is important. Liver biopsy is often helpful in the differential diagnosis. It is very important to freeze part of the biopsy specimen in liquid nitrogen for biochemical, molecular, and enzymatic studies and to submit another part for electron microscopy.

Pathologic Features

Hereditary and metabolic disorders often exhibit diffuse changes of hepatocytes such as glycogenosis, microvesicular and macrovesicular steatosis, and various degrees of portal or sinusoidal fibrosis. In contrast to nonmetabolic liver disease, there is minimal or no hepatocellular necrosis and inflammation.

Bile ducts are normal, and cholestasis is mild or absent except in AAT deficiency, cystic fibrosis, and abnormal bile salt metabolism. Hepatocytes and/or macrophages in sinusoids and portal tracts may contain abnormal metabolic products as a result of the inborn error of metabolism. These storage disorders may be diagnosed by special stains, immunohistochemical stains, or electron microscopy. Biochemical and enzyme determinations on frozen liver tissue in specialty laboratories are often diagnostic. Wilson disease, hereditary hemochromatosis, and AAT deficiency are discussed in Chapter 3.

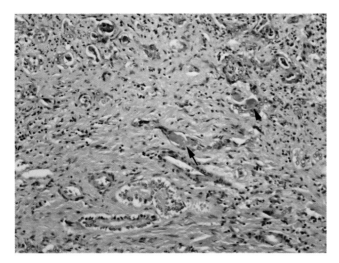

Figure 6.8.1 Cystic fibrosis with dilated bile ducts and ductules containing inspissated mucous (arrow) and bile concretion (arrowhead).

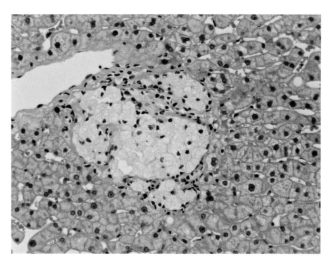

Figure 6.8.2 Gaucher disease showing clusters of pale macrophages with finely striated cytoplasm.

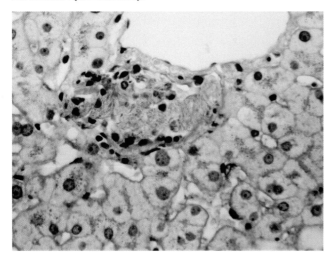

Figure 6.8.3 PAS-positive diastase-resistant cerebrosides in macrophages of Gaucher disease.

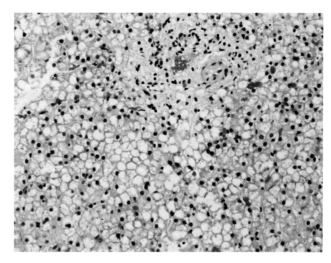

Figure 6.8.4 Hurler disease with distended hepatocytes containing mucopolysaccharide.

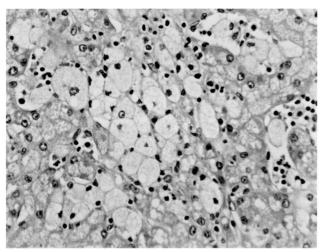

Figure 6.8.5 Niemann-Pick disease with swollen pale hepatocytes, recognized by the presence of prominent nucleoli, and macrophages containing sphyngomyelin.

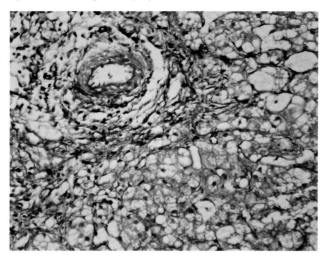

Figure 6.8.6 Niemann-Pick disease with extensive pericellular fibrosis (trichrome stain).

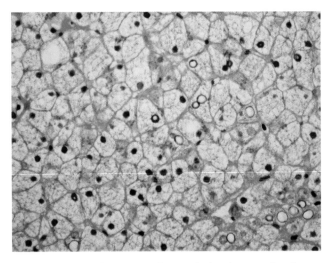

Figure 6.8.7 Glycogenosis type I showing swollen hepatocytes with pale cytoplasm containing glycogen and fat.

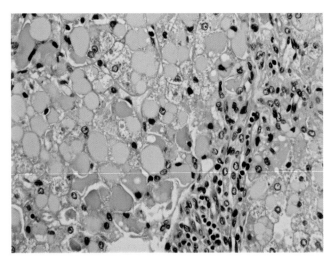

Figure 6.8.8 Glycogenosis type IV with round lighter and darker eosinophilic cytoplasmic inclusion, often occupying the entire cytoplasm.

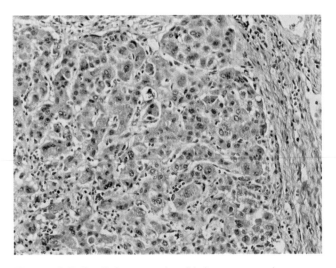

Figure 6.8.9 Galactosemia with hepatocyte degeneration, siderosis, and fibrosis.

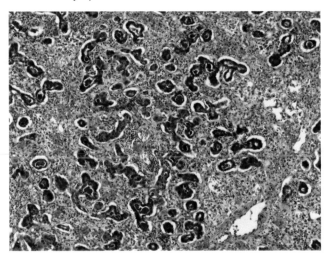

Figure 6.8.10 Tyrosinemia with ductular structures, cholestasis, and fibrosis.

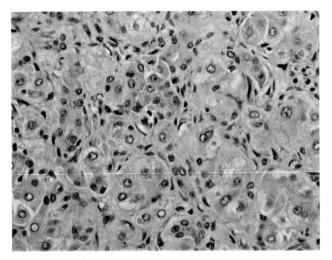

Figure 6.8.11 Tyrosinemia in an older child with hepatocyte differentiation of the ductular structures. Iron deposits are seen.

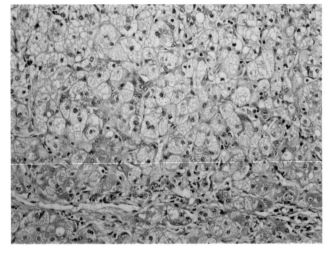

Figure 6.8.12 Pale swollen hepatocytes with microvesicular steatosis and thin fibrous septum in argininemia.

Table 6.8.1 Common Hereditary and Metabolic Liver Disorders

Disorders	Major Findings	Special or Immunohistochemical Stains	Electron Microscopy
α-1-Antitrypsin deficiency	Neonatal cholestatic hepatitis or chronic hepatitis and cirrhosis	Immunostain and PAS-positive diastase-resistant hyalin globules	Finely granular material in dilated endoplasmic reticulum of hepatocytes or in membrane-bound vacuoles
Cystic fibrosis	Inspissated mucus and bile in dilated bile ducts and ductular reaction surrounded by fibrosis and inflammatory infiltrate	PAS-positive inspissated mucus	Filamentous intraluminal material in bile ducts
Gaucher disease	Macrophages with finely striated cytoplasm resembling wrinkled paper	PAS-positive diastase resistant cerebrosides in macrophages	Tubular inclusions in lysosomes of macrophages.
Mucopolysaccharidoses (Hurler, Hunter, Sanfillippo, etc.)	Distended hepatocytes with rarefied cytoplasm	Colloidal iron stain reveals mucopolysaccharide in hepatocytes and Kupffer cells	Flocculent or fibrillar material in membrane-bound inclusions in the cytoplasm of hepatocytes, Kupffer cells, and hepatic stellate cells
Sphingomyelin lipidosis (Niemann-Pick)	Swollen and foamy hepatocytes and macrophages	Giemsa stain reveals sea blue sphingomyelin accumulation in hepatocytes, bile duct epithelial cells, and macrophages	Myelin-like figures in lysosomes
Wolman and cholesterol ester storage diseases	Foamy hepatocytes and macrophages. Lipid accumulation is birefringent	Lipids are PAS-negative, positive by Schultz's stain for cholesterol and by Sudan IV stain for neutral lipids	Lipid droplets and liposomes in hepatocytes and Kupffer cells, and cholesterol clefts in Kupffer cells
Glycogenosis type II	Abnormal glycogen accumulation is highly soluble and difficult to demonstrate	PAS-positive, diastase sensitive glycogen accumulation in hepatocytes	Glycogen accumulation in lysosomes
Glycogenosis types I and III	Pale swollen hepatocytes due to accumulation of fat and glycogen.	PAS-positive, diastase-sensitive glycogen in the cytoplasm of hepatocytes	Glycogen accumulation in cytoplasm and nuclei of hepatocytes
Glycogenosis type IV	Faintly basophilic inclusion in the cytoplasm of hepatocytes	PAS-positive, partially diastase digested glycogen in cytoplasm	Abnormal glycogen appears as nonbranched filaments in cytoplasm
Galactosemia, tyrosinemia, hereditary fructose intolerance	Hepatocyte degeneration with steatosis, cholestasis, siderosis and replacement by ductular reaction. The ductular structures are accompanied by fibrosis and progressively replace the parenchyma leading to cirrhosis. Tyrosinemia causes remarkable variegated parenchymal nodules	No stainable inclusion	Fat accumulation, increased number of mitochondria
Urea cycle defects and argininemia	Pale swollen hepatocytes due to accumulation of fat and glycogen. Microvesicular steatosis and fibrosis (argininemia)	No stainable inclusion	Dilatation of endoplasmic reticulum and megamitochondria

6.9 Pediatric Liver Tumors

Hepatoblastoma

Hepatoblastoma is the most common primary hepatic malignancy in childhood and must be differentiated primarily from hepatocellular carcinoma in children. Most of the cases occur in the first 2 years of life and rarely in children older than 5 years. This is in contrast to hepatocellular carcinoma, which rarely occurs in children younger than 5 years old. The incidence of hepatoblastoma in boys is twice that in girls. Cirrhosis and other risks factors are absent.

Patients present with progressive enlargement of the abdomen, anorexia, weight loss, and failure to thrive. An abdominal mass is easily palpable and may show calcification on abdominal x-ray examination. The serum α-fetoprotein levels are markedly elevated. Sexual precocity may be present due to the synthesis of ectopic gonadotropin. Because of rapid growth, death can occur from rupture and hemorrhage.

Hepatoblastoma consists of malignant liver cells at various stages of maturation and a variable mesenchymal component (Figures 6.9.1 to 6.9.8). The epithelial component always predominates and consists of 2 types of cells: "embryonal"-type cells, which are small, basophilic, darkly stained with uniform, hyperchromatic nuclei and scanty cytoplasm, arranged in sheets, ribbons, rosettes, acini, or tubules; and "fetal"-type cells, resembling hepatocytes with central round to oval nuclei and abundant granular or clear cytoplasm depending on the amount of glycogen or fat. These cells are larger, eosinophilic, and lighter stained than the embryonal-type cells and arranged in trabeculae or plates. They are separated by sinusoids and may form bile canaliculi. Extramedullary hematopoiesis is often present in the sinusoids. The variation of darker- and lighter-stained cells is characteristic of hepatoblastoma. When the biopsy specimen is small and contains only fetal-type cells, the distinction from well-differentiated hepatocellular carcinoma may be difficult.

The presence of a mesenchymal component, most commonly osteoid tissue and rarely cartilage, rhabdomyoblasts, or neural elements, rules out hepatocellular carcinoma. α-Fetoprotein is almost always demonstrable in the cytoplasm of the epithelial cell component by immunohistochemical staining.

Tumors composed of pure fetal cells carry a better prognosis than embryonal or mixed epithelial-mesenchymal hepatoblastomas. Resection of the tumor combined with chemotherapy and/or radiation results in a better prognosis than for hepatocellular carcinoma.

Hepatocellular Carcinoma

Hepatocelullar carcinoma accounts for a quarter of pediatric hepatic malignancies. Predisposing conditions include hepatic fibrosis and cirrhosis secondary to metabolic liver disease, viral hepatitis B, extrahepatic biliary atresia, TPN, and chemotherapy-induced fibrosis (Figures 6.9.9 and 6.9.10). The morphology of hepatocellular carcinoma in the pediatric population is similar to that in the adult population but sometimes may resemble hepatoblastoma due to its origin from hepatic progenitor cells. Fibrolamellar carcinoma does not occur in the pediatric population.

Hemangioma and Infantile Hemangioendothelioma

Hemangiomas are the most common benign liver tumors in children and commonly occur within the first 6 months of life. Hemangiomas are composed of cavernous spaces lined by hyperchromatic endothelial cells with scant cytoplasm, similar to those seen in adult cavernous hemangioma (see Chapter 5).

Infantile hemangioendothelioma is a subtype of hemangioma that is typically found in infants and more commonly in females. It is composed of intercommunicating vascular channels lined by a single layer of plump endothelial cells, surrounded by scanty fibrous stroma (Figures 6.9.11 and 6.9.12). The center of the lesion may have cavernous spaces that can undergo thrombosis and infarction. The tumor periphery is usually well demarcated, but sinusoidal extension entrapped hepatocytes can often be seen. Extramedullary hematopoiesis is often present. Spontaneous involution is common. Surgical resection is curative in confined tumor. A large tumor may cause high-output heart failure or liver failure. The latter may require liver transplantation.

Mesenchymal Hamartoma

Mesenchymal hamartoma is a rare benign liver tumor in children, usually in children younger than 2 years. It is considered to be more of a malformation than true neoplasm. It usually grows during the first few months of life, then stabilizes or regresses, and is commonly found in the right lobe of the liver. It is commonly multicystic, heterogenous, and often asymptomatic. The α-fetoprotein levels may be variably elevated.

Mesenchymal hamartoma is composed of large, serous fluid cysts surrounded by loose mesenchymal tissue containing a mixture of bile ducts, hepatocyte cords, and clusters of vessels (Figures 6.9.5 to 6.9.13). The mesenchymal tissue consists of scattered stellate-shaped cells in a matrix rich in mucopolysaccharide. Loose mesenchymal area may be surrounded by areas with collagen deposition. The cysts are either unlined or lined by cuboidal epithelium.

Complete surgical excision is the treatment of choice for mesenchymal hamartoma.

Embryonal Sarcoma

Embryonal sarcoma, also known as undifferentiated sarcoma, is a primitive malignant tumor unique to the liver. It occurs in childhood, with the majority between 6 and 10 years old. Radiologically, it appears as a tumor with solid and cystic features, usually located in the right lobe, and the differentiation from mesenchymal hamartoma is difficult.

Embryonal sarcoma is composed of stellate or spindle-shaped pleomorphic tumor cells in compactly or loosely arranged stroma with abundant mucopolysaccharide matrix (Figure 6.9.16). A characteristic feature is the presence of multiple, varying-sized PAS with diastase-positive eosinophilic globules (Figure 6.9.17). Entrapped dilated bile ducts and cords of hepatocytes are often seen in the periphery of the lesion.

Combined modality treatment of resection and chemotherapy prolonged the survival of patients who otherwise have a poor prognosis.

Yolk Sac Tumor

Yolk sac tumor or endodermal sinus tumor usually arises in the gonads but can sometimes arise in extragonadal sites including the liver. In the liver, it has been reported in children and adults. The typical presentation is abdominal enlargement and pain due to rapidly enlarging tumor.

Yolk sac tumor is composed of α-fetoprotein–positive epithelial cells. The epithelial cells form Schiller-Duval bodies, consisting of papillary structure with central thin-walled blood vessel surrounded by hobnail-shaped cells (Figure 6.9.18). The PAS-positive hyalin globules can be found.

Combined modality treatment of resection and chemotherapy is required.

Metastatic Tumors

Hepatic metastases are more common in the pediatric population than primary tumors and may arise from various primary malignancies, including neuroblastoma, Wilms tumor, rhabdomyosarcoma, rhabdoid tumor, non-Hodgkin lymphoma, and adrenal cortical carcinoma. The role of surgical resection of these lesions is extremely limited.

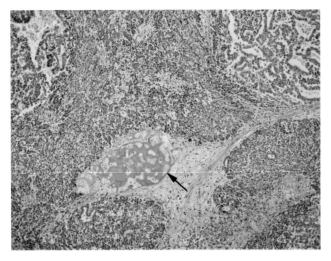

Figure 6.9.1 Hepatoblastoma consisting of malignant cells similar to hepatocellular carcinoma, with mesenchymal "osteoid" component (arrow).

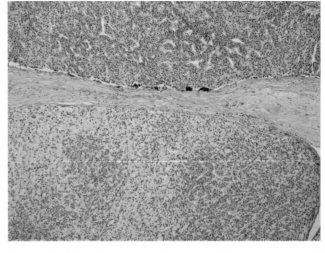

Figure 6.9.2 The hepatoblastoma nodules are separated by dense fibrous septum. Variable amount of glycogen and fat within the cells impart a "light and dark" pattern of the tumor (lower field).

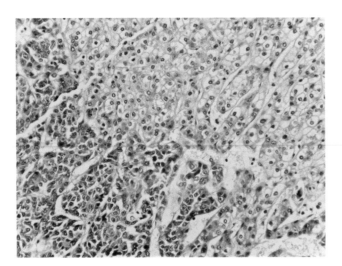

Figure 6.9.3 Fetal (right, light staining) and embryonal (left, dark staining) cell types, producing intermittent dark-light areas characteristic of hepatoblastoma.

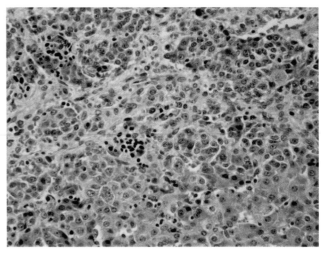

Figure 6.9.4 Dark staining clusters of erythroid precursors representing extramedullary hematopoiesis are often seen in hepatoblastoma.

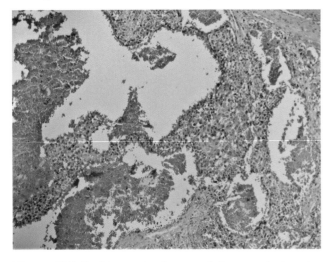

Figure 6.9.5 Hemorrhagic or peliotic area in hepatoblastoma often demonstrates immature embryonal cells.

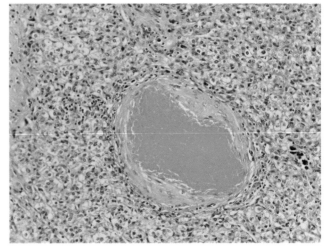

Figure 6.9.6 Large vessels are often encountered in hepatoblastoma.

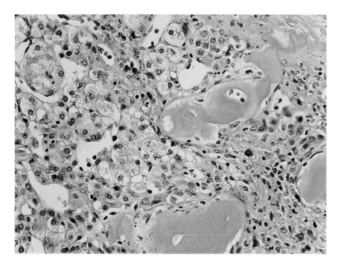

Figure 6.9.7 Osteoid mesenchymal component in hepatoblastoma. The surrounding cells are neoplastic hepatoblastoma cells.

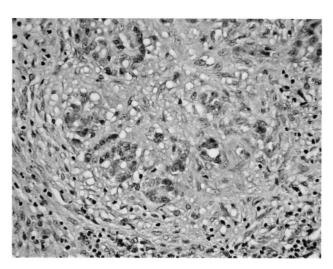

Figure 6.9.8 Ductular structures in the background of cartilaginous stroma in hepatoblastoma.

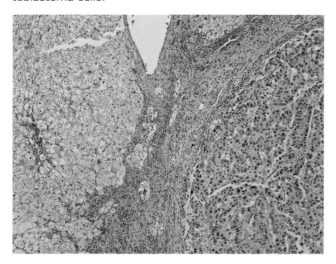

Figure 6.9.9 Hepatocellular carcinoma in a patient with glycogen storage disease type 1A.

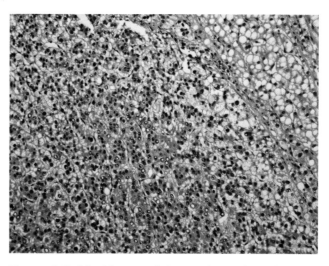

Figure 6.9.10 Hepatocellular carcinoma in a child with hepatitis B cirrhosis. The tumor exhibits fat and glycogen accumulation.

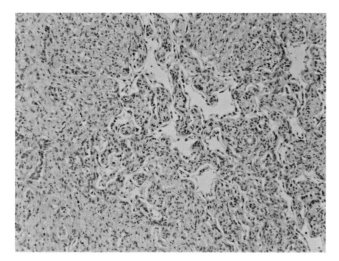

Figure 6.9.11 Infantile hemangioendothelioma composed of intercommunicating vascular channels lined by plump endothelial cells.

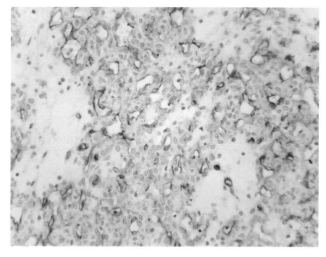

Figure 6.9.12 The endothelial cells in infantile hemangioendothelioma are positive for CD34 immunostain.

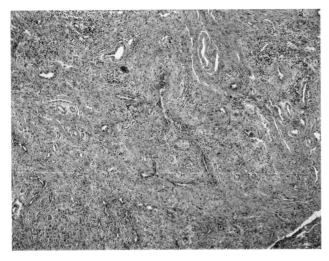

Figure 6.9.13 Section from the wall of cystic lesion of mesenchymal hamartoma showing loose mesenchymal tissue containing mixture of ductular structures and vessels.

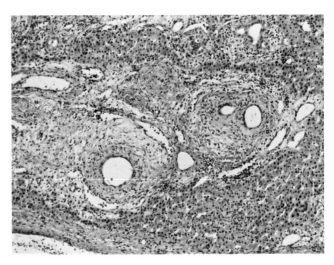

Figure 6.9.14 Mesenchymal hamartoma showing bile ductular structures surrounded by loose mesenchymal tissue admixed with vessels and hepatocytes.

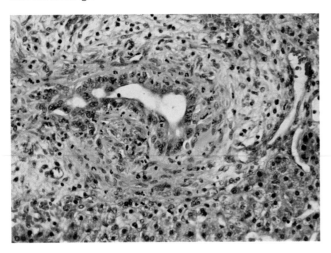

Figure 6.9.15 Loose mesenchymal stroma around bile duct in mesenchymal hamartoma.

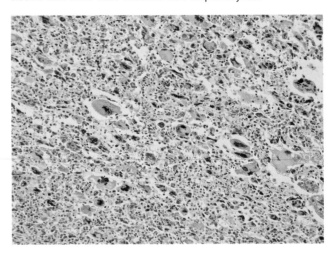

Figure 6.9.16 Embryonal sarcoma composed of pleomorphic undifferentiated cells.

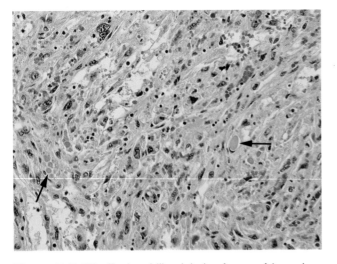

Figure 6.9.17 Eosinophilic globules (arrows) in embryonal sarcoma.

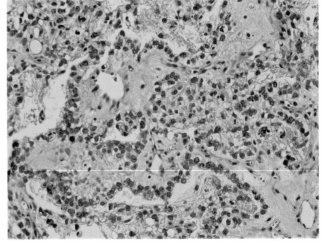

Figure 6.9.18 Yolk sac tumor showing papillary structure with central thin-walled blood vessel surrounded by hobnail-shaped cells referred as Schiller-Duval bodies.

SUGGESTED READINGS

Chapter 1

1.1 Approach to Liver Specimens

Campbell MS, Reddy KR. Review article: the evolving role of liver biopsy. *Aliment Pharmacol Ther.* 2004;20(3):249–259.

Colloredo G, Guido M, Sonzogni A, Leandro G. Impact of liver biopsy size on histological evaluation of chronic viral hepatitis: the smaller the sample, the milder the disease. *J Hepatol.* 2003;39(2):239–244.

Siegel CA, Silas AM, Suriawinata AA, van Leeuwen DJ. Liver biopsy 2005: when and how? *Cleve Clin J Med.* 2005;72(3):199–201, 206, 208.

Suriawinata AA, Antonio LB, Thung SN. Liver tissue processing and normal histology. In: Odze RD, Goldblum JR, eds. *Surgical Pathology of the GI Tract, Liver, Biliary Tract, and Pancreas.* Philadelphia: Saunders-Elsevier; 2009:963–978.

Van Leeuwen DJ, Balabaud C, Crawford JM, Bioulac-Saqe P, Dhillon AP. A clinical and histopathologic perspective on evolving noninvasive and invasive alternatives for liver biopsy. *Clin Gastroenterol Hepatol.* 2008;6(5):491–496.

1.2 Routine and Special Stains

Chejfec G. Liver biopsy: special histologic techniques including immunopathology. *Lab Res Methods Biol Med.* 1983;7:509–514, C13–C16.

Lefkowitch JH. Special stains in diagnostic liver pathology. *Semin Diagn Pathol.* 2006;23(3–4):190–198.

Prophet EB, Mills B, Arrington JB, Sobin LH, eds. *Laboratory Methods in Histotechnology.* Washington, DC: American Registry of Pathology; 1992.

Suriawinata AA, Antonio LB, Thung SN. Liver tissue processing and normal histology. In: Odze RD, Goldblum JR, eds. *Surgical Pathology of the GI Tract, Liver, Biliary Tract, and Pancreas.* Philadelphia: Saunders-Elsevier; 2009;963–978.

1.3 Immunohistochemistry

Chu PG, Ishizawa S, Wu E, Weiss LM. Hepatocyte antigen as a marker of hepatocellular carcinoma: an immunohistochemical comparison to carcinoembryonic antigen, CD10, and alpha-fetoprotein. *Am J Surg Pathol.* 2002;26(8):978–988.

Durnez A, Verslype C, Nevens F, et al. The clinicopathological and prognostic relevance of cytokeratin 7 and 19 expression in hepatocellular carcinoma. A possible progenitor cell origin. *Histopathology.* 2006;49(2):138–151.

Gerber MA, Thung SN. The diagnostic value of immunohistochemical demonstration of hepatitis viral antigens in the liver. *Hum Pathol.* 1987;18(8):771–774.

Van Eyken P, Desmet VJ. Cytokeratins and the liver. *Liver.* 1993;13(3):113–122.

Wieczorek TJ, Pinkus JL, Glickman JN, et al. Comparison of thyroid transcription factor-1 and hepatocyte antigen immunohistochemical analysis in the differential diagnosis of hepatocellular carcinoma, metastatic adenocarcinoma, renal cell carcinoma, and adrenal cortical carcinoma. *Am J Clin Pathol.* 2002;118(6):911–921.

1.4 Molecular Studies and Electron Microscopy

Ishak KG. Hepatic morphology in the inherited metabolic diseases. *Semin Liver Dis.* 1986;6(3):246–258.

Ishak KG. Applications of scanning electron microscopy to the study of liver disease. *Prog Liver Dis.* 1986;8:1–32.

Llovet JM, Chen Y, Wurmbach E, et al. A molecular signature to discriminate dysplastic nodules from early hepatocellular carcinoma in HCV cirrhosis. *Gastroenterology*. 2006;131(6):1758–1767.

Monga SPS, Behari J. Molecular basis of liver disease. In: Coleman WB, Tsongalis GJ, eds. *Essential Concepts in Molecular Pathology*. Burlington: Academic Press-Elsevier; 2010:263–278.

Scott JD, Gretch DR. Molecular diagnostics of hepatitis C virus infection: a systematic review. *JAMA*. 2007; 297(7):724–732.

1.5 Normal Liver

Crawford AR, Lin XZ, Crawford JM. The normal adult human liver biopsy: a quantitative reference standard. *Hepatology*. 1998;28(2):323–331.

International Group. Hepatic stellate cell nomenclature. *Hepatology*. 1996;23(1):193.

Kudryavtsev BN, Kudryavtseva MV, Sakuta GA, et al. Human hepatocyte polyploidization kinetics in the course of life cycle. *Virchows Arch B Cell Pathol Incl Mol Pathol*. 1993;64(6):387–393.

Roskams TA, Theise ND, Balabaud C, et al. Nomenclature of the finer branches of the biliary tree: canals, ductules, and ductular reactions in human livers. *Hepatology*. 2004;39(6):1739–1745.

Suriawinata AA, Thung SN. Liver. In: Mills SE, editor. *Histology for Pathologists*. Philadelphia: Lippincott Williams & Wilkins; 2007:685–704.

1.6 Hepatocyte Degeneration, Death and Regeneration

Akazawa Y, Gores GJ. Death receptor-mediated liver injury. *Semin Liver Dis*. 2007;27(4):327–338.

Curado S, Stainier DY. deLiver'in regeneration: injury response and development. *Semin Liver Dis*. 2010;30(3):288–295.

Fausto N. Liver regeneration and repair: hepatocytes, progenitor cells, and stem cells. Hepatology. 2004;39(6):1477–1487.

Fausto N, Campbell JS, Riehle KJ. Liver regeneration. *Hepatology*. 2006;43(2)(suppl 1):S45–S53.

1.7 Nonspecific Reactive Hepatitis, Mild Acute Hepatitis, and Residual Hepatitis

Geraghty JM, Goldin RD. Liver changes associated with cholecystitis. *J Clin Pathol*. 1994;47(5):457–460.

Gerber MA, Thung SN. Histology of the liver. *Am J Surg Pathol*. 1987;11(9):709–722.

Matsumoto T, Yoshimine T, Shimouchi K, et al. The liver in systemic lupus erythematosus: pathologic analysis of 52 cases and review of Japanese Autopsy Registry Data. *Hum Pathol*. 1992;23(10):1151–1158.

Rubio-Tapia A, Murray JA. Liver involvement in celiac disease. *Minerva Med*. 2008;99(6):595–604.

1.8 Portal and Vascular Problems

Bioulac-Sage P, Le Bail B, Bernard PH, Balabaud C. Hepatoportal sclerosis. *Semin Liver Dis*. 1995;15(4):329–339.

Nakanuma Y, Tsuneyama K, Ohbu M, Katayanagi, K. Pathology and pathogenesis of idiopathic portal hypertension with an emphasis on the liver. *Pathol Res Pract*. 2001;197(2):65–76.

Okudaira M, Ohbu M, Okuda K. Idiopathic portal hypertension and its pathology. *Semin Liver Dis*. 2002;22(1):59–72.

Thung SN, Gerber MA, Bodenheimer HC Jr. Nodular regenerative hyperplasia of the liver in a patient with diabetes mellitus. *Cancer*. 1982;49(3):543–546.

Tublin ME, Towbin AJ, Federle MP, Nalesnik MA. Altered liver morphology after portal vein thrombosis: not always cirrhosis. *Dig Dis Sci*. 2008;53(10):2784–2788.

1.9 Brown Pigments in the Liver

Jung T, Bader N, Grune T. Lipofuscin: formation, distribution, and metabolic consequences. *Ann N Y Acad Sci*. 2007;1119:97–111.

Batts KP. Iron overload syndromes and the liver. *Mod Pathol*. 2007;20 Suppl 1:S31–S39.

Ludwig J, Moyer TP, Rakela J. The liver biopsy diagnosis of Wilson's disease. Methods in pathology. *Am J Clin Pathol*, 1994;102(4):443–446.

Zimniak P. Dubin-Johnson and Rotor syndromes: molecular basis and pathogenesis. *Semin Liver Dis*. 1993;13(3): 248–260.

Chapter 2

2.1 Acute Hepatitis

Ishak KG. Light microscopic morphology of viral hepatitis. *Am J Clin Pathol*. 1976;65(5)(suppl):787–827.

Ramachandran R, Kakar S. Histological patterns in drug-induced liver disease. *J Clin Pathol*. 2009;62(6):481–492.

Suriawinata AA, Thung SN. Acute and chronic hepatitis. *Semin Diagn Pathol*. 2006;23(3–4):132–148.

2.2 Acute Hepatotropic Viral Hepatitis

Geller SA. Hepatitis B and hepatitis C. *Clin Liver Dis*. 2002;6(2):317–334, v.

Kobayashi K, Hashimoto E, Ludwig J, Hisamitsu T, Obata H. Liver biopsy features of acute hepatitis C compared with hepatitis A, B, and non-A, non-B, non-C. *Liver*. 1993;13(2):69–72.

Popper H, Thung SN, Gerber MA, et al. Histologic studies of severe delta agent infection in Venezuelan Indians. *Hepatology*. 1983;3(6):906–912.

Sciot R, Van Damme B, Desmet VJ. Cholestatic features in hepatitis A. *J Hepatol*, 1986;3(2):172–181.

Teixeira MR Jr, Weller IV, Murray A, et al. The pathology of hepatitis A in man. *Liver*. 1982;2(1):53–60.

2.3 Acute Nonhepatotropic Viral Hepatitis

Devaney K, Goodman ZD, Ishak KG. Postinfantile giant-cell transformation in hepatitis. *Hepatology*. 1992;16(2):327–333.

Ishak KG, Walker DH, Coetzer JA, Gardner JJ, Gorelkin L. Viral hemorrhagic fevers with hepatic involvement: pathologic aspects with clinical correlations. *Prog Liver Dis*. 1982;7:495–515.

Pinna AD, Rakela J, Demetris AJ, Fung JJ. Five cases of fulminant hepatitis due to herpes simplex virus in adults. *Dig Dis Sci*. 2002;47(4):750–754.

Snover DC, Horwitz CA. Liver disease in cytomegalovirus mononucleosis: a light microscopical and immunoperoxidase study of six cases. *Hepatology*. 1984;4(3):408–412.

Wang WH, Wang HL. Fulminant adenovirus hepatitis following bone marrow transplantation. A case report and brief review of the literature. *Arch Pathol Lab Med*. 2003;127(5):e246–e248.

2.4 Acute Hepatitis With Massive Hepatic Necrosis

Bernal W, Auzinger G, Dhawan A, Wendon J. Acute liver failure. *Lancet*. 2010;376(9736):190–201.

Craig CE, Quaglia A, Selden C, Lowdell M, Hodgson H, Dhillon AP. The histopathology of regeneration in massive hepatic necrosis. *Semin Liver Dis*. 2004;24(1):49–64.

Lefkowitch JH, Mendez L. Morphologic features of hepatic injury in cardiac disease and shock. *J Hepatol*. 1986;2(3):313–327.

Rubin EM, Martin AA, Thung SN, Gerber MA. Morphometric and immunohistochemical characterization of human liver regeneration. *Am J Pathol*. 1995;147(2):397–404.

2.5 Granulomatous Inflammation

Aderka D, Kraus M, Avidor I, Sidi Y, Weinberger A, Pinkhas J. Hodgkin's and non-Hodgkin's lymphomas masquerading as "idiopathic" liver granulomas. *Am J Gastroenterol*. 1984;79(8):642–644.

Fiel MI, Shukla D, Saraf N, Xu R, Schiano TD. Development of hepatic granulomas in patients receiving pegylated interferon therapy for recurrent hepatitis C virus post liver transplantation. *Transpl Infect Dis*. 2008;10(3):184–189.

Ishak KG, Zimmerman HJ. Drug-induced and toxic granulomatous hepatitis. *Baillieres Clin Gastroenterol*, 1988;2(2):463–480.

Kahi CJ, Saxena R, Temkit M, et al. Hepatobiliary disease in sarcoidosis. *Sarcoidosis Vasc Diffuse Lung Dis*, 2006;23(2):117–123.

Wilkins MJ, Lindley R, Dourakis SP, Goldin RD. Surgical pathology of the liver in HIV infection. *Histopathology*. 1991;18(5):459–464.

2.6 Acute Cholestasis

Ballonoff A, Kavanagh B, Nash R, et al. Hodgkin lymphoma-related vanishing bile duct syndrome and idiopathic cholestasis: statistical analysis of all published cases and literature review. *Acta Oncol*. 2008;47(5):962–970.

Brown SJ, Desmond PV. Hepatotoxicity of antimicrobial agents. *Semin Liver Dis*. 2002;22(2):157–167.

Chitturi S, George J. Hepatotoxicity of commonly used drugs: nonsteroidal anti-inflammatory drugs, antihypertensives, antidiabetic agents, anticonvulsants, lipid-lowering agents, psychotropic drugs. *Semin Liver Dis*. 2002;22(2):169–183.

Pauli-Magnus C, Meier PJ, Stieger B. Genetic determinants of drug-induced cholestasis and intrahepatic cholestasis of pregnancy. *Semin Liver Dis*. 2010;30:147–59.

Paulusma CC, Elferink RP, Jansen PL. Progressive familial intrahepatic cholestasis type 1. *Semin Liver Dis*. 2010;30(2):117–124.

2.7 Alcoholic Hepatitis

Guigui B, Perrot S, Berry JP, et al. Amiodarone-induced hepatic phospholipidosis: a morphological alteration independent of pseudoalcoholic liver disease. *Hepatology*. 1988;8(5):1063–1068.

Popper H, Thung SN, Gerber MA. Pathology of alcoholic liver diseases. *Semin Liver Dis*. 1981;1(3):203–216.

Sougioultzis S, Dalakas E, Hayes PC, Plevris JN. Alcoholic hepatitis: from pathogenesis to treatment. *Curr Med Res Opin*. 2005;21(9):1337–1334.

Stromeyer FW, Ishak KG. Histology of the liver in Wilson's disease: a study of 34 cases. *Am J Clin Pathol*. 1980;73(1):12–24.

Zatloukal K, French SW, Stumptner C, et al. From Mallory to Mallory-Denk bodies: what, how and why? *Exp Cell Res*. 2007;313(10):2033–2049.

2.8 Drug-Induced Liver Injury

Brown SJ, Desmond PV. Hepatotoxicity of antimicrobial agents. *Semin Liver Dis*. 2002;22(2):157–167.

Chitturi S, George J. Hepatotoxicity of commonly used drugs: nonsteroidal anti-inflammatory drugs, antihypertensives, antidiabetic agents, anticonvulsants, lipid-lowering agents, psychotropic drugs. *Semin Liver Dis*. 2002;22(2):169–83.

Farrell GC. Drugs and steatohepatitis. *Semin Liver Dis*. 2002;22(2):185–194.

Kleiner DE. The pathology of drug-induced liver injury. *Semin Liver Dis*. 2009;29:364–372.

Russo MW, Scobey M, Bonkovsky HL. Drug-induced liver injury associated with statins. *Semin Liver Dis*. 2009;29(4):412–422.

Stedman C. Herbal hepatotoxicity. *Semin Liver Dis*. 2002;22(2):195–206.

2.9 Bacterial, Fungal, and Parasitic Infection

Greenstein AJ, Sachar DB. Pyogenic and amebic abscesses of the liver. *Semin Liver Dis.* 1988;8(3):210–217.

Kaplan KJ, Goodman ZD, Ishak KG. Eosinophilic granuloma of the liver: a characteristic lesion with relationship to visceral larva migrans. *Am J Surg Pathol.* 2001;25(10):1316–1321.

Lewis JH, Patel HR, Zimmerman HJ. The spectrum of hepatic candidiasis. *Hepatology,* 1982;2(4):479–487.

Lucas SB. Other viral and infectious diseases and HIV-related liver disease. In: Burt AD, Portmann BC, Ferrell LD, eds. *MacSween's Pathology of the Liver.* Philadelphia: Churchill Livingstone – Elsevier; 2007:443–492.

2.10 Sepsis

Banks JG, Foulis AK, Ledingham IM, Macsween RN. Liver function in septic shock. *J Clin Pathol.* 1982;35(11):1249–1252.

Christoffersen P, Poulsen H, Skeie E. Focal liver cell necroses accompanied by infiltration of granulocytes arising during operation. *Acta Hepatosplenol.* 1970;17(4):240–245.

Franson TR, Hierholzer WJ Jr, LaBrecque DR. Frequency and characteristics of hyperbilirubinemia associated with bacteremia. *Rev Infect Dis.* 1985;7(1):1–9.

Kosters A, Karpen SJ. The role of inflammation in cholestasis: clinical and basic aspects. *Semin Liver Dis.* 2010; 30(2):186–194.

Lefkowitch JH. Bile ductular cholestasis: an ominous histopathologic sign related to sepsis and "cholangitis lenta". *Hum Pathol.* 1982;13(1):19–24.

2.11 Large Bile Duct Obstruction

Christoffersen P, Poulsen H. Histological changes in human liver biopsies following extrahepatic biliary obstruction. *Acta Pathol Microbiol Scand Suppl.* 1970;212: Suppl 212:150+.

Lefkowitch JH. Histological assessment of cholestasis. *Clin Liver Dis.* 2004;8(1):27–40.

Lefkowitch JH. Bile ductular cholestasis: an ominous histopathologic sign related to sepsis and "cholangitis lenta". *Hum Pathol.* 1982;13(1):19–24.

Scheuer PJ. Ludwig Symposium on biliary disorders–part II. Pathologic features and evolution of primary biliary cirrhosis and primary sclerosing cholangitis. *Mayo Clin Proc.* 1998;73(2):179–183.

2.12 Liver Disease in Pregnancy

Joshi D, James A, Quaglia A, et al. Liver disease in pregnancy. *Lancet.* 2010;375(9714):594–605.

Pauli-Magnus C, Meier PJ, Stieger B. Genetic determinants of drug-induced cholestasis and intrahepatic cholestasis of pregnancy. *Semin Liver Dis.* 2010;30:147–159.

Rolfes DB, Ishak KG. Acute fatty liver of pregnancy: a clinicopathologic study of 35 cases. *Hepatology.* 1985;5(6): 1149–1158.

Rolfes DB, Ishak KG. Liver disease in toxemia of pregnancy. *Am J Gastroenterol.* 1986;81(12):1138–1144.

Chapter 3

3.1 Chronic Hepatitis

Hytiroglou P, Thung SN, Gerber MA. Histological classification and quantitation of the severity of chronic hepatitis: keep it simple! *Semin Liver Dis.* 1995;15(4):414–421.

Sherman KE, Goodman ZD, Sullivan ST, Faris-Young S; GILF Study Group. Liver biopsy in cirrhotic patients. *Am J Gastroenterol.* 2007;102(4):789–793.

Siegel CA, Silas AM, Suriawinata AA, et al. Liver biopsy 2005: when and how? *Cleve Clin J Med.* 2005;72(3):199–201, 206, 208.

Suriawinata AA, Thung SN. Acute and chronic hepatitis. *Semin Diagn Pathol.* 2006;23(3–4):132–148.

3.2 Chronic Viral Hepatitis

Kleiner DE. The liver biopsy in chronic hepatitis C: a view from the other side of the microscope. *Semin Liver Dis.* 2005;25(1):52–64.

Mani H, Kleiner DE. Liver biopsy findings in chronic hepatitis B. *Hepatology.* 2009;49(5)(suppl):S61–S71.

Gerber MA. Histopathology of HCV infection. *Clin Liver Dis.* 1997;1(3):529–541, vi.

Gerber MA, Thung SN. The diagnostic value of immunohistochemical demonstration of hepatitis viral antigens in the liver. *Hum Pathol.* 1987;18(8):771–774.

Sterling RK, Sulkowski MS. Hepatitis C virus in the setting of HIV or hepatitis B virus coinfection. *Semin Liver Dis.* 2004;24 Suppl 2:61–68.

3.3 Grading and Staging of Chronic Viral Hepatitis

Brunt EM. Grading and staging the histopathological lesions of chronic hepatitis: the Knodell histology activity index and beyond. *Hepatology.* 2000;31(1):241–246.

Colloredo G, Guido M, Sonzogni A, Leandro G. Impact of liver biopsy size on histological evaluation of chronic viral hepatitis: the smaller the sample, the milder the disease. *J Hepatol,* 2003;39(2):239–244.

Ishak K, Baptista A, Bianchi L, et al. Histological grading and staging of chronic hepatitis. *J Hepatol.* 1995;22(6): 696–699.

Schiano TD, Azeem S, Bodian CA, et al. Importance of specimen size in accurate needle liver biopsy evaluation of patients with chronic hepatitis C. *Clin Gastroenterol Hepatol.* 2005;3(9):930–935.

Van Leeuwen DJ, Balabaud C, Crawford JM, Bioulac-Sage P, Dhillon AP. A clinical and histopathologic perspective on evolving noninvasive and invasive alternatives for liver biopsy. *Clin Gastroenterol Hepatol.* 2008;6(5):491–496.

3.4 Nonalcoholic Fatty Liver Disease

Brunt EM. Pathology of nonalcoholic steatohepatitis. *Hepatol Res.* 2005;33(2):68–71.

Diehl AM, Goodman Z, Ishak KG. Alcohollike liver disease in nonalcoholics. A clinical and histologic comparison with alcohol-induced liver injury. *Gastroenterology.* 1988;95(4):1056–1062.

Kleiner DE, Brunt EM, Van Natta M, et al; Nonalcoholic Steatohepatitis Clinical Research Network. Design and validation of a histological scoring system for nonalcoholic fatty liver disease. *Hepatology.* 2005;41(6):1313–1321.

Neuschwander-Tetri BA. Hepatic lipotoxicity and the pathogenesis of nonalcoholic steatohepatitis: the central role of nontriglyceride fatty acid metabolites. *Hepatology.* 2010;52(2):774–788.

Schwimmer JB, Behling C, Newbury R, et al. Histopathology of pediatric nonalcoholic fatty liver disease. *Hepatology.* 2005;42(3):641–649.

Tiniakos DG, Vos MB, Brunt EM. Nonalcoholic fatty liver disease: pathology and pathogenesis. *Annu Rev Pathol.* 2010;5:145–147.

3.5 Alcoholic Liver Disease

Goodman ZD, Ishak KG. Occlusive venous lesions in alcoholic liver disease. A study of 200 cases. *Gastroenterology.* 1982;83(4):786–796.

Ishak KG, Zimmerman HJ, Ray MB. Alcoholic liver disease: pathologic, pathogenetic and clinical aspects. *Alcohol Clin Exp Res.* 1991;15(1):45–66.

Nasrallah SM, Nassar VH, Galambos JT. Importance of terminal hepatic venule thickening. *Arch Pathol Lab Med.* 1980;104(2):84–86.

Popper H, Thung SN, Gerber MA. Pathology of alcoholic liver diseases. *Semin Liver Dis.* 1981;1(3):203–216.

Strnad P, Zatloukal K, Stumptner C, et al. Mallory-Denk bodies: lessons from keratin-containing hepatic inclusion bodies. *Biochim Biophys Acta.* 2008;1782(12):764–774.

3.6 Autoimmune Hepatitis

Bach N, Thung SN, Schaffner F. The histological features of chronic hepatitis C and autoimmune chronic hepatitis: a comparative analysis. *Hepatology,* 1992;15(4):572–577.

Hennes EM, Zeniya M, Czaja AJ, et al; International Autoimmune Hepatitis Group. Simplified criteria for the diagnosis of autoimmune hepatitis. *Hepatology.* 2008;48(1):169–176.

Mieli-Vergani G, Vergani D. Autoimmune hepatitis in children: what is different from adult AIH? *Semin Liver Dis.* 2009;29(3):297–306.

Wiegard C, Schramm C, Lohse AW. Scoring systems for the diagnosis of autoimmune hepatitis: past, present, and future. *Semin Liver Dis.* 2009;29(3):254–261.

3.7 Primary Biliary Cirrhosis

Ludwig J, Dickson ER, McDonald GS. Staging of chronic nonsuppurative destructive cholangitis (syndrome of primary biliary cirrhosis). *Virchows Arch A Pathol Anat Histol.* 1978;379(2):103–112.

Mendes F, Lindor KD. Antimitochondrial antibody-negative primary biliary cirrhosis. *Gastroenterol Clin North Am.* 2008;37(2):479–478.

Nakanuma Y, Zen Y, Harada K, et al. Application of a new histological staging and grading system for primary biliary cirrhosis to liver biopsy specimens: Interobserver agreement. *Pathol Int.* 2010;60(3):167–174.

Neuberger J, Bradwell AR. Anti-mitochondrial antibodies in primary biliarycirrhosis. *J Hepatol.* 2002;37(6):712–716.

Poupon R. Primary biliary cirrhosis: a 2010 update. *J Hepatol.* 2010;52(5):745–758.

Wiesner RH, LaRusso NF, Ludwig J, Dickson ER. Comparison of the clinicopathologic features of primary sclerosing cholangitis and primary biliary cirrhosis. *Gastroenterology.* 1985;88:108–114.

3.8 Primary Sclerosing Cholangitis

Broomé U, Bergquist A. Primary sclerosing cholangitis, inflammatory bowel disease, and colon cancer. *Semin Liver Dis.* 2006;26(1):31–41.

Deltenre P, Valla DC. Ischemic cholangiopathy. *Semin Liver Dis.* 2008;28(3):235–246.

Nakanuma Y, Harada K, Katayanagi K, Tsuneyama K, Sasaki M. Definition and pathology of primary sclerosing cholangitis. *J Hepatobiliary Pancreat Surg.* 1999;6(4):333–342.

Nakanuma Y, Zen Y. Pathology and immunopathology of immunoglobulin G4-related sclerosing cholangitis: The latest addition to the sclerosing cholangitis family. *Hepatol Res.* 2007;37 Suppl 3:S478–S486.

Vitellas KM, Keogan MT, Freed KS, et al. Radiologic manifestations of sclerosing cholangitis with emphasis on MR cholangiopancreatography. *Radiographics.* 2000;20(4):959–975.

3.9 Overlap Syndromes

Al-Chalabi T, Portmann BC, Bernal W, McFarlane IG, Heneghan MA. Autoimmune hepatitis overlap syndromes: an evaluation of treatment response, long-term outcome and survival. *Aliment Pharmacol Ther.* 2008;28(2):209–220.

Kumagi T, Alswat K, Hirschfield GM, Heathcote J. New insights into autoimmune liver diseases. *Hepatol Res.* 2008;38(8):745–761.

Silveira MG, Lindor KD. Overlap syndromes with autoimmune hepatitis in chronic cholestatic liver diseases. *Expert Rev Gastroenterol Hepatol.* 2007;1(2):329–340.

Twaddell WS, Lefkowitch J, Berk PD. Evolution from primary biliary cirrhosis to primary biliary cirrhosis/autoimmune hepatitis overlap syndrome. *Semin Liver Dis.* 2008;28(1):128–134.

Washington MK. Autoimmune liver disease: overlap and outliers. *Mod Pathol.* 2007;20 Suppl 1:S15–S30.

3.10 Chronic Drug-Induced Injury

Björnsson E. The natural history of drug-induced liver injury. *Semin Liver Dis.* 2009;29(4):357–363.

Goldstein NS, Bayati N, Silverman AL, Gordon SC. Minocycline as a cause of drug-induced autoimmune hepatitis. Report of four cases and comparison with autoimmune hepatitis. *Am J Clin Pathol.* 2000;114(4):591–598.

Kleiner DE. The pathology of drug-induced liver injury. *Semin Liver Dis.* 2009;29(4):364–372.

Mitchell JR, Zimmerman HJ, Ishak KG, et al. Isoniazid liver injury: clinical spectrum, pathology, and probable pathogenesis. *Ann Intern Med.* 1976;84(2):181–192.

Raja K, Thung SN, Fiel MI, Chang C. Drug-induced steatohepatitis leading to cirrhosis: long-term toxicity of amiodarone use. *Semin Liver Dis.* 2009;29(4):423–428.

3.11 Hereditary Metabolic Diseases

Brunt EM. Pathology of hepatic iron overload. *Semin Liver Dis.* 2005;25(4):392–401.

Davies SE, Williams R, Portmann B. Hepatic morphology and histochemistry of Wilson's disease presenting as fulminant hepatic failure: a study of 11 cases. *Histopathology.* 1989;15(4):385–394.

Ombiga J, Adams LA, Tang K, Trinder D, Olynyk JK. Screening for HFE and iron overload. *Semin Liver Dis.* 2005;25(4):402–410.

Ludwig J, Moyer TP, Rakela J. The liver biopsy diagnosis of Wilson's disease. Methods in pathology. *Am J Clin Pathol.* 1994;102(4):443–446.

Perlmutter DH. α-1-antitrypsin deficiency. *Semin Liver Dis.* 1998;18(3):217–225.

3.12 Diagnosis of Cirrhosis

Chang CY, Martin P, Fotiadu A, Hytiroglou P. A patient with chronic hepatitis B and regression of fibrosis during treatment. *Semin Liver Dis.* 2010;30(3):296–301.

Ferrell L. Liver pathology: cirrhosis, hepatitis, and primary liver tumors. Update and diagnostic problems. *Mod Pathol.* 2000;13(6):679–704.

Gieling RG, Burt AD, Mann DA. Fibrosis and cirrhosis reversibility – molecular mechanisms. *Clin Liver Dis.* 2008;12(4):915–937.

Nakanuma Y. Non-neoplastic nodular lesions in the liver. *Pathol Int.* 1995;45(10):703–714.

Sciot R, Staessen D, Van Damme B, et al. Incomplete septal cirrhosis: histopathological aspects. *Histopathology.* 1988;13(6):593–603.

3.13 Fibropolycystic Disease of the Liver

Desmet VJ. Congenital diseases of intrahepatic bile ducts: variations on the theme "ductal plate malformation". *Hepatology.* 1992;16(4):1069–1083.

Jordon D, Harpaz N, Thung SN. Caroli's disease and adult polycystic kidney disease: a rarely recognized association. *Liver.* 1989;9(1):30–35.

Nakanuma Y, Harada K, Sato Y, Ikeda H. Recent progress in the etiopathogenesis of pediatric biliary disease, particularly Caroli's disease with congenital hepatic fibrosis and biliary atresia. *Histol Histopathol.* 2010;25(2):223–235.

Nakanuma Y. Non-neoplastic nodular lesions in the liver. *Pathol Int.* 1995;45(10):703–714.

Tsui WM. How many types of biliary hamartomas and adenomas are there? *Adv Anat Pathol.* 1998;5(1):16–20.

3.14 Outflow Problem

DeLeve LD. Hepatic microvasculature in liver injury. *Semin Liver Dis.* 2007;27(4):390–400.

Lohse AW, Dienes HP, Wölfel T, Meyer zum Büschenfelde KH, Dippold W. Veno-occlusive disease of the liver in Hodgkin's disease prior to and resolution following chemotherapy. *J Hepatol.* 1995;22(3):378.

Myers RP, Cerini R, Sayegh R, et al. Cardiac hepatopathy: clinical, hemodynamic, and histologic characteristics and correlations. *Hepatology.* 2003;37(2):393–400.

Plessier A, Valla DC. Budd-Chiari syndrome. *Semin Liver Dis.* 2008;28(3):259–269.

Tanaka M, Wanless IR. Pathology of the liver in Budd-Chiari syndrome: portal vein thrombosis and the histogenesis of veno-centric cirrhosis, veno-portal cirrhosis, and large regenerative nodules. *Hepatology.* 1998;27(2):488–496.

3.15 Intracytoplasmic Inclusions

Gerber MA, Thung SN. Hepatic oncocytes. Incidence, staining characteristics, and ultrastructural features. *Am J Clin Pathol.* 1981;75:498–503.

Hadziyannis S, Gerber MA, Vissoulis C, Popper H. Cytoplasmic hepatitis B antigen in "ground-glass" hepatocytes of carriers. *Arch Pathol.* 1973;96(5):327–330.

Klatt EC, Koss MN, Young TS, Macauley L, Martin SE. Hepatic hyaline globules associated with passive congestion. *Arch Pathol Lab Med.* 1988;112(5):510–513.

Lefkowitch JH, Lobritto SJ, Brown RS Jr, et al. Ground-glass, polyglucosan-like hepatocellular inclusions: A "new" diagnostic entity. *Gastroenterology.* 2006;131(3):713–718.

Ng IO, Sturgess RP, Williams R, Portmann B. Ground-glass hepatocytes with Lafora body like inclusions–histochemical, immunohistochemical and electronmicroscopic characterization. *Histopathology.* 1990;17(2):109–115.

Pamperl H, Gradner W, Fridrich L, Pointer H, Denk H. Influence of long-term anticonvulsant treatment on liver ultrastructure in man. *Liver.* 1984;4(5):294–300.

Qizilbash A, Young-Pong O. alpha-1-antitrypsin liver disease differential diagnosis of PAS-positive, diastase-resistant globules in liver cells. *Am J Clin Pathol.* 1983; 79(6):697–702.

Stewart RV, Dincsoy HP. The significance of giant mitochondria in liver biopsies as observed by light microscopy. *Am J Clin Pathol.* 1982;78(3):293–298.

Strnad P, Zatloukal K, Stumptner C, Kulaksiz H, Denk H. Mallory-Denk-bodies: lessons from keratin-containing hepatic inclusion bodies. *Biochim Biophys Acta.* 2008; 1782(12):764–774.

Chapter 4

4.1 Donor Liver Evaluation

Alkofer B, Samstein B, Guarrera JV, et al. Extended-donor criteria liver allografts. *Semin Liver Dis.* 2006;26(3): 221–233.

Demetris AJ, Crawford JM, Minervini MI, et al. Transplantation pathology of the liver. In: *Surgical Pathology of the GI Tract, Liver, Biliary Tract, and Pancreas.* Philadelphia: Saunders-Elsevier; 2009:1169–1230.

Kakizoe S, Yanaga K, Starzl TE, Demetris AJ. Frozen section of liver biopsy for the evaluation of liver allografts. *Transplant Proc.* 1990;22:416–417.

Marcos A, Fisher RA, Ham JM, et al. Selection and outcome of living donors for adult to adult right lobe transplantation. *Transplantation.* 2000;69:2410–2415.

Testa G, Goldstein RM, Netto G, et al. Long-term outcome of patients transplanted with livers from hepatitis C-positive donors. *Transplantation.* 1998;65:925–929.

Zamboni F, Franchello A, David E, et al. Effect of macrovesicular steatosis and other donor and recipient characteristics on the outcome of liver transplantation. *Clin Transplant.* 2001;15:53–57.

4.2 Preservation Injury

Adeyi O, Fischer SE, Guindi M. Liver allograft pathology: approach to interpretation of needle biopsies with clinicopathological correlation. *J Clin Pathol.* 2010;63(1): 47–74.

Batts KP. Acute and chronic hepatic allograft rejection: pathology and classification. *Liver Transpl Surg.* 1999;5(4)(suppl 1):S21–S29.

Bilzer M, Gerbes AL. Preservation injury of the liver: Mechanisms and novel therapeutic strategies. *J Hepatol.* 2000; 32:508–515.

D'Alessandro AM, Kalayoglu M, Sollinger HW, et al. The predictive value of donor liver biopsies on the development of primary nonfunction after orthotopic liver transplantation. *Transplant Proc.* 1991;23:1536–1537.

Teoh NC, Farrell GC. Hepatic ischemia reperfusion injury: pathogenic mechanisms and basis for hepatoprotection. *J Gastroenterol Hepatol.* 2003;18:891–902.

4.3 Vascular and Biliary Tract Complications

Ayata G, Pomfret E, Pomposelli JJ, et al. Adult-to-adult live donor liver transplantation: a short-term clinicopathologic study. *Hum Pathol.* 2001;32:814–822.

Cameron AM, Busuttil RW. Ischemic cholangiopathy after liver transplantation. *Hepatobiliary Pancreat Dis Int.* 2005;4:495–501.

Demetris AJ, Kelly DM, Eghtesad B, et al. Pathophysiologic observations and histopathologic recognition of the portal hyperperfusion or small-for-size syndrome. *Am J Surg Pathol.* 2006;30:986–993.

Pascher A, Neuhaus P. Bile duct complications after liver transplantation. *Transpl Int.* 2005;18:627–642.

Nishizaki T, Ikegami T, Hiroshige S, et al. Small graft for living donor liver transplantation. *Ann Surg.* 2001;233:575–580.

4.4 Acute Rejection

Banff schema for grading liver allograft rejection: an international consensus document. *Hepatology.* 1997;25(3):658–663.

Neuberger J. Incidence, timing, and risk factors for acute and chronic rejection. *Liver Transpl Surg.* 1999;5(4)(suppl 1): S30–S361.

International Working Party. Terminology for hepatic allograft rejection. *Hepatology.* 1995;22(2):648–654.

4.5 Chronic Rejection

Demetris A, Adams D, Bellamy C, et al. Update of the International Banff Schema for Liver Allograft Rejection: working recommendations for the histopathologic staging and reporting of chronic rejection. An International Panel. *Hepatology.* 2000;31:792–799.

Neil DA, Hubscher SG. Histologic and biochemical changes during the evolution of chronic rejection of liver allografts. *Hepatology.* 2002;35:639–651.

4.6 Acute Hepatitis

Douglas DD, Rakela J, Wright TL, Krom RA, Wiesner RH. The clinical course of transplantation-associated de novo hepatitis B infection in the liver transplant recipient. *Liver Transpl Surg.* 1997;3:105–111.

Hytiroglou P, Lee R, Sharma K, et al. FK506 versus cyclosporine as primary immunosuppressive agent for orthotopic liver allograft recipients. Histologic and immunopathologic observations. *Transplantation.* 1993;56(6):1389–1394.

Sterneck M, Wiesner R, Ascher N, et al. Azathioprine hepatotoxicity after liver transplantation. *Hepatology.* 1991;14: 806–810.

McCaughan GW, Torzillo PJ. Hepatitis A, liver transplants and indigenous communities. *Med J Aust.* 2000;172:6–7.

4.7 Recurrent Diseases

Bäckman L, Gibbs J, Levy M, et al. Causes of late graft loss after liver transplantation. *Transplantation.* 1993;55:1078–1082.

Burke A, Lucey MR. Non-alcoholic fatty liver disease, non-alcoholic steatohepatitis and orthotopic liver transplantation. *Am J Transplant.* 2004;4:686–693.

Burra P, Mioni D, Cecchetto A, et al. Histological features after liver transplantation in alcoholic cirrhotics. *J Hepatol.* 2001;34:716–722.

Dixon LR, Crawford JM. Early histologic changes in fibrosing cholestatic hepatitis C. *Liver Transpl.* 2007;13:219–226.

Faust TW. Recurrent primary biliary cirrhosis, primary sclerosing cholangitis, and autoimmune hepatitis after transplantation. *Liver Transpl.* 2001;7(11)(suppl 1):S99–S108.

Gautam M, Cheruvattath R, Balan V. Recurrence of autoimmune liver disease after liver transplantation: a systematic review. *Liver Transpl.* 2006;12:1813–1824.

Hubscher SG. Recurrent autoimmune hepatitis after liver transplantation: diagnostic criteria, risk factors, and outcome. *Liver Transpl.* 2001;7:285–291.

Slapak GI, Saxena R, Portmann B, et al. Graft and systemic disease in long-term survivors of liver transplantation. *Hepatology.* 1997;25:195–202.

Thung SN. Histologic findings in recurrent HBV. *Liver Transpl.* 2006;12(11)(suppl 2):S50–S53.

4.8 Immune-Mediated Hepatitis and Other Findings in Late Posttransplant Biopsies

Evans HM, Kelly DA, McKiernan PJ, Hübscher S. Progressive histological damage in liver allografts following pediatric liver transplantation. *Hepatology.* 2006;43:1109–1117.

Gane E, Portmann B, Saxena R, Wong P, Ramage J, Williams R. Nodular regenerative hyperplasia of the liver graft after liver transplantation. *Hepatology.* 1994;20:88–94.

Salcedo M, Vaquero J, Bañares R, et al. Response to steroids in de novo autoimmune hepatitis after liver transplantation. *Hepatology.* 2002;35:349–356.

Shaikh OS, Demetris AJ. Idiopathic posttransplantation hepatitis? *Liver Transpl.* 2007;13:943–946.

Slapak GI, Saxena R, Portmann B, et al. Graft and systemic disease in long-term survivors of liver transplantation. *Hepatology.* 1997;25:195–202.

4.9 Opportunistic Infections

Kusne S, Schwartz M, Breinig MK, et al. Herpes simplex virus hepatitis after solid organ transplantation in adults. *J Infect Dis.* 1991;163:1001–1007.

Saad RS, Demetris AJ, Lee RG, Kusne S, Randhawa PS. Adenovirus hepatitis in the adult allograft liver. *Transplantation.* 1997;64:1483–1485.

Snow AL, Martinez OM. Epstein-Barr virus: Evasive maneuvers in the development of PTLD. *Am J Transplant.* 2007;7:271–277.

Theise ND, Conn M, Thung SN. Localization of cytomegalovirus antigens in liver allografts over time. *Hum Pathol.* 1993;24:103–108.

4.10 Posttransplant Lymphoproliferative Disorder

Harris NL, Swerdlow SH, Frizzera G, et al. Post-transplant lymphoproliferative disorders. In: Jaffe ES, Harris NL, Stein H, Vardiman JW, eds. *World Health Organization Classification of Tumours. Pathology and Genetics of Tumours of Haematopoietic and Lymphoid Tissues.* Lyon: IARC Press; 2001:264–269.

Lones MA, Shintaku IP, Weiss LM, Thung SN, Nichols WS, Geller SA. Posttransplant lymphoproliferative disorder in liver allograft biopsies: a comparison of three methods for the demonstration of Epstein-Barr virus. *Hum Pathol.* 1997;28(5):533–539.

Randhawa P, Blakolmer K, Kashyap R, et al. Allograft liver biopsy in patients with Epstein-Barr virus-associated posttransplant lymphoproliferative disease. *Am J Surg Pathol.* 2001;25(3):324–330.

4.11 Bone Marrow Transplantation

Knapp AB, Crawford JM, Rappeport JM, Gollan JL. Cirrhosis as a consequence of graft-versus-host disease. *Gastroenterology.* 1987;92:513–519.

Quaglia A, Duarte R, Patch D, Ngianga-Bakwin K, Dhillon AP. Histopathology of graft versus host disease of the liver. *Histopathology.* 2007;50:727–738.

Shulman HM, Fisher LB, Schoch HG, Henne KW, McDonald GB. Veno-occlusive disease of the liver after marrow transplantation: Histological correlates of clinical signs and symptoms. *Hepatology.* 1994;19:1171–1181.

Snover DC. Acute and chronic graft versus host disease: Histopathological evidence for two distinct pathogenetic mechanisms. *Hum Pathol.* 1984;15:202–205.

Chapter 5

5.1 Hepatic Granulomas

Alvarez SZ. Hepatobiliary tuberculosis. *J Gastroenterol Hepatol.* 1998;13(8):833–839.

Bhardwaj SS, Saxena R, Kwo PY. Granulomatous liver disease. *Curr Gastroenterol Rep.* 2009;11(1):42–49.

Kahi CJ, Saxena R, Temkit M, et al. Hepatobiliary disease in sarcoidosis. *Sarcoidosis Vasc Diffuse Lung Dis.* 2006;23(2):117–123.

Lamps LW. Hepatic granulomas, with an emphasis on infectious causes. *Adv Anat Pathol.* 2008;15(6):309–318.

Petersen P, Christoffersen P. Ultrastructure of lipogranulomas in human fatty liver. *Acta Pathol Microbiol Scand A.* 1979;87(1):45–49.

5.2 Ductular Proliferative Lesions

Allaire GS, Rabin L, Ishak KG, Sesterhenn IA. Bile duct adenoma. A study of 152 cases. *Am J Surg Pathol.* 1988;12(9):708–715.

Craig CE, Quaglia A, Selden C, Lowdell M, Hodgson H, Dhillon AP. The histopathology of regeneration in massive hepatic necrosis. *Semin Liver Dis.* 2004;24(1):49–64.

Hughes NR, Goodman ZD, Bhathal PS. An immunohistochemical profile of the so-called bile duct adenoma: clues to pathogenesis. *Am J Surg Pathol.* 2010;34(9):1312–1318.

Roskams TA, Theise ND, Balabaud C, et al. Nomenclature of the finer branches of the biliary tree: canals, ductules, and ductular reactions in human livers. *Hepatology.* 2004;39(6):1739–1745.

Tsui WM. How many types of biliary hamartomas and adenomas are there? *Adv Anat Pathol.* 1998;5(1):16–20.

5.3 Cysts of the Liver

Colombari R, Tsui WM. Biliary tumors of the liver. *Semin Liver Dis.* 1995;15(4):402–413.

Ishak KG, Willis GW, Cummins SD, Bullock AA. Biliary cystadenoma and cystadenocarcinoma: report of 14 cases and review of the literature. *Cancer.* 1977;39(1): 322–338.

Kerkar N, Norton K, Suchy FJ. The hepatic fibrocystic diseases. *Clin Liver Dis.* 2006;10(1):55–71.

Nakanuma Y. Peribiliary cysts: a hitherto poorly recognized disease. *J Gastroenterol Hepatol.* 2001;16(10):1081–1083.

Vick DJ, Goodman ZD, Deavers MT, et al. Ciliated hepatic foregut cyst: a study of six cases and review of the literature. *Am J Surg Pathol.* 1999;23(6):671–677.

5.4 Hepatic Abscess, Inflammatory Pseudotumor, and Hydatid Cysts

Koide H, Sato K, Fukusato T, et al. Spontaneous regression of hepatic inflammatory pseudotumor with primary biliary cirrhosis: case report and literature review. *World J Gastroenterol.* 2006;12(10):1645–1648.

Mortelé KJ, Segatto E, Ros PR. The infected liver: radiologic-pathologic correlation. *Radiographics.* 2004;24(4): 937–955.

Teitz S, Guidetti-Sharon A, Manor H, Halevy A. Pyogenic liver abscess: warning indicator of silent colonic cancer. Report of a case and review of the literature. *Dis Colon Rectum.* 1995;38(11):1220–1223.

Yamaguchi J, Sakamoto Y, Sano T, et al. Spontaneous regression of inflammatory pseudotumor of the liver: report of three cases. *Surg Today.* 2007;37(6):525–529.

Zen Y, Fujii T, Sato Y, Masuda S, Nakanuma Y. Pathological classification of hepatic inflammatory pseudotumor with respect to IgG4-related disease. *Mod Pathol.* 2007;20(8): 884–894.

5.5 Benign Hepatocellular Tumors

Bioulac-Sage P, Balabaud C, Bedossa P, et al; Laennec and Elves groups. Pathological diagnosis of liver cell adenoma and focal nodular hyperplasia: Bordeaux update. *J Hepatol.* 2007;46(3):521–527.

Bioulac-Sage P, Balabaud C, Zucman-Rossi J. Subtype classification of hepatocellular adenoma. *Dig Surg.* 2010;27(1): 39–45.

Farges O, Ferreira N, Dokmak S, et al. Changing trends in malignant transformation of hepatocellular adenoma. *Gut.* 2011;60(1):85–89.

Paradis V, Benzekri A, Dargère D, et al. Telangiectatic focal nodular hyperplasia: a variant of hepatocellular adenoma. *Gastroenterology.* 2004;126(5):1323–1329

Wanless IR, Albrecht S, Bilbao J, et al. Multiple focal nodular hyperplasia of the liver associated with vascular malformations of various organs and neoplasia of the brain: a new syndrome. *Mod Pathol.* 1989;2(5):456–462.

Wanless IR, Mawdsley C, Adams R. On the pathogenesis of focal nodular hyperplasia of the liver. *Hepatology.* 1985;5(6):1194–1200.

5.6 Nodules in Cirrhosis

Hytiroglou P, Park YN, Krinsky G, Theise ND. Hepatic precancerous lesions and small hepatocellular carcinoma. *Gastroenterol Clin North Am.* 2007;36(4):867–887.

International Consensus Group for Hepatocellular Neoplasia. The International Consensus Group for Hepatocellular Neoplasia. Pathologic diagnosis of early hepatocellular carcinoma: a report of the international consensus group for hepatocellular neoplasia. *Hepatology.* 2009;49(2):658–664.

Llovet JM, Chen Y, Wurmbach E, et al. A molecular signature to discriminate dysplastic nodules from early hepatocellular carcinoma in HCV cirrhosis. *Gastroenterology.* 2006;131(6):1758–1767.

Roskams T, Kojiro M. Pathology of early hepatocellular carcinoma: conventional and molecular diagnosis. *Semin Liver Dis.* 2010;30(1):17–25.

Suriawinata A, Thung SN. Molecular signature of early hepatocellular carcinoma. *Oncology.* 2010;78 Suppl 1:36–39.

5.7 Hepatocellular Carcinoma

Durnez A, Verslype C, Nevens F, et al. The clinicopathological and prognostic relevance of cytokeratin 7 and 19 expression in hepatocellular carcinoma. A possible progenitor cell origin. *Histopathology.* 2006;49(2):138–151.

Kakar S, Gown AM, Goodman ZD, Ferrell LD. Best practices in diagnostic immunohistochemistry: hepatocellular carcinoma versus metastatic neoplasms. *Arch Pathol Lab Med.* 2007;131(11):1648–1654.

Theise ND, Yao JL, Harada K, et al. Hepatic 'stem cell' malignancies in adults: four cases. *Histopathology.* 2003; 43(3):263–271.

Wakasa T, Wakasa K, Shutou T, et al. A histopathological study on combined hepatocellular and cholangiocarcinoma: cholangiocarcinoma component is originated from hepatocellular carcinoma. *Hepatogastroenterology.* 2007;54(74):508–513.

Ward SC, Huang J, Tickoo SK, Thung SN, Ladanyi M, Klimstra DS. Fibrolamellar carcinoma of the liver exhibits immunohistochemical evidence of both hepatocyte and bile duct differentiation. *Mod Pathol.* 2010;23(9): 1180–1190.

5.8 Cholangiocarcinoma

Chen TC, Nakanuma Y, Zen Y, et al. Intraductal papillary neoplasia of the liver associated with hepatolithiasis. *Hepatology.* 2001;34(4Pt 1):651–658.

Komuta M, Spee B, Vander Borght S, et al. Clinicopathological study on cholangiolocellular carcinoma suggesting hepatic progenitor cell origin. *Hepatology.* 2008;47(5): 1544–1556.

Nakanuma Y, Sasaki M, Ikeda H, et al. Pathology of peripheral intrahepatic cholangiocarcinoma with reference to tumorigenesis. *Hepatol Res.* 2008;38(4):325–334.

Nakanuma Y, Zen Y, Harada K, et al. Tumorigenesis and phenotypic characteristics of mucin-producing bile duct tumors: an immunohistochemical approach. *J Hepatobiliary Pancreat Sci.* 2010;17(3):211–222.

Sempoux C, Jibara G, Ward SC, et al. Intrahepatic cholangiocarcinoma: New insights in pathology. *Semin Liver Dis.* 2011;31:49–60.

Zen Y, Adsay NV, Bardadin K, et al. Biliary intraepithelial neoplasia: an international interobserver agreement study and proposal for diagnostic criteria. *Mod Pathol.* 2007; 20(6):701–709.

5.9 Vascular Lesions

Falk H, Thomas LB, Popper H, Ishak KG. Hepatic angiosarcoma associated with androgenic-anabolic steroids. *Lancet.* 1979;2(8152):1120–1123.

Kim GE, Thung SN, Tsui WM, et al. Hepatic cavernous hemangioma: underrecognized associated histologic features. *Liver Int.* 2006;26(3):334–338.

Makhlouf HR, Ishak KG. Sclerosed hemangioma and sclerosing cavernous hemangioma of the liver: a comparative clinicopathologic and immunohistochemical study with emphasis on the role of mast cells in their histogenesis. *Liver.* 2002;22(1):70–78.

Makhlouf HR, Ishak KG, Goodman ZD. Epithelioid hemangioendothelioma of the liver: a clinicopathologic study of 137 cases. *Cancer.* 1999;85(3):562–582.

Telles NC, Thomas LB, Popper H, Ishak KG, Falk H. Evolution of thorotrast-induced hepatic angiosarcomas. *Environ Res.* 1979;18(1):74–87.

5.10 Lipomatous Lesions

Battaglia DM, Wanless IR, Brady AP, Mackenzie RL. Intrahepatic sequestered segment of liver presenting as focal fatty change. *Am J Gastroenterol.* 1995;90(12):2238–2239.

Moreno GE, Seoane GJB, Bercedo MJ, et al. Hepatic myelolipoma: new case and review of the literature. *Hepatogastroenterology.* 1991;38(1):60–63.

Nguyen TT, Gorman B, Shields D, Goodman Z. Malignant hepatic angiomyolipoma: report of a case and review of literature. *Am J Surg Pathol.* 2008;32(5):793–798.

Quinn AM, Guzman-Hartman G. Pseudolipoma of Glisson capsule. *Arch Pathol Lab Med.* 2003;127(4):503–504.

Tsui WM, Colombari R, Portmann BC, et al. Hepatic angiomyolipoma: a clinicopathologic study of 30 cases and delineation of unusual morphologic variants. *Am J Surg Pathol.* 1999;23(1):34–48.

5.11 Other Mesenchymal Tumors

Gen E, Kusuyama Y, Saito K, et al. Primary fibrosarcoma of the liver with hypoglycemia. *Acta Pathol Jpn.* 1983;33:177–182.

Govender D, Rughubar KN. Primary hepatic osteosarcoma: case report and literature review. *Pathology.* 1998;30:323–325.

Hytiroglou P, Linton P, Klion F, Schwartz M, Miller C, Thung SN. Benign schwannoma of the liver. *Arch Pathol Lab Med.* 1993;117:216–218.

Nelson V, Fernandes NF, Woolf GM, Geller SA, Petrovic LM. Primary liposarcoma of the liver: a case report and review of literature. *Arch Pathol Lab Med.* 2001;125:410–412.

Urizono Y, Ko S, Kanehiro H, et al. Primary leiomyoma of the liver: report of a case. *Surg Today.* 2006;36:629–632.

5.12 Lymphoma and Leukemia

Scoazec JY, Degott C, Brousse N, et al: Non-Hodgkin's lymphoma presenting as a primary tumor of the liver: presentation, diagnosis and outcome in eight patients. *Hepatology.* 1991;13:870–875.

Silvestri F, Pipan C, Barillari G, et al. Prevalence of hepatitis C virus infection in patients with lymphoproliferative disorders. *Blood.*1996;87:4296–4301.

Suriawinata A, Thung SN. Hepatitis C virus and malignancy. *Hepatol Res.* 2007;37:397–401.

Vega F, Medeiros LJ, Gaulard P. Hepatosplenic and other gammadelta T-cell lymphomas. *Am J Clin Pathol.* 2007;127:869–880.

Ye MQ, Suriawinata A, Black C, Min AD, Strauchen J, Thung SN. Primary hepatic marginal zone B-cell lymphoma of mucosa-associated lymphoid tissue type in a patient with primary biliary cirrhosis. *Arch Pathol Lab Med.* 2000;124:604–608.

5.13 Metastatic Tumors

Chu PG, Ishizawa S, Wu E, Weiss LM. Hepatocyte antigen as a marker of hepatocellular carcinoma: an immunohistochemical comparison to carcinoembryonic antigen, CD10, and alpha-fetoprotein. *Am J Surg Pathol.* 2002;26(8):978–988.

Kandil DH, Cooper K. Glypican-3: a novel diagnostic marker for hepatocellular carcinoma and more. *Adv Anat Pathol.* 2009;16(2):125–129.

Lau SK, Prakash S, Geller SA, Alsabeh R. Comparative immunohistochemical profile of hepatocellular carcinoma, cholangiocarcinoma, and metastatic adenocarcinoma. *Hum Pathol.* 2002;33(12):1175–1181.

Morrison C, Marsh W Jr, Frankel WL. A comparison of CD10 to pCEA, MOC-31, and hepatocyte for the distinction of malignant tumors in the liver. *Mod Pathol.* 2002;15(12):1279–1287.

Pang Y, von Turkovich M, Wu H, et al. The binding of thyroid transcription factor-1 and hepatocyte paraffin 1 to mitochondrial proteins in hepatocytes: a molecular and immunoelectron microscopic study. *Am J Clin Pathol.* 2006;125(5):722–726.

5.14 Tumor-Associated Changes

Gerber MA, Thung SN, Bodenheimer HC Jr, Kapelman B, Schaffner F. Characteristic histologic triad in liver adjacent to metastatic neoplasm. *Liver.* 1986;6(2):85–88.

Grossholz M, Terrier F, Rubbia L, et al. Focal sparing in the fatty liver as a sign of an adjacent space-occupying lesion. *AJR Am J Roentgenol.* 1998;171(5):1391–1395.

Li MK, Crawford JM. The pathology of cholestasis. *Semin Liver Dis.* 2004;24(1):21–42.

Takeshita A, Yamamoto K, Fujita A, Hanafusa T, Yasuda E, Shibayama Y. Focal hepatic steatosis surrounding a metastatic insulinoma. *Pathol Int.* 2008;58:59–63.

Chapter 6

6.1 Pediatric Liver Biopsy

Crawford JM: Development of the intrahepatic biliary tree. *Semin Liver Dis.* 2002;22:213–226.

Silver MM, Valberg LS, Cutz E, Lines LD, Phillips MJ. Hepatic morphology and iron quantitation in perinatal hemochromatosis: Comparison with a large perinatal control population, including cases with chronic liver disease. *Am J Pathol.* 1993;143:1312–1325.

Suriawinata AA, Thung SN. Liver. In: Mills SE, ed. *Histology for Pathologists.* Philadelphia: Lippincott Williams & Wilkins; 2007:685–704.

6.2 Neonatal Hepatitis Syndrome

Amarapurkar A, Somers S, Knisely AS, et al. Steatosis of periportal hepatocytes is associated with α-1-antitrypsin storage disorder at presentation in infancy. *Lab Invest.* 2002;82:309A–310A.

Phillips MJ, Blendis LM, Poucell S, et al. Syncytial giant-cell hepatitis: Sporadic hepatitis with distinctive pathological features, a severe clinical course, and paramyxoviral features. *N Engl J Med.* 1991;324:455–460.

Reubner B. The pathology of neonatal hepatitis. *Am J Pathol.* 1960;36:151–163.

Roberts EA. Neonatal hepatitis syndrome. *Semin Neonatol.* 2003;8:357–374.

6.3 Extrahepatic Biliary Atresia and Paucity of Intrahepatic Bile Duct

Alagille D, Estrada A, Hadchouel M, Gautier M, Odièvre M, Dommergues JP. Syndromic paucity of interlobular bile ducts. *J Pediatr.* 1987;110:195–200.

Balistreri WF, Grand R, Hoofnagle JH, et al. Biliary atresia: current concepts and research directions: Summary of a symposium. *Hepatology.* 1996;23:1682–1692.

Libbrecht L, Spinner NB, Moore EC, Cassiman D, Van Damme-Lombaerts R, Roskams T. Peripheral bile duct paucity and cholestasis in the liver of a patient with Alagille syndrome: Further evidence supporting a lack of postnatal bile duct branching and elongation. *Am J Surg Pathol.* 2005;29:820–826.

Mack CL. The pathogenesis of biliary atresia: evidence for a virus-induced autoimmune disease. *Semin Liver Dis.* 2007;27:233–242.

Raweily EA, Gibson AA, Burt AD: Abnormalities of intrahepatic bile ducts in extrahepatic biliary atresia. *Histopathology.* 1990;17:521–527.

Sinha J, Magid MS, VanHuse C, Thung SN, Suchy F, Kerkar N. Bile duct paucity in infancy. *Semin Liver Dis.* 2007;27(3):319–23.

6.4 Fatty Liver Disease

Brunt EM. Pathology of nonalcoholic fatty liver disease. *Nat Rev Gastroenterol Hepatol.* 2010;7(4):195–203.

Brown RE, Ishak KG. Hepatic zonal degeneration and necrosis in Reye syndrome. *Arch Pathol Lab Med.* 1976;100(3):123–126.

Chalasani N, Wilson L, Kleiner DE, et al; NASH Clinical Research Network. Relationship of steatosis grade and zonal location to histological features of steatohepatitis in adult patients with non-alcoholic fatty liver disease. *J Hepatol.* 2008;48(5):829–834.

Patton HM, Lavine JE, Van Natta ML, et al; Nonalcoholic Steatohepatitis Clinical Research Network. Clinical correlates of histopathology in pediatric nonalcoholic steatohepatitis. *Gastroenterology.* 2008;135(6):1961–1971.

Schwimmer JB, Behling C, Newbury R, et al. Histopathology of pediatric nonalcoholic fatty liver disease. *Hepatology.* 2005;42(3):641–649.

6.5 Total Parenteral Nutrition–Induced Cholestatic Liver Disease

Mullick FG, Moran CA, Ishak KG. Total parenteral nutrition: a histopathologic analysis of the liver changes in 20 children. *Mod Pathol.* 1994;7(2):190–194.

Moss RL, Das JB, Raffensperger JG. Total parenteral nutrition-associated cholestasis: clinical and histopathologic correlation. *J Pediatr Surg.* 1993;28(10):1270–1274.

Quigley EM, Marsh MN, Shaffer JL, Markin RS. Hepatobiliary complications of total parenteral nutrition. *Gastroenterology.* 1993;104(1):286–301.

6.6 Congenital Hepatic Fibrosis

Alvarez F, Bernard O, Brunelle F, et al. Congenital hepatic fibrosis in children. *J Pediatr* 1981;99:370–375.

Averback P. Congenital hepatic fibrosis: asymptomatic adults without renal anomaly. *Arch Pathol Lab Med.* 1977;101:260–261.

Desmet VJ: What is congenital hepatic fibrosis? *Histopathology.* 1992;20:465–477.

Hoevenaren IA, Wester R, Schrier RW, et al. Polycystic liver: clinical characteristics of patients with isolated polycystic liver disease compared with patients with polycystic liver and autosomal dominant polycystic kidney disease. *Liver Int.* 2008;28:264–270.

Jordon D, Harpaz N, Thung SN. Caroli's disease and adult polycystic kidney disease: a rarely recognized association. *Liver.* 1989;9:30–35.

Kaczorowski JM, Halterman JS, Spitalnik P, et al. Congenital hepatic fibrosis and autosomal dominant polycystic kidney disease. *Pediatr Pathol Mol Med.* 2001;20:245–248.

6.7 Progressive Familial Intrahepatic Cholestasis

Davit-Spraul A, Gonzales E, Baussan C, Jacquemin E. The spectrum of liver diseases related to ABCB4 gene mutations: pathophysiology and clinical aspects. *Semin Liver Dis.* 2010;30(2):134–146.

deVree JM, Jacquemin E, Sturm E, et al. Mutations in the MDR3 gene cause progressive familial intrahepatic cholestasis. *Proc Natl Acad Sci U S A.* 1998;95:282–287.

Lam P, Soroka CJ, Boyer JL. The bile salt export pump: clinical and experimental aspects of genetic and acquired cholestatic liver disease. *Semin Liver Dis.* 2010;30(2):125–133.

Lucena JF, Herrero JI, Quiroga J, et al. A multidrug resistance 3 gene mutation causing cholelithiasis, cholestasis of pregnancy, and adulthood biliary cirrhosis. *Gastroenterology.* 2003;124:1037–1042.

Morotti RA, Suchy FJ, Magid MS. Progressive familial intrahepatic cholestasis (PFIC) type 1, 2 & 3: A review of the liver pathologic findings. *Semin Liver Dis.* 2011; 31(1):3–10.

Paulusma CC, Elferink RP, Jansen PL. Progressive familial intrahepatic cholestasis type 1. *Semin Liver Dis.* 2010; 30(2):117–124.

6.8 Hereditary and Metabolic Liver Disorder

Callea F, Brisigotti M, Fabbretti G, et al. Hepatic endoplasmic reticulum storage diseases. *Liver.* 1992;12(6): 357–362.

Desai PK, Astrin KH, Thung SN, et al. Cholesteryl ester storage disease: pathologic changes in an affected fetus. *Am J Med Genet.* 1987;26(3):689–698.

Dumontel C, Girod C, Dijoud F, et al. Fetal Niemann-Pick disease type C: ultrastructural and lipid findings in liver and spleen. *Virchows Arch A Pathol Anat Histopathol.* 1993; 422(3):253–259.

Portmann BC, Thompson RJ, Roberts EA, et al. Genetic and metabolic liver disease. In: Burt AD, Portmann BC, Ferrell LD, eds. *MacSween's Pathology of the Liver.* Philadelphia: Churchill Livingstone–Elsevier, 2007:147–198.

Resnick JM, Whitley CB, Leonard AS, et al. Light and electron microscopic features of the liver in mucopolysaccharidosis. *Hum Pathol.* 1994;25(3):276–286.

Xu R, Mistry P, McKenna G, et al. Hepatocellular carcinoma in type 1 Gaucher disease: a case report with review of the literature. *Semin Liver Dis.* 2005;25(2): 226–229.

6.9 Pediatric Liver Tumors

Finegold MJ, Egler RA, Goss JA, et al. Liver tumors: pediatric population. *Liver Transpl.* 2008;14(11):1545–1556.

Franco LM, Krishnamurthy V, Bali D, et al. Hepatocellular carcinoma in glycogen storage disease type Ia: A case series. *J Inherit Metab Dis.* 2005; 28:153–162.

Stocker JT. An approach to handling pediatric liver tumors. *Am J Clin Pathol.* 1998;109(4 Suppl 1):S67–72.

Ward SC, Thung SN, Lim KH, et al. Hepatic progenitor cells in liver cancers from Asian children. *Liver Int.,* 2010;30(1):102–111.

Index